Gastroenterology and Hepatology

Lecture Notes

This new edition is also available as an e-book. For more details, please see www.wiley.com/buy/9781118728123 or scan this QR code:

Gastroenterology and Hepatology
Lecture Notes

Stephen Inns

MBChB FRACP
Senior Lecturer
Clinical Lecturer in Gastroenterology
Otago School of Medicine, Wellington
Consultant Gastroenterologist
Hutt Valley Hospital, Wellington
New Zealand

Anton Emmanuel

BSc MD FRCP
Senior Lecturer in Neurogastroenterology
and Consultant Gastroenterologist
University College Hospital
London, UK

Second Edition

WILEY Blackwell

Contents

Part IV Study Aids and Revision

Part V Self-Assessment: Answers

Key to the important aspects icons

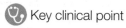 Key clinical point

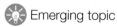 Emerging topic

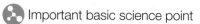 Important basic science point

Preface to the second edition

He who studies medicine without books sails an uncharted sea, but he who studies medicine without patients does not go to sea at all.
William Osler 1849–1919

Let the young know they will never find a more interesting, more instructive book than the patient himself.

Giorgio Baglivi 1668–1707

With the first edition of *Lecture notes in Gastroenterology and Hepatology* we strove to create a book that read just as we teach, incorporating the important and pertinent parts of anatomy, physiology and pathology into the structure of the lesson. In this way the building blocks of clinical understanding can illuminate rather than distract, or worse yet bore, the student or aspiring gastroenterologist. With this edition we have attempted to augment and clarify this concept by using a very uniform structure. Each section, where it is at all appropriate, is divided into subsections on the epidemiology, causes, clinical features, investigation, treatment and prognosis of the condition being considered. We hope this will help with understanding the material and integrating it into practice, as well as improve the textbook as a reference source or revision aid. Icons that alert the reader to those aspects of a disease that we believe are especially important, whether it be from a basic science, clinical or emerging topic perspective, have been added to focus the reader further.

This textbook is intended as a source of information and advice for all who are starting out in the important work of assisting people with disturbances of gastroenterological and hepatological function, from the most junior of medical students to those preparing for specialist exams. To this end we have added 'key point' summaries to each chapter, as an aid to revision and understanding. We have also added an extensive 'best answer' multi-choice question section, in the style of the MRCP and FRACP examinations. These questions remain very clinically focused and draw heavily on our own clinical experiences. We believe that those early in their training will find them just as illuminating as those further along will find them challenging. Additionally, we have added further line diagrams and clinical images, with the aim of illustrating the important concepts without cluttering the book.

We firmly believe that our patients are the people who teach us the most. However, guidance from our colleagues and sources such as this book help light the path that each of us must walk to become the best clinician we can. We hope this book guides you in the same way that writing it has us.

Stephen Inns and Anton Emmanuel

Preface to the first edition

Science is the father of knowledge, but opinion breeds ignorance.

Hippocrates 460–357 BCE

Specialised knowledge will do a man no harm if he also has common sense; but if he lacks this he can only be more dangerous to his patients.

Oliver Wendell Holmes 1809–94

The content of any textbook has, by definition, got to be factual. There are two potential consequences of this. The first, and most important, is that medical fact is based on science, and we have based this book on the anatomical, physiological and pathological basis of gastrointestinal practice. The second potential consequence of a factual focus is that the text can become rather dry and list like. To limit this we have tried to present the information from a clinical perspective – as the patients present in outpatients or casualty.

Gastroenterology is well suited to such an approach. It is a fundamentally practical speciality, with a strong emphasis on history, examination and endoscopy. The importance of integrating clinical assessment with investigation – both anatomical and physiological – is emphasised by the curiously limited range of symptoms despite the complexity of the gastrointestinal tract. The gut contains about three-quarters of the body's immune cells; it produces a wider range of hormones than any single endocrine organ; it has almost as many nerves as the spinal cord; it regulates the daily absorption of microgram quantities of vitamins simultaneously with macronutrients in 100 million times that amount.

We have tried to combine a didactic approach to facts alongside recurrently occurring themes to aid memory. For example, we have referred to the principles of embryology of the gut to give a common-sense reminder of how abdominal pain is referred and how the blood supply can be understood; approached lists of investigations by breaking them down to tests which establish the condition, the cause or the complications; approached aetiological lists by breaking down into predisposing, precipitating and perpetuating ones. We have eschewed 'introductory chapters' on anatomy, physiology and biochemistry as these are frequently skipped by readers who are often studying gastroenterology alongside some other subject. Rather, we have included preclinical material in the practical context of relevant disease areas (fluid absorption physiology in the section on diarrhoea, haemoglobin biochemistry in that on jaundice, etc.). Ultimately, we hope the reader uses this book as a source of material to help understand a fascinating speciality, pass exams in it, but above all be able to get as much as possible out of each patient seen with a gastrointestinal complaint.

Anton Emmanuel and Stephen Inns

About the companion website

Gastroenterology and Hepatology Lecture Notes is accompanied by a companion website, featuring 16 in-depth case studies:

www.lecturenoteseries.com/gastroenterology

Part I

Clinical Basics

Approach to the patient with abdominal pain

In gastroenterological practice, patients commonly present complaining of abdominal pain. The clinician's role is to undertake a full history and examination, in order to discern the most likely diagnosis and to plan safe and cost-effective investigation. This chapter describes an approach to this process. The underlying diagnoses and pathological mechanisms encountered in chronic pain are often quite different from those seen in acute pain, and for this reason each is considered in turn here.

Chronic abdominal pain

Anatomy and physiology of abdominal pain

Pain within the abdomen can be produced in two main ways: irritation of the parietal peritoneum or disturbance of the function and/or structure of the viscera (Box 1.1). The latter is mediated by autonomic innervation to the organs, which respond primarily to distension and muscular contraction. The resulting pain is dull and vague. In contrast, chemical, infectious or other irritation of the parietal peritoneum results in a more localised, usually sharp or burning pain. The location of the pain correlates more closely with the location of the pathology and may give important clues as to the diagnosis. However, once peritonitis develops, the pain becomes generalised and the abdomen typically becomes rigid (guarding).

Referred pain occurs due to the convergence of visceral afferent and somatic afferent neurons in the spinal cord. Examples include right scapula pain related to gallbladder pain and left shoulder region pain from a ruptured spleen or pancreatitis.

Clinical features

History taking

Initially the approach to the patient should use *open-ended* questions aimed at eliciting a full description of the pain and its associated features. Useful questions or enquiries include:

- 'Can you describe your pain for me in more detail?'
- 'Please tell me everything you can about the pain you have and anything you think might be associated with it.'
- 'Please tell me more about the pain you experience and how it affects you.'

Only following a full description of the pain by the patient should the history taker ask closed questions designed to complete the picture.

In taking the history it is essential to elucidate the presence of warning or 'alarm' features (Box 1.2). These are indicators that increase the likelihood that an organic condition underlies the pain. The alarm features guide further investigation.

Historical features that it is important to elicit include those in the following sections.

Onset

- **Gradual or sudden?** Pain of acute onset may result from an acute vascular event, obstruction of a viscus or infection. Pain resulting from chronic inflammatory processes and functional causes is more likely to be gradual in onset.

Gastroenterology and Hepatology: Lecture Notes, Second Edition. Stephen Inns and Anton Emmanuel.
© 2017 John Wiley & Sons, Ltd. Published 2017 by John Wiley & Sons, Ltd.
Companion website: www.lecturenoteseries.com/gastroenterology

---

Box 1.1 Character of visceral versus somatic pain

Visceral
- Originates from internal organs and visceral peritoneum
- Results from stretching, inflammation or ischaemia
- Described as dull, crampy, burning or gnawing
- Poorly localised

Somatic
- Originates from the abdominal wall or parietal peritoneum
- Sharper and more localised

Box 1.2 Alarm features precluding a diagnosis of irritable bowel syndrome (IBS)

History
- Weight loss
- Older age
- Nocturnal wakening
- Family history of cancer or IBD

Examination
- Abnormal examination
- Fever

Investigations
- Positive faecal occult blood
- Anaemia
- Leucocytosis
- Elevated ESR or CRP
- Abnormal biochemistry

Box 1.3 Characteristic causes of different patterns of abdominal pain

Chronic intermittent pain
- Mechanical:
  - Intermittent intestinal obstruction (hernia, intussusception, adhesions, volvulus)
  - Gallstones
  - Ampullary stenosis
- Inflammatory:
  - Inflammatory bowel disease
  - Endometriosis/endometritis
  - Acute relapsing pancreatitis
  - Familial Mediterranean fever
- Neurological and metabolic:
  - Porphyria
  - Abdominal epilepsy
  - Diabetic radiculopathy
  - Nerve root compression or entrapment
  - Uraemia
- Miscellaneous:
  - Irritable bowel syndrome
  - Non-ulcer dyspepsia
  - Chronic mesenteric ischaemia

Chronic constant pain
- Malignancy (primary or metastatic)
- Abscess
- Chronic pancreatitis
- Psychiatric (depression, somatoform disorder)
- Functional abdominal pain

Frequency and duration

- **Colicky pain (which progresses and remits in a crescendo–decrescendo pattern)?** Usually related to a viscus (e.g. intestinal, renal and biliary colic), whereas constant intermittent pain may relate to solid organs (Box 1.3).
- **How long has the pain been a problem?** Pain that has been present for weeks is unlikely to have an acutely threatening illness underlying it and very longstanding pain is unlikely to be related to malignant pathology.

Location: Radiation or referral (Figure 1.1 right)

- **Poorly localised?** Usually related to a viscus (e.g. intestinal, renal and biliary colic).
- **Located to epigastrium?** Disorders related to the liver, pancreas, stomach and proximal small bowel (from the embryological foregut).
- **Located centrally?** Disorders related to the small intestine and proximal colon (from the embryological midgut).
- **Located to suprapubic area?** Disorders related to the colon, renal tract and female reproductive organs (from the embryological hindgut).

Radiation of pain may be useful in localising the origin of the pain. For example, renal colic commonly radiates from the flank to the groin and pancreatic pain through to the back.

Referred pain (Figure 1.1 left) occurs as a result of visceral afferent neurons converging with somatic afferent neurons in the spinal cord and sharing second-order neurons. The brain then interprets the transmitted pain signal to be somatic in nature and localises it to the origin of the somatic afferent, distant from the visceral source.

Character and nature

- **Dull, crampy, burning or gnawing?** Visceral pain: related to internal organs and the visceral peritoneum.

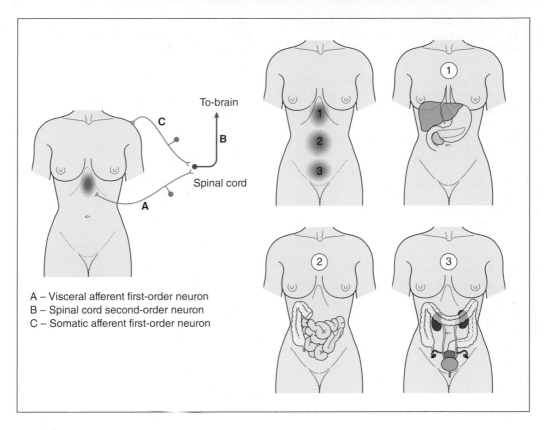

Figure 1.1 *Left*: Mechanism of referred pain. *Right*: Location of pain in relation to organic pathology. Source: Frederick H. Millham, in Feldman M, Friedman L, Brandt L (eds) (2010) *Sleisenger and Fordtran's Gastrointestinal and Liver Disease*, 9th edn, Philadelphia, PA: Saunders, Figure 10.1. Reproduced with permission of Elsevier.

- **Sharp, pricking?** Somatic pain: originates from the abdominal wall or parietal peritoneum (Box 1.1).

One process can cause both features, the classic example being appendicitis, which starts with a poorly localised central abdominal aching visceral pain; as the appendix becomes more inflamed and irritates the parietal peritoneum, it progresses to sharp somatic-type pain localised to the right lower quadrant.

Exacerbating and relieving features

Patients should be asked if there are any factors that 'bring the pain on or make it worse' and conversely 'make the pain better'. Specifically:

- **Any dietary features, including particular foods or the timing of meals?** Patients with chronic abdominal pain frequently attempt dietary manipulation to treat the pain. Pain consistently developing soon after a meal, particularly when associated with upper abdominal bloating and nausea or

vomiting, may indicate gastric or small intestinal pathology or sensitivity.
- **Relief of low abdominal pain by the passage of flatus or stool?** This indicates rectal pathology or increased rectal sensitivity.
- **The effect of different forms of analgesia or antispasmodic when used may give clues as to the aetiology of the pain.** Simple analgesics such as paracetamol may be more effective in treating musculoskeletal or solid organ pain, whereas antispasmodics such as hyoscine butylbromide (Buscopan) or mebeverine may be more beneficial in treating pain related to hollow organs.
- **Pain associated with twisting or bending?** More likely related to the abdominal wall than intra-abdominal structures.
- **Pain severity** may be affected by stress in functional disorders, but increasing evidence shows that psychological stress also plays a role in the mediation of organic disease, such as inflammatory bowel disease (IBD).

Any associated symptoms?

The presence of associated symptoms may be instrumental in localising the origin of the pain.

- **Relationship to bowel habit: frequency, consistency, urgency, blood, mucus and any association of changes in the bowel habit with the pain are important.** Fluctuation in the pain associated with changes in bowel habit is indicative of a colonic process and is typical of irritable bowel syndrome (IBS).
- **Vomiting or upper abdominal distension?** Suggestive of small bowel obstruction or ileus.
- **Haematuria?** Indicates renal colic.
- **Palpable lump in the area of tenderness?** Suggests an inflammatory mass related to transmural inflammation of a viscus, but may simply be related to colonic loading of faeces.

Examination technique

The physical examination begins with a careful **general inspection**.

- **Does the patient look unwell?** Obvious weight loss or cachexia is an indicator of malabsorption or undernourishment.
- **Is the patient comfortable? If in acute pain, are they adopting a position to ease the pain?** The patient lying stock still in bed with obvious severe pain may well have peritonitis, whereas a patient moving about the bed, unable to get comfortable, is more likely to have visceral pain such as obstruction of a viscus.

- **Observation of the skin** may demonstrate jaundice, pallor associated with anaemia, erythema ab igne (reticular erythematous hyperpigmentation caused by repeated skin exposure to moderate heat used to relieve pain) or specific extraintestinal manifestations of disease (Table 1.1). Leg swelling may be an indicator of decreased blood albumin related to liver disease or malnutrition.
- **Observe the abdomen** for visible abdominal distension (caused by either ascites or distension of viscus by gas or fluid).
- **Vital signs, including the temperature**, should be noted.
- **Examination of the hands** may reveal clues to intra-abdominal disease. Clubbing may be related to chronic liver disease, IBD or other extra-abdominal disease with intra-abdominal consequences. Pale palmar creases may be associated with anaemia. Palmar erythema, asterixis, Dupytren's contractures and spider naevi on the arms may be seen in chronic liver disease.
- **Inspection of the face** may reveal conjunctival pallor in anaemia, scleral yellowing in jaundice, or periorbital corneal arcus indicating hypercholesterolaemia and an increased risk of vascular disease or pancreatitis.
- **Careful cardiac and respiratory examinations** may reveal abnormalities associated with intra-abdominal disease. For example, peripheral vascular disease may indicate that a patient is at risk for intestinal ischaemia; congestive heart failure is

Table 1.1 Extraintestinal manifestations of hepatogastrointestinal diseases.

Disease	Dermatological	Musculoskeletal
Inflammatory bowel disease:		
• Crohn's disease	Erythema nodosum, pyoderma gangrenosum	Axial arthritis more common
• Ulcerative colitis	Erythema nodosum, pyoderma gangrenosum	Axial and peripheral arthritis similar in frequency
Enteric infections (Shigella, Salmonella, Yersinia, Campylobacter)	Keratoderma blennorrhagica	Reactive arthritis
Malabsorption syndromes:		
• Coeliac sprue	Dermatitis herpetiformis	Polyarthralgia
Viral hepatitis:		
• Hepatitis B	Jaundice (hepatitis), livedo reticularis, skin ulcers (vasculitis)	Prodrome that includes arthralgias; mononeuritis multiplex
• Hepatitis C	Jaundice (hepatitis), palpable purpura	Can develop positive rheumatoid factor
Henoch–Schönlein purpura	Palpable purpura over buttocks and lower extremities	Arthralgias

associated with congestion of the liver, the production of ascites and gut oedema; and pain from cardiac ischaemia or pleuritis in lower-lobe pneumonia may refer to the abdomen.

- **Examination of the gastrointestinal (GI) system per se begins with careful inspection of the mouth with the aid of a torch and tongue depressor**. The presence of numerous or large mouth ulcers or marked swelling of the lips may be associated with IBD. Angular stomatitis occurs in iron deficiency. Glossitis may develop in association with vitamin B_{12} deficiency caused by malabsorption.
- **Examination of the thyroid is followed by examination of the neck and axilla** for lymphadenopathy.
- **Careful inspection of the abdomen is repeated and the abdominal examination is completed as described in Part IV, taking great care to avoid causing undue additional discomfort**. The examiner must be careful to ask first whether there are any tender spots in the abdomen before laying on a hand. Special care should be taken, starting with very light palpation, asking the patient to advise the examiner of any discomfort felt and by watching the patient's expression at all times. Only if light palpation is tolerated in an area of the abdomen should deep palpation be undertaken in that area. A useful additional sign to elicit when areas of localised tenderness are found is Carnett's sign. While the examiner palpates over the area of tenderness, the patient is asked to raise their head from the bed against the resistance provided by the examiner's free hand on their forehead. If the palpation tenderness continues or intensifies during this manoeuvre, it is likely to be related to the abdominal wall rather than to intra-abdominal structures.

Approach to differential diagnosis of pain and directed investigation

Following a careful history and examination, the clinician should be able to develop an idea of which organ(s) is/are likely to be involved and what the likely pathogenesis might be considering the demographics of the patient and the nature of the pain. It is important to list the most likely diagnoses based on these factors first. The differential can then be expanded by the application of a surgical sieve (as described in Part IV) to add the less likely possibilities.

Most patients should have a minimal blood panel to rule out warning features and to make any obvious diagnoses. These would include full blood count (FBC); urea, creatinine and electrolytes; liver function tests (LFTs); and coeliac antibodies, especially if there is any alteration of bowel habit. Further testing should be directed at each of the most likely diagnoses in the list of differential diagnoses. The clinician should attempt to choose the range of investigations that will most cost-effectively examine for the greatest number of likely diagnoses with the greatest sensitivity and specificity (see Clinical example 1.1).

 CLINICAL EXAMPLE 1.1

HISTORY Ms AP is a 37-year-old woman who describes 1 year of intermittent right lower quadrant abdominal pain. She is Caucasian, her body mass index is 19 kg/m² and she smokes 20 cigarettes/day. The pain first came on following an illness associated with vomiting and diarrhoea. She saw her GP and was given antibiotics, but stool culture revealed no pathogens. The diarrhoea settled spontaneously and she currently opens her bowels three times a day to soft-to-loose stool with no blood or mucus. The pain is aching and intermittent, but seems to be worse during periods of life stress. It often occurs about half an hour after meals and is associated with abdominal bloating and on occasion nausea, but no vomiting. It lasts 30 minutes to some hours at a time. There is no position in which she can get comfortable and she describes herself as 'writhing around' with the pain.

She has reduced the size of her meals and avoids excess fibre, which seems to help. No specific foods contribute to the symptoms. Opening her bowels does not relieve the pain. She has trialled no medications. She has lost 5 kg in weight in the last year. The pain does not wake her at night and there is no nocturnal diarrhoea. There has been no change in the menstrual cycle and no association of the pain with menses. There has been no haematuria and she has never passed stones with the urine. She is on no regular medication. There is no significant family history.

EXAMINATION Observation reveals a thin woman with no hand or face signs of gastrointestinal disease; in particular, no pallor, skin lesions, angular stomatitis, mouth ulceration or tongue swelling. The abdomen is not distended. There is localised tenderness in the right lower quadrant. No mass is palpable. Carnett's sign is negative (the tenderness disappears when the patient lifts her head from the bed). There is no organomegaly. Bowel sounds are normal.

SYNTHESIS (SEE TABLE 1.2) In considering the differential diagnosis and investigation plan, one must first consider which organ(s) might be involved, then what the possible pathologies in those organs might be, before considering the investigations that are useful for each possible pathology in each organ system. This will allow a tailored approach to directed investigation that is cost-effective and limits the potential harm to the patient.

Likely organ involved In considering the differential diagnosis, one must first consider which organ(s) might be involved. The central and aching nature of the pain, as well as the fact that it causes the patient to writhe around, suggest that it is originating in a hollow organ, perhaps the small bowel or proximal colon. The localised tenderness further localises the pain to the distal small bowel or proximal colon. The onset was associated with a probable gastroenteritis and the bowel habit is mildly disturbed, also suggesting an intestinal cause. The lack of association with menses and the absence of other urinary symptoms make conditions of the reproductive system and renal tract less likely.

Likely pathology The most likely diagnoses in this setting are inflammatory bowel disease and functional GI disease (IBS). Most patients with gastrointestinal symptoms require serological testing for coeliac disease, as it is very common and its symptoms commonly mimic other diseases. Use of a surgical sieve applied to the distal small bowel and proximal colon expands the list to include infection, neoplasia (including benign neoplasia resulting in intermittent intussusceptions) and, although unlikely in a young woman, intestinal ischaemia. Less likely causes in other organ systems include biliary colic, ovarian pain and renal colic.

Investigation plan Initial investigation reveals a microcytic anaemia but no abnormality of the renal and liver tests and negative coeliac antibodies. Stool culture and examination for ova, cysts and parasites are negative. Urine dipstick shows no blood. Warning features in the form of weight loss and anaemia prompt further investigation. The investigation of choice to rule out inflammatory disease in the terminal ileum and colon is ileocolonoscopy and biopsy. The standard investigation for the remaining small bowel is computed tomography (CT) or magnetic resonance imaging (MRI) enterography. This will also effectively investigate for biliary disease, ovarian disease and renal disease. More expensive and invasive investigations designed to examine for the less likely diagnoses are not utilised in the first instance (see Chapter 6).

At colonoscopy the caecum and terminal ileum are seen to be inflamed and ulcerated. Biopsies show chronic inflammation, ulceration and granuloma formation, suggestive of Crohn's disease. CT shows no disease of the ovaries, kidneys or biliary tree, but does suggest thickening and inflammation of the terminal ileum and caecum. There is no significant lymphadenopathy. A diagnosis of probable Crohn's disease is made and the patient treated accordingly.

Acute abdominal pain

The patient presenting with acute abdominal pain is a particular challenge to the clinician. Pain production within the abdomen is such that a wide range of diagnoses can present in an identical manner. However, a thorough history and examination still constitute the cornerstone of assessment. It is essential to have an understanding of the mechanisms of pain generation. Equally, it is important to recognise the alarm symptoms and initial investigative findings that help to determine which patients may have a serious underlying disease process, who therefore warrant more expeditious evaluation and treatment.

Clinical features
History taking

The assessment of the patient with abdominal pain proceeds in the same way whatever the severity of the pain; however, in the acute setting, assessment and management may need to proceed simultaneously and almost invariably involve consultation with a surgeon. Much debate has centred on the pros and cons of opiate analgesia in patients with severe abdominal pain, as this may affect assessment. The current consensus is that while judicious use of opiate analgesia may affect the examination findings, it does not adversely affect the outcome for the patient and is preferable to leaving a patient in severe pain.

Table 1.2 Approach to differential diagnosis and directed investigation for Ms AP.

Likely organ involved	Likely pathology	Investigation choices	Investigation plan
Small bowel and colon	Inflammatory bowel disease	Ileocolonoscopy CT/MRI enterography US small bowel Capsule endoscopy	Stool test Ileocolonoscopy CT (or MRI) enterography
	Irritable bowel syndrome	Suggestive symptom complex in the absence of other diagnoses	
	Infection	Stool culture and examination for *C. difficile*, ova, cysts and parasites Specific parasitic serology if peripheral eosinophilia	
	Neoplasia	Ileocolonoscopy and enterography (CT/MRI) or capsule endoscopy	
	Ischaemia	Angiography	
Biliary system	Biliary stones, neoplasia	Ultrasound abdomen MRCP Endoscopic ultrasound ERCP	
Ovary	Ovarian cyst, torted ovary	Ultrasound pelvis CT pelvis	
Renal	Renal stones	Ultrasound abdomen CT urogram	

US, ultrasound; MRI, magnetic resonance imaging; MRCP, magnetic resonance cholangiopancreatography; ERCP, endoscopic retrograde cholangiopancreatography; CT, computed tomography scan.

The history (Table 1.3) gives vital clues as to the diagnosis and should include questions regarding the location (Figure 1.2), character, onset and severity of the pain, any radiation or referral, any past history of similar pain, and any associated symptoms.

Careful exclusion of past or chronic health problems that may have progressed to, or be associated with, the current condition is important. A patient with chronic dyspepsia may now be presenting with perforation of a duodenal ulcer. The patient with severe peripheral vascular disease, or who has had recent vascular intervention, might have acute mesenteric ischaemia. A binge drinker with past episodes of alcohol-related pain is at risk for acute pancreatitis, as is the patient with known cholelithiasis. Patients with past multiple abdominal surgeries are at risk for intestinal obstruction.

Questioning regarding current and past prescribed, illicit and complementary medicine use is necessary. The patient using non-steroidal anti-inflammatory drugs (NSAIDs) is at risk of peptic ulceration; use of anticoagulants increases the risk of haemorrhagic conditions; prednisone or immunosuppressants may blunt the inflammatory response to perforation or peritonitis, resulting in less pain than expected.

Examination

Initial assessment is aimed at determining the seriousness of the illness. A happy, comfortable-appearing patient rarely has a serious problem, unlike one who is anxious, pale, sweaty or in obvious pain. Vital signs, state of consciousness and other indications of peripheral perfusion must be evaluated.

- **Examination of the non-abdominal organ systems** is aimed at determining any evidence for an extra-abdominal cause for the pain:
  - Abdominal wall tenderness and swelling with rectus muscle haematoma. Extremely tender, sometimes red and swollen scrotum with testicular torsion.
  - Resolving (sometimes completely resolved) rash in post-herpetic pain.
  - Ketones on the breath in diabetic ketoacidosis.
  - Pulmonary findings in pneumonia and pleuritis.

Table 1.3 Historical features in acute abdominal pain examination.

Where is the pain?	See Figure 1.2
Character of the pain?	Acute waves of sharp constricting pain that 'take the breath away' (renal or biliary colic)
	Waves of dull pain with vomiting (intestinal obstruction)
	Colicky pain that becomes steady (appendicitis, strangulating intestinal obstruction, mesenteric ischaemia)
	Sharp, constant pain, worsened by movement (peritonitis)
	Tearing pain (dissecting aneurysm)
	Dull ache (appendicitis, diverticulitis, pyelonephritis)
Past similar pain?	'Yes' suggests recurrent problems such as ulcer disease, gallstone colic, diverticulitis or mittelschmerz
Onset?	Sudden: 'like a thunderclap' (perforated ulcer, renal stone, ruptured ectopic pregnancy, torsion of ovary or testis, some ruptured aneurysms)
	Less sudden: most other causes
Severity of the pain?	Severe pain (perforated viscus, kidney stone, peritonitis, pancreatitis)
	Pain out of proportion to physical findings (mesenteric ischaemia)
Radiation/referral?	Right scapula (gallbladder pain)
	Left shoulder region (ruptured spleen, pancreatitis)
	Pubis or vagina (renal pain)
	Back (ruptured aortic aneurysm)
Relieving factors?	Antacids (peptic ulcer disease)
	Lying as quietly as possible (peritonitis)
Associated symptoms?	Vomiting precedes pain and is followed by diarrhoea (gastroenteritis)
	Delayed vomiting, absent bowel movement and flatus (acute intestinal obstruction; the delay increases with a lower site of obstruction)
	Severe vomiting precedes intense epigastric, left chest or shoulder pain (emetic perforation of the intra-abdominal oesophagus)

- **Examination of the abdomen** focuses on the detection of peritonitis, any intra-abdominal masses or organomegaly, and localisation of the underlying pathology:
  ○ Distension of the abdomen may be associated with intestinal obstruction.
  ○ Bruising at the flanks (Grey Turner's sign) and periumbilically (Cullen's sign) is occasionally seen in acute haemorrhagic pancreatitis.
  ○ Absent bowel sounds is indicative of ileus and in the presence of severe pain suggests peritonitis.
  ○ High-pitched or overactive bowel sounds might indicate intestinal obstruction.
- **Palpation** should start with very light examination well away from the area of greatest pain. Guarding, rigidity and rebound indicate peritoneal irritation. Guarding is a slow and sustained involuntary contraction of the abdominal muscles, rather than the flinching that is observed with sensitive or anxious patients. Careful exclusion of hernias at the inguinal canals and over surgical scars, as well as pelvic and rectal examination, is essential.

Investigation

Most patients will have an FBC, urea, creatinine and electrolytes, and dipstick urinalysis performed, although the results from these tests are neither sensitive nor specific. Serum lipase, however, is useful in detecting acute pancreatitis. It is essential that erect chest and abdomen and supine abdominal X-rays are performed when there is the possibility of intestinal perforation or obstruction. If the patient cannot sit up, the left lateral position may be used.

Modern imaging can detect the underlying pathology in acute abdominal pain with high sensitivity and specificity. While ultrasound examination has the benefits of portability and avoidance of radiation exposure, it is most useful in detecting disease of the

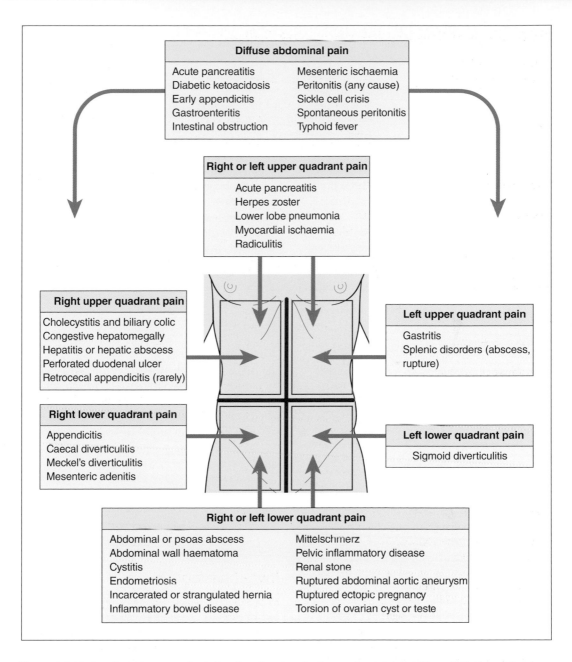

Diffuse abdominal pain

Acute pancreatitis	Mesenteric ischaemia
Diabetic ketoacidosis	Peritonitis (any cause)
Early appendicitis	Sickle cell crisis
Gastroenteritis	Spontaneous peritonitis
Intestinal obstruction	Typhoid fever

Right or left upper quadrant pain

Acute pancreatitis
Herpes zoster
Lower lobe pneumonia
Myocardial ischaemia
Radiculitis

Right upper quadrant pain

Cholecystitis and biliary colic
Congestive hepatomegally
Hepatitis or hepatic abscess
Perforated duodenal ulcer
Retrocecal appendicitis (rarely)

Left upper quadrant pain

Gastritis
Splenic disorders (abscess, rupture)

Right lower quadrant pain

Appendicitis
Caecal diverticulitis
Meckel's diverticulitis
Mesenteric adenitis

Left lower quadrant pain

Sigmoid diverticulitis

Right or left lower quadrant pain

Abdominal or psoas abscess	Mittelschmerz
Abdominal wall haematoma	Pelvic inflammatory disease
Cystitis	Renal stone
Endometriosis	Ruptured abdominal aortic aneurysm
Incarcerated or strangulated hernia	Ruptured ectopic pregnancy
Inflammatory bowel disease	Torsion of ovarian cyst or teste

Figure 1.2 Likely pathologies according to location of acute pain. Source: Frederick H. Millham, in Feldman M, Friedman L, Brandt L (eds) (2010) *Sleisenger and Fordtran's Gastrointestinal and Liver Disease*, 9th edn, Philadelphia, PA: Saunders, Figure 10.3. Reproduced with permission of Elsevier.

gallbladder, and gynaecological and obstetric conditions. CT has emerged as the dominant imaging tool for evaluation of the patient with severe acute abdominal pain. This has come about with the frequent advent of easy access to helical CT within or adjacent to the emergency department. The proper execution and interpretation of CT in this setting have been shown to reduce the need for exploratory laparotomy and hence morbidity, mortality and medical expense.

Management and prognosis

The management and prognosis of both acute and chronic abdominal pain very much depend on the underlying cause. The management and prognosis of the individual diseases that cause abdominal pain (see Box 1.3 and Figure 1.2) are dealt with in each of the individual disease chapters of this book (Chapters 7 to 30).

 KEY POINTS

- Peritoneal pain localizes to the area affected, whereas visceral pain tends to be felt in the upper abdomen – foregut; central abdomen – midgut; or lower abdomen – hindgut.
- Mode of onset, time course, location and radiation, character and exacerbants/relievers are essential to determining the cause of abdominal pain.

- Symptoms associated with the pain are invaluable in further localising the disease process.
- Develop a wide-ranging list of differential diagnoses first, then tailor the investigative strategy to that list and other factors that affect the individual patient.

 SELF-ASSESSMENT QUESTION

(The answer to this question is given on p. 265)

A 45-year-old woman presents acutely with vague, cramping, right upper quadrant, epigastric and right shoulder blade pain. She has experienced similar pain on a few previous occasions over the last year, but never this severe. In the past the pain has been exacerbated by fatty meals, as on this occasion. She cannot get comfortable with the pain; it tends to come in waves but never completely abates. When it is present she finds breathing more difficult. She has taken paracetamol with minimal relief.

With regard to your initial approach to this patient, which of the following is most true?

(a) The localisation of her pain to one area indicates that there is irritation of the parietal peritoneum.

(b) Her scapular pain indicates that there is retroperitoneal involvement.

(c) Her description of the pain makes a hollow organ the likely source.

(d) The epigastric and right upper quadrant location of her pain indicate that it is likely to be coming from the midgut.

(e) She is describing radiation of the pain to the back, which makes a pancreatic cause more likely.

2

Approach to the patient with liver disease

Patients with liver disease can present with a wide range of complaints, and the clinician must remain alert at all times to the possibility of hepatic involvement in disease. Increasingly commonly, asymptomatic patients will present because of liver test abnormalities discovered incidentally. Once the presence of hepatic dysfunction has been established, the not always straightforward task of defining the underlying pathology is critical to planning appropriate management.

Epidemiology

The exact epidemiology of hepatic disease in the world is largely unknown. However, most estimates show that it is increasing out of proportion to many other chronic diseases. This is largely driven by increasing rates of obesity and non-alcoholic fatty liver disease, as well as of alcohol consumption and hepatitis B and C. Some sense of the burden of disease is given by the rates of cirrhosis and liver cancer, as they represent the end stage of liver pathology. Even across Europe the incidence of cirrhosis varies widely, with 1 in 1000 Hungarian males dying of cirrhosis each year compared with 1 in 100,000 Greek females. The World Health Organization (WHO) estimates that liver cancer is responsible for around 47,000 deaths per year in the European Union (EU).

Clinical features

History taking

Liver disease can present in a variety of ways:

- **Non-specific symptoms** include fatigue, anorexia, nausea and, occasionally, vomiting.
- **Loose, fatty stools (steatorrhoea)** can occur if cholestasis interrupts bile flow to the small intestine.
- **Fever (due to liver pyrogens)** may be the first feature in viral or alcoholic hepatitis.
- **Jaundice** becomes visible when the serum bilirubin reaches 34–43 μmol/l (2–2.5 mg/dl). While jaundice may be related to hepatic dysfunction, equally it can be a result of bilirubin overproduction. Mild jaundice without dark urine suggests unconjugated hyperbilirubinaemia (most often caused by haemolysis or Gilbert's syndrome).

The historical features that it is important to elicit include those in the following sections.

Onset and duration

- **Did the symptoms come on gradually or suddenly? How long have the symptoms been a problem?** Symptoms of acute onset may result from an acute vascular event, toxic cause, obstruction of the biliary system or acute infection.

Gastroenterology and Hepatology: Lecture Notes, Second Edition. Stephen Inns and Anton Emmanuel.
© 2017 John Wiley & Sons, Ltd. Published 2017 by John Wiley & Sons, Ltd.
Companion website: www.lecturenoteseries.com/gastroenterology

Symptoms resulting from chronic inflammatory processes are more likely to be of gradual onset. The development of dark urine (bilirubinuria) due to increased serum bilirubin, from hepatocellular or cholestatic causes, often precedes the onset of visible jaundice.

- **Identify precipitating events** related to the onset of the symptoms. Direct questions often need to be asked regarding exposure to common causes (BOX 2.1), in particular:

  - Any association with pain that might relate to biliary obstruction?
  - Any use of medicines – prescribed, complementary or illicit? (NB: Antibiotic-related disease may take up to two weeks to present)
  - Any trauma or major stress, including surgery?
  - Any association with starvation (important in Gilbert's syndrome; see Chapter 20)?
  - Any history of marked weight loss or gain?
  - Any association with vascular events or hypotension?
  - Any possible infectious contact or exposure?

Perpetuating and exacerbating features

Patients should be asked if there are any factors that 'bring on or make the symptoms worse or better'. Pain of a colicky nature that is exacerbated by eating, in particular fatty meals, may indicate a biliary cause for jaundice. A relapsing and remitting course associated with any toxic or medicinal exposure must be carefully sought. The use of immunosuppressive medications for other conditions may improve chronic inflammatory conditions, but conversely may exacerbate infectious causes.

Associated symptoms

The presence of associated symptoms can help localise the origin of symptoms:

- Onset of nausea and vomiting prior to jaundice is associated with acute hepatitis or common bile duct obstruction by a stone.
- Presence of pale stool, bilirubinuria and generalised pruritus is indicative of cholestasis. If this is associated with fevers and rigors, an extrahepatic cause is more likely.
- Central abdominal pain radiating to the back might indicate a pancreatic cause for obstruction.
- Gradual onset of anorexia and malaise commonly occurs in alcoholic liver disease, chronic hepatitis and cancer.

Box 2.1 Common causes of liver disease

Infectious liver disease
- Hepatitis A
- Hepatitis B
- Hepatitis C
- Hepatitis D
- Hepatitis E
- Epstein–Barr virus

Drug-induced hepatitis or cholestasis
Vascular disease
- Ischaemic hepatitis
- Portal vein thrombosis
- Budd–Chiari syndrome
- Nodular regenerative hyperplasia
- Veno-occlusive disease of the liver

Immune hepatitis
- Autoimmune hepatitis
- Granulomatous hepatitis

Deposition diseases
- Wilson's disease
- Haemochromatosis
- Alpha-1-antitrypsin deficiency

Alcoholic liver disease
Fatty liver
- Non-alcoholic fatty liver disease
- Non-alcoholic steatohepatitis
- Focal fatty liver

Tumours and lesions of the liver
- Hepatocellular carcinoma
- Liver secondaries
- Hepatic adenoma
- Focal nodular hyperplasia of the liver
- Hepatic cyst/polycystic liver disease
- Hepatic haemangioma

Congenital liver disease
- Congenital hepatic fibrosis
- Gilbert's syndrome
- Dubin–Johnson syndrome
- Crigler–Najjar syndrome

Liver disease of pregnancy
- Hyperemesis gravidarum
- Cholestasis of pregnancy
- Acute fatty liver of pregnancy
- HELLP syndrome

Cryptogenic cirrhosis

- Disturbances of consciousness, personality changes, intellectual deterioration and changes in speech might indicate hepatic encephalopathy.

Past medical and family history

The importance of a thorough past medical history, social history, family history and list of medicines, including complementary treatments, cannot be stressed enough in the evaluation of liver disease.

- Any history of vascular disease, in particular thromboembolic disease, might point to a vascular cause for hepatic dysfunction.
- Previous or concomitant autoimmune disease increases the possibility of autoimmune hepatitis.
- Pregnancy is associated with a particular set of hepatic problems (see Chapter 29).
- Past carcinoma raises the concern of metastatic liver disease.
- A history of obesity, in particular in association with other features of the metabolic syndrome, increases the risk of steatohepatitis.
- Patients should be carefully questioned regarding the presence of liver disease in the family. Inheritable liver conditions present uncommonly in adulthood, but haemochromatosis and Wilson's disease should be considered. Hepatitis viruses, in particular hepatitis B, may be contracted congenitally. The metabolic syndrome shows a familial tendency and increases the risk of fatty liver disease.

Lifestyle history

- A careful alcohol history, past and present, is essential when interviewing a patient with liver disease.
- Risk factors for infectious hepatitis also need to be carefully questioned in all patients (intravenous drug use, transfusion history including blood products, and close contacts with hepatitis).
- The occupational history may reveal exposure to hepatotoxins (employment involving alcohol, but also carbon tetrachloride, benzene derivatives and toluene).
- A complete list of exposure to medicines, prescribed and illicit, conventional and complementary, must be sought. It must be remembered that in drug-induced liver disease the temporal association may appear obscure, as the interval between exposure and development of symptomatic disease is variable (usually within 5–90 days).

Mental status assessment

It is important to document the mental state of all patients with known hepatic dysfunction, in particular cirrhosis. The Glasgow Coma Scale should be completed (Table 2.1), as it gives prognostically useful information. In the absence of disturbances of consciousness, early encephalopathy interferes with visual spatial awareness, demonstrated as a constructional apraxia, elicited by asking the patient to reproduce simple designs, most commonly a five-pointed star, or deterioration in the quality of handwriting.

Examination technique

The physical examination begins with a careful general inspection – the importance of observing for the stigmata of chronic liver disease (Table 2.2) relates to making the diagnosis, and identifying aetiology and decompensation.

- **Careful inspection of the abdomen is repeated and the abdominal examination is completed as described in Part IV.** Particular care should be taken to define the liver edges by percussion, and the position, texture and consistency of the lower liver edge by palpation. The normal liver span is less than 12.5 cm. The normal liver edge may be pushed

Table 2.1 Glasgow Coma Scale.

	6	5	4	3	2	1
Eyes	N/A	N/A	Opens eyes spontaneously	Opens eyes in response to voice	Opens eyes in response to painful stimuli	Does not open eyes
Verbal	N/A	Oriented, converses normally	Confused, disoriented	Utters inappropriate words	Incomprehensible sounds	Makes no sounds
Motor	Obeys commands	Localises painful stimuli	Withdraws from painful stimuli	Abnormal flexion to painful stimuli	Extension to painful stimuli	Makes no movements

Table 2.2 Stigmata of chronic liver disease (progressing through the hands, face, abdomen and legs).

Diagnosis	Aetiology	Decompensation
Palmar erythema	Dupuytren's contracture (alcohol)	Leuconychia (synthetic function)
Clubbing	Skin discoloration (haemochromatosis)	Multiple bruises (synthetic function)
Excoriation	Tattoos (viral hepatitis)	Asterixis (encephalopathy)
Spider naevi (in distribution of superior vena cava)	Peripheral neuropathy (alcohol)	Drowsiness (encephalopathy)
Conjunctival pallor (anaemia)	Kayser–Fleisher rings (Wilson's)	Jaundice (excretory function)
Gynaecomastia	Parotidomegaly (alcohol)	Hyperventilation (encephalopathy and acidosis)
Female pattern body hair	Cerebellar signs: nystagmus, intention tremor (alcohol and Wilson's)	Ascites (portal hypertension and synthetic function)
Caput medusa (recanalised umbilical vein)	Chronic pulmonary disease (α-1-antitrypsin deficiency, cystic fibrosis)	Pedal/sacral oedema (synthetic function and right heart failure)
Distended abdominal veins	Obesity (non-alcoholic fatty liver disease)	
Testicular atrophy	Diffuse lymphadenopathy (lymphoproliferative disease)	

Table 2.3 Differential diagnosis based on features of the liver examination.

Diagnosis	Characteristics of the liver edge	Degree of hepatomegaly
Metastases	Irregular	Mild to massive
Fatty infiltration due to alcoholic liver disease, myeloproliferative disease	Smooth	
Right heart failure	Smooth Tender if rapid liver enlargement Pulsatile in tricuspid regurgitation	
Hepatocellular cancer	Smooth, tender and occasionally pulsatile	
Haemochromatosis, haematological disease (e.g. chronic leukaemia, lymphoma), fatty liver, infiltration (e.g. amyloid), granuloma (e.g. sarcoid)	Smooth	Mild to moderate
Hepatitis	Smooth and tender	Mild
Biliary obstruction	Smooth	
Hydatid disease, cysts	Firm and irregular	
Hepatic abscess	Smooth and tender	None to mild
Vascular abnormalities	May be smooth or irregular, may be pulsatile	
Cirrhosis from any cause	Firm and irregular	Small liver to mild hepatomegaly

down by pulmonary hyperinflation in emphysema or asthma and with a Riedel's lobe, which is a tongue-like projection from the right lobe's inferior surface. Not all diseased livers are enlarged; a small liver is common in cirrhosis. Cachexia and an unusually hard or lumpy liver more often indicate metastases than cirrhosis. A tender liver suggests hepatitis, hepatocellular cancer or hepatic abscess, but may occur with rapid liver enlargement, e.g. in right heart failure (Table 2.3).

- **Careful examination for the spleen is essential.** While enlargement of the spleen and liver might suggest chronic liver disease with portal hypertension, hepatosplenomegaly without other signs of chronic liver disease may be caused by an infiltrative disorder (e.g. lymphoma, amyloidosis or, in endemic areas, schistosomiasis or malaria), although jaundice is usually minimal or absent in such disorders.

- **Shifting dullness** is elicited by demonstrating flank dullness to percussion that moves with repositioning of the patient. Very rarely it is possible for intraabdominal cystic masses to cause 'pseudo-ascites'; hence if shifting dullness is found, it should be confirmed bilaterally to ensure that it is due to ascitic fluid shift.

Investigation

Following a careful history and examination, the likely pathological processes relevant to the patient should be identifiable. The most likely diagnoses should be listed first and these can then be expanded by the application of a surgical sieve (as described in Part IV).

All patients should have routine biochemistry, haematology and coagulation tests performed. Serial liver enzyme assays give a picture of the course of the illness. In **hepatitis** an initial diagnostic serological screen should examine for the commoner causes. These would commonly include:

- Hepatitis A, B and C serology.
- Autoimmune screen to include antinuclear antibodies (ANA), antimitochondrial antibodies (AMA), smooth muscle antibodies (SMA) and liver/kidney microsomal antibody type 1 in the younger patient.
- Serum immunoglobulin (Ig) levels are also commonly performed: there is some diagnostic sensitivity for elevated IgA in alcoholic liver disease and IgM in primary biliary cirrhosis.
- As reports of occult coeliac disease as a cause of LFT abnormalities are increasing, testing for antiendomysial (EMA) or antitissue transglutaminase (tTG) may be beneficial, particularly in the patient with GI disturbance.
- Fasting blood sugars and lipids should be tested where fatty liver disease is suspected.
- In the young patient the rare genetic causes, Wilson's disease (serum caeruloplasmin), hereditary haemochromatosis (serum ferritin and transferrin saturation) and alpha-1-antitrypsin deficiency (AAT concentrations), can be screened for.

Investigation of the liver architecture and hepatic vasculature by ultrasound is generally indicated.

Box 2.2 Indications for liver biopsy

- Diagnose unexplained liver enzyme abnormalities
- Diagnose and assess alcoholic liver disease
- Diagnose and assess non-alcoholic steatosis
- Diagnose and stage chronic hepatitis (viral and autoimmune)
- Diagnose storage disorders (iron, copper)
- Diagnose hepatomegaly of unknown cause
- Diagnose unexplained intrahepatic cholestasis
- Monitor use of hepatotoxic drugs (e.g. methotrexate)
- Obtain histology of suspicious lesions
- Obtain histology or culture in systemic illnesses
- Following liver transplant: suspected rejection
- Prior to liver transplant to assess donor

Due to its low cost and the absence of ionising radiation, ultrasound can be considered the imaging modality of first choice. However, ultrasound may be difficult in the obese or gaseous patient, in those with a high-lying liver completely covered by the rib margin and in postoperative patients with dressings or painful scars. CT and MRI are useful second-line modalities and have largely replaced radioisotope scanning.

Liver biopsy is not usually required for the diagnosis of acute hepatitis. Its use is typically reserved for the assessment of chronic liver disease in order to inform prognosis and management, and following hepatic transplantation. Liver biopsy can, however, be useful in confirming deposition diseases of the liver and where a clear diagnosis as to the cause of hepatitis has not been forthcoming after a complete serological work-up. Biopsy of possible malignant tumours has to be weighed against the risk of tumour seeding (Box 2.2). Biopsy may be undertaken through percutaneous, transjugular or rarely laparoscopic approaches.

Because of the risk from liver biopsy (1 in 100 risk of bleeding or perforation), non-invasive means of determining the degree of liver damage (fibrosis) have been developed, in order to predict prognosis and guide treatment for diseases such as Hepatitis B and C. One such tool is the Fibroscan®. This uses a mechanical pulse, generated at the skin surface and propagated through the liver. The velocity of the wave generated is measured by ultrasound and directly correlates with the stiffness of the liver: the stiffer the liver, the greater the degree of fibrosis.

Assessment of the severity of liver disease

Where chronic liver disease is confirmed, some assessment of the severity of hepatic dysfunction should be made. The commonest scoring system used is the Child–Turcotte–Pugh score (Table 2.4).

This score is calculated using the total bilirubin, serum albumin, international normalised ratio (INR), degree of ascites and grade of hepatic encephalopathy. Based on this score, patients are grouped into three severity levels: A, B and C.

These Child–Turcotte–Pugh 'classes' are predictive of prognosis and useful in determining the required strength of treatment and the necessity of liver transplantation (Table 2.5). Another specialised pretransplantation assessment is the Model for End-stage Liver Disease (MELD) score (Table 2.6).

Table 2.4 Child–Turcotte–Pugh scoring system.

Measure	1 point	2 points	3 points
Bilirubin (total) (µmol/l [mg/dl])	<34 [<2]	34–50 [2–3]	>50 [>3]
Serum albumin	>35	28–35	<28
INR	<1.7	1.71–2.20	>2.20
Ascites	None	Suppressed with medication	Refractory
Hepatic encephalopathy	None	Grade I–II (or suppressed with medication)	Grade III–IV (or refractory)

INR, international normalised ratio.

Table 2.5 Prognosis related to Child–Turcotte–Pugh scoring system.

Points	Class	1-year survival (%)	2-year survival (%)
5–6	A	100	85
7–9	B	81	57
10–15	C	45	35

Table 2.6 Model for End-stage Liver Disease (MELD) score.

MELD score	3-Month mortality (% hospitalised patients)
≤9	4
10–19	27
20–29	76
30–39	83
≥40	100

 KEY POINTS

- Jaundice becomes visible when the serum bilirubin is about 35 micromol/L.
- Jaundice in the absence of dark urine suggests unconjugated hyperbilirubinaemia (Gilbert's or haemolysis).
- Pale stool and jaundice may suggest biliary obstruction; the presence of urinary bilirubin (conjugated) in the absence of urinary urobilinogen confirms this.
- A careful medication history is essential – antibiotics particularly can take up to two weeks to cause their effect on the liver.
- The 'signs of chronic liver disease' are most useful for just that – determining whether liver disease is likely to be chronic or not.

- It is useful to have a 'standard hepatitis screen' in mind, including hepatitis B and C (A if acute), ANA, AMA, SMA (LKM1 if young), serum immunoglobulins and EMA/tTG. Also serum copper and caeruloplasmin, ferritin and transferrin, and alpha1 antitrypsin levels in the young or those with a family history of hepatitis.
- Liver biopsy is rarely used for diagnostic purposes and its value in assessing the severity of fibrosis is slowly being replaced by non-invasive alternatives.

SELF-ASSESSMENT QUESTION

(The answer to this question is given on p. 265)

A 66-year-old woman presents with visible jaundice over the last week. She has been feeling non-specifically unwell for about 1 week with fatigue and nausea. She has noticed that her urine has become darker than usual. Her stool is unchanged. She has not been exposed to anyone with hepatic disease and has made no changes to her medications in the last two weeks.

Regarding her clinical presentation, which of the following statements is most correct?

(a) Dark urine and jaundice make biliary obstruction very likely in this case.

(b) Wilson's disease is extremely unlikely in this situation.

(c) For jaundice to occur, the serum bilirubin must be above 65 micromol/L.

(d) The fact that she has not had any new medicines in the last 2 weeks makes drug-induced liver disease unlikely.

(e) Ultrasound is unlikely to be helpful in this situation and she should proceed to liver biopsy to gain a definitive diagnosis.

3

Approach to the patient with luminal disease

This chapter provides both a basis to structure revision and details of a practical approach to patients presenting in gastroenterology wards and clinics. Abdominal pain is dealt with in Chapter 1. The other common presenting problem of GI bleeding is dealt with in Chapters 7 and 8.

Dysphagia

Dysphagia is defined as difficulty in swallowing, distinct from odynophagia, which means pain on swallowing. It also needs to be distinguished from globus, which is a functional syndrome of the sensation of a lump in the throat in the absence of an organic cause. In taking a history, one needs to differentiate one of three general causes – oropharyngeal or oesophageal mechanical or oesophageal dysmotility (Table 3.1).

Causes

For the causes of dysphagia, see Table 3.2.

Epidemiology

In a population study in Australia, approximately 16% of people experienced dysphagia at some time.

Clinical features

History

See Table 3.1.

Investigation

- **Condition and cause**:
  - Endoscopy: first-choice investigation, allows biopsy and/or dilatation of strictures; may be performed after barium swallow to allow exclusion of pharyngeal pouch, which could be perforated by the unsuspecting endoscopist.
  - Barium swallow (irregular stricture = malignant; smooth stricture = benign).
  - Chest X-ray (hilar lymphadenopathy = oesophageal malignancy).
  - Videofluoroscopy (if oropharyngeal cause suspected).
  - ENT (Ear, Nose and Throat) opinion (if oropharyngeal cause suspected).
  - Systemic sclerosis antibodies.
- **Complications**:
  - FBC (anaemia = oesophageal malignancy, malnutrition, Plummer–Vinson syndrome).
  - LFTs (stage oesophageal malignancy).

Management

Specific management depends on the underlying cause (see appropriate sections).

Prognosis

Prognosis very much depends on the underlying diagnosis. Because of its association with oesophageal carcinoma, particularly in older patients, dysphagia is considered an indication for urgent endoscopy.

Gastroenterology and Hepatology: Lecture Notes, Second Edition. Stephen Inns and Anton Emmanuel.
© 2017 John Wiley & Sons, Ltd. Published 2017 by John Wiley & Sons, Ltd.
Companion website: www.lecturenoteseries.com/gastroenterology

Table 3.1 Historical features of help in identifying the cause of dysphagia.

Clinical features	Oropharyngeal	Oesophageal mechanical cause	Oesophageal dysmotility cause
Initiating swallow	Difficult	Unaffected	Unaffected
Interval to dysphagia after swallow	Instant	Few seconds	Few seconds
Progression	Variable	Progressively worsening	Intermittent
Type of food	Liquids	Solids	Liquids and solids
Associated symptoms	Choking, nasal regurgitation, drooling	Weight loss, prior heartburn	Odynophagia
Associated signs	Cranial nerve signs	Cervical lymph nodes, anaemia	Systemic sclerosis?

Table 3.2 Causes of dysphagia, classified by frequency of occurrence.

	Oropharyngeal	Oesophageal
Common	Stroke Candidiasis Globus sensation	Benign (peptic) stricture Oesophageal carcinoma Oesophagitis
Less common	Pharyngeal pouch Motor neurone disease Xerostomia	Dysmotility (achalasia > spasm > systemic sclerosis) Webs and rings External pressure (hilar nodes, lung cancer)
Rare	Oral tumours Severe aphthous ulcers Muscular dystrophy	Oesophageal infections Retrosternal goitre Corrosive stricture

Nausea and vomiting

Vomiting is the violent expulsion of gastric and intestinal content induced by contraction of the abdominal musculature and diaphragm. It is distinct from **regurgitation**, which is the passive passage of gastric content without abdominal contraction and may reflect oesophageal or gastric disease. **Nausea** is the perceptual component of vomiting.

Causes

The list of potential causes is enormous, but can be classified as in Box 3.1. More than one cause is often present.

Epidemiology

Nausea and vomiting are common complaints that affect most of us at some point. In an Australian population study, 1.6% of visits to GPs were for nausea and vomiting.

Clinical features

History

- **Timing**: acute cases (see later) need to be distinguished from chronic, as causation is quite different:
  - If shortly after meals, suggests a gastric cause.
  - If long after meals, suggests distal intestinal cause.
  - If unrelated to meals, suggests non-GI cause.
  - If mostly on waking, suggests central nervous system (CNS) cause.
- **Amount of vomitus**:
  - Large volumes suggest obstruction or gastric cause.
  - Small volumes suggest a functional problem.
- **Content of vomitus**:
  - If bile (bitter brown liquid) present, then pylorus is patent, and gastroparesis is unlikely.
  - If undigested food is present many hours after being eaten, then a gastric cause is likely.

Box 3.1 Causes of vomiting

Gastrointestinal

- Functional disorders:
  - Functional dyspepsia syndromes
  - IBS
- Obstructive:
  - Achalasia
  - Gastric outlet obstruction
    - Pyloric stenosis
    - Gastroparesis
  - Small bowel obstruction
- Organic luminal disease:
  - Peptic ulcers
  - Upper GI cancers
  - Gastroenteritis
- Organic hepato-pancreato-biliary disease:
  - Hepatitis: acute and chronic
  - Pancreatitis: acute and chronic
  - Cholecystitis: acute and chronic

Neurological

- Vestibular disorders
- Raised intracranial pressure
- Migraine
- Demyelinating disorders

Psychogenic

- Bulimia nervosa > anorexia nervosa
- Psychogenic vomiting
- Cyclical vomiting syndrome

Alcohol

Drugs – almost any, but especially:

- Opiates
- Antibiotics, especially erythromycin
- Chemotherapy agents
- NSAIDs
- Anticonvulsants

Metabolic

- Uraemia
- Diabetic ketoacidosis
- Addison's disease

Pregnancy

- **Associated features**:
  - If isolated, almost always functional.
  - Drug history (see causes).
  - Neurological symptoms (see causes).
- **Assessment**:
  - Signs of dehydration (*complication*).
  - Signs of sepsis (*cause*).
  - Signs of visible peristalsis and hernia (*cause*).
  - Sucussion splash (*condition*).

- Dental enamel erosions (*cause* – gastro-oesophageal reflux disease [GORD] or bulimia).
- Neurological signs (*cause*).

Investigation

The investigation of vomiting needs to be focused by consideration of causes (see Box 3.1).

Management

This should, where possible, be directed at treating the underlying cause (as per Box 3.1). Symptomatic relief may be obtained as follows.

- **Centrally acting antiemetics**:
  - Phenothiazines (prochlorperazine, haloperidol):
    - Antidopamine effect.
    - Best for neurological, drug-induced and metabolic nausea.
    - Side effects: sedation, orthostatic hypotension.
  - 5-HT_3 antagonists (ondansetron):
    - Antihistamine effect at chemoreceptor trigger zone.
    - Best for drug-induced nausea.
    - Well tolerated, but expensive.
  - 5-HT_1 antagonists (diphenhydramine):
    - Antihistamine effect at chemoreceptor trigger zone.
    - Best for neurological causes of nausea.
    - Well tolerated, but limited efficacy.
- **Peripherally acting antiemetics**:
  - Prokinetic agents (domperidone, metoclopramide):
    - Best for GI causes of vomiting.
    - Side effects: gynaecomastia, extrapyramidal effects.
  - Motilin analogues (erythromycin):
    - Especially useful in gastroparesis.
- **Centrally and peripherally acting agents**:
  - Steroids (dexamethasone).
  - Benzodiazepines (lorazepam).

Prognosis

Prognosis is completely dependant on the underlying cause. Refer to the specific disease chapters of this book.

Constipation

Constipation is defined in purely symptomatic terms (in contrast to diarrhoea, which is defined as stool weight >200 g). Implicit in this is the fact that constipation is merely a symptom, not a diagnosis.

Table 3.3 Secondary causes of constipation.

Primary pathology	Examples
Endocrine conditions	Hypothyroidism* Hyperparathyroidism Diabetes mellitus* Glucagonoma
Neurological conditions	Multiple sclerosis Autonomic neuropathy Parkinson's disease* Spinal injury*
Psychogenic conditions	Affective disorders* Eating disorders* Dementia or learning difficulty
Metabolic	Hypercalcaemia Uraemia Hypokalaemia Porphyria Amyloidosis Lead poisoning
Colonic	Stricture Tumour* Ischaemia Diverticular disease*
Anal	Fissure* Polyp Tumour
Physiological	Pregnancy* Old age*
Drugs (all of which lead to prolongation of transit)	Opiates Anticholinergics Anticonvulsants Tricyclic antidepressants Antacids (aluminium- and calcium-containing ones) NSAIDs Iron Antihypertensives

*Most common.

Functional constipation is distinct from **irritable bowel syndrome (IBS)**, in that abdominal pain is not necessarily associated with bowel dysfunction. Constipation is defined as infrequent stools (<3 per week), passage of hard stools (>25% of the time), straining to empty the rectum (>25% of the time) or a sensation of incomplete evacuation (>25% of the time). See Box 3.2.

Epidemiology

Constipation is one of the most common GI complaints. It affects about 25% of the population at some time, being more common in women and the elderly.

Causes

Constipation is mostly idiopathic. It is, however, important to be able to recognise the secondary causes, the most important of which are listed in Table 3.3.

Classification

Constipation can be classified as primary or secondary to other disorders, and it is often multifactorial. The distinction is important as it will direct management.

Primary causes can be due to constipation with a colon of normal diameter or with a dilated colon, but this is a clinically important distinction to make, and can be assessed on abdominal X-ray or barium study.

Constipation with a colon of normal diameter

Patients who have constipation with a colon of normal diameter can be classified into three subgroups:

- **Normal transit constipation**. This is the commonest type of constipation. It is characterised by a normal rate of stool movement through the colon, but the patient feels constipated. It is usually secondary to perceived difficulty with defaecation and hard stools. Symptoms may overlap with those of constipation-predominant IBS, since pain and bloating are common.

- **Slow transit constipation**. Most common in young women, with symptoms dating back to childhood. Characterised by infrequent bowel movements and slow movement of stool through the colon. Bloating, abdominal pain and an infrequent urge to defaecate are commonly associated with this condition. There may be underlying neural changes in the colon, although these may be secondary to the condition itself.
- **Disordered defaecation**. Usually due to dysfunction of the pelvic floor or anal sphincters. Patients typically report an inability to defaecate despite feeling an urge to do so, and need to use digital manipulation per vagina or per anum. Most often there is incoordination of the pelvic floor and anal sphincters, resulting in non-propulsion of stool from the rectum; this may have been triggered by deliberately suppressing the urge to defaecate. Alternatively there may be structural abnormalities, such as a rectocoele (a bulging of the rectum into the posterior wall of the vagina) or rectal intussusception (telescoping of the rectum into itself during straining), which cause an 'obstruction' to defaecation.

Constipation with a dilated colon

Severe constipation with gut dilatation is secondary to neuromuscular disorders of the colon:

- Hirschsprung's disease (see Chapter 16).
- Idiopathic megacolon (see Chapter 16).
- Chronic intestinal pseudo-obstruction (see Chapter 15).

Clinical features

History

- **Stool frequency and consistency**: hard stools suggest delayed transit; normal stools suggest normal transit; loose stools may relate to laxative use.
- **Need to strain or digitally extract stool?** Suggests defaecatory disorder.
- **What is the urge frequency?** Daily suggests normal transit; every two days or less suggests slow transit.
- **Any clear precipitants to onset?** Abdominal or pelvic surgery, childbirth or emotional trauma.
- **Faecal impaction and faecal soiling?** Suggests idiopathic megacolon.
- **Alarm symptoms** needing urgent imaging:
  - Rectal bleeding.
  - Recent onset of symptoms.
  - Weight loss.
  - Family history of colon cancer.
- **Comorbid medical history: thyroid disease, diabetes or renal impairment?**
- **Drug history** (see Table 3.3).
- **Dietary history**: specifically meal frequency and fibre intake.

Investigation

- **Blood tests**:
  - FBC: for anaemia if colon cancer is the cause of constipation.
  - Urea and electrolyte (U&E): uraemia as a cause of constipation.
  - Thyroid function tests: hypothyroidism as a cause of constipation.
  - Calcium: hypercalcaemia as a cause of constipation.
  - Glucose: diabetes, of which constipation is the commonest GI manifestation.
- **Imaging**:
  - Colonic imaging to exclude cancer if there are any alarm symptoms, or in patients over 50 years of age who have a new onset of symptoms: colonoscopy or CT colonography (for details, see Chapter 6).
  - Evacuation proctography (by barium or MRI contrast) allows study of anorectal morphology and dynamics during defaecation. It detects:
    - Functional abnormalities such as incoordination of the pelvic floor and anal sphincters.
    - Structural abnormalities of rectal emptying such as intussusception, rectal prolapse and rectocoele.
  - Radio-opaque marker study of whole gut transit – a useful measure of the motor function of the whole gut (Figure 3.1). Whole gut transit can be measured by performing an abdominal X-ray after the ingestion of radio-opaque markers; it primarily reflects colonic transit, given that intestinal transit time is mostly colonic.
  - Plain abdominal X-ray is *not* a sensitive diagnostic test of constipation.
- **Anorectal physiological tests**. These are only needed in the minority of patients who do not respond to lifestyle advice or brief laxative use:
  - Recto-anal inhibitory reflex: presence excludes Hirschsprung's disease.
  - Anorectal sensory testing: to detect whether there is loss of rectal sensation (in patients with multiple sclerosis, Parkinson's disease etc.).

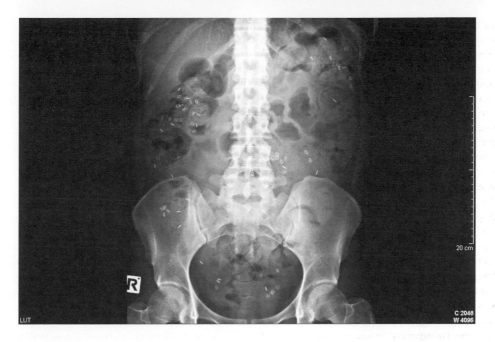

Figure 3.1 Shape study for colonic transit. The number of shapes and where they are in the colon 4 and 7 days after ingestion are added up to give a transit time across the colon.

Management

- **Diet**: in general, patients with normal transit need to augment dietary fibre and liquid intake. Only if they cannot manage this through normal diet should they be prescribed fibre supplements. Patients with slow transit, by contrast, need less fibre in their diet, since fibre tends to exacerbate bloating and does not help accelerate transit.
- **Laxatives**:
  - Stimulant laxatives (senna, bisacodyl) are probably best used on an as-required basis rather than regularly. Longstanding concerns regarding laxative dependence have largely been discounted by recent studies, however, and patients should not be denied these alternatives if they find that this is the most beneficial option.
  - Stool softeners (docusate) are primarily used as adjuvant agents.
  - Osmotic agents (magnesium [Mg] salts, lactulose) are effective in slow transit and allow dose adjustment according to response, but may be unpalatable. Polyethylene glycol is a very effective osmotic and can be beneficial in intractable slow transit constipation.
- **Biofeedback**: behavioural therapy with biofeedback is an effective alternative to laxatives for patients who want to avoid long-term dependence on drugs.
- **Surgery**: while rectocoele or pelvic floor repairs may help some patients with structural rectal or pelvic abnormalities, colonic resection surgery for constipation has mostly fallen out of favour (due to poor long-term results and the frequent need for re-operation).
- **Psychological therapy**: some patients with constipation have the symptom as a consequence of significant psychological distress, and in these situations specific psychological help can be helpful.

Prognosis

The mortality associated with constipation is low. There is no association between colorectal cancer and constipation, and constipation is very rarely the sole presenting complaint for someone with colorectal cancer.

Diarrhoea

Diarrhoea is strictly defined as an increase in stool weight above 200 g – mostly occurring as a result of an increase in stool water content. An alternative definition is a change in bowel habit to more than three stools a day. It is not the frequent passage of formed stool.

Table 3.4 Physiology of fluid fluxes in the gut.

Fluids into lumen		Fluids out of lumen	
Food in	*2000 ml*	Small bowel reabsorption	5350 ml
Saliva	250 ml	Colonic reabsorption	2000 ml
Gastric secretions	2000 ml	*Stool volume*	*150 ml*
Small intestinal secretions	3250 ml		
TOTAL	7500 ml	TOTAL	7500 ml

Table 3.4 illustrates the approximate fluid fluxes in the gut in a healthy, well-nourished individual. It illustrates the principle that two-thirds of the reabsorption of liquid is accomplished during the rapid period of transit (approximately 2–4 hours) through the small bowel. This leaves approximately 2 l of material entering the caecum each day, which gets progressively dehydrated in its passage through the colon over approximately 24 hours. It is readily appreciable, therefore, that small changes in colonic function will alter stool volume: a 10% reduction in colonic reabsorption will leave an extra 200 ml of liquid in the lumen, and more than double the stool volume.

Epidemiology

The prevalence of chronic diarrhoea (>4 weeks of symptoms) is approximately 4% in the community population in the UK.

Causes

While a comprehensive list of causes of diarrhoea is given in Table 3.5 (for examination revision purposes), it is easier to remember this list by considering the potential causes of diarrhoea. Many disorders cause a mixture of the three basic mechanisms.

Mechanisms of diarrhoea

Osmotic diarrhoea

- **Principle**: persistence of non-absorbed osmotically active compounds (typically carbohydrates or fat) that retain fluid in the lumen exceeding the colonic capacity to reabsorb.
- **Characteristic**: 'porridgy' stool; symptoms resolve on fasting.
- **Investigation**: rarely needed, but physiologically gratifying. Identifies an increased faecal osmotic gap: $290 - 2 \times ([\text{faecal Na}^+] + [\text{faecal K}^+])$; a gap >125 mOsm/kg is diagnostic.

- **Causes**:
  - Laxative misuse (lactulose or other osmotic laxatives).
  - Lactose intolerance (most commonly as part of another intestinal disorder, such as Crohn's disease, coeliac disease).
  - Bacterial overgrowth (due to production of osmotically active compounds by small bowel bacterial colonisation).
  - Steatorrhoea causes (chronic pancreatitis, small bowel disease).

Secretory diarrhoea

- **Principle**: small bowel secretion abnormally stimulated by a peptide (vasoactive intestinal peptide [VIP] or gastrin) or a toxin (*Escherichia. coli* enterotoxin, *Vibrio cholera* toxin). The causative agents act on cyclic nucleotide release within enterocytes, resulting in ion secretion and water loss into the lumen.
- **Characteristic**: 'watery' stool in huge volumes; does not settle with fasting.
- **Investigation**: rarely needed, but stool volumes usually >500 ml/day, with normal faecal osmotic gap (<50 mOsm/kg).
- **Causes**:
  - Toxins (*E. coli, V. cholera, Clostridium*).
  - Tumour (VIPoma, Zollinger–Ellison, bile acid malabsorption, villous adenoma).

Dysmotility diarrhoea

- **Principle**: accelerated transit leaves less time for reabsorption in small and/or large bowel.
- **Characteristic**: stool consistency varies day to day.
- **Investigation**: none, other than an accurate history.
- **Causes**:
  - IBS.
  - Post-GI resection.
  - Drugs (stimulant laxatives).

Table 3.5 Causes of diarrhoea.

Condition	Comments	Frequency
Gastroenteritis	Virus	Commonest
	Bacterial (*Campylobacter*, *Salmonella*)	Common
	Toxin (*E. coli*, *Shigella*)	Common
	Parasite (*Giardia*)	Rare
Inflammatory bowel disease		Common
Drug-induced	Many, including alcohol, antibiotics, Mg-containing antacids, proton pump inhibitors (PPIs), NSAIDs	Common
Colorectal carcinoma	Left sided > right sided	Common
Irritable bowel syndrome (IBS)	Diarrhoea-predominant IBS may complicate prior gastroenteritis in 25% of cases	Common
Coeliac disease	>50% of patients report diarrhoea	Unusual
Microscopic colitis	Diagnosis depends on correct colon histology	Unusual
Laxative misuse	High level of suspicion needed to avoid unnecessary investigation	Unusual
Bacterial overgrowth	Usually as comorbidity of another disorder	Unusual
Uncommon gut disorders	Pseudo-membranous colitis	Unusual
	Post-gastric or ileal resection or vagotomy	Unusual
	Ischaemic colitis	Unusual
	Lactose intolerance	Unusual
	Bile acid malabsorption	Rare
	Whipple's disease	Rare
	Gastrinoma/VIPoma	Rare
	Carcinoid	Rare
Non-intestinal disease	Chronic pancreatitis	Unusual
	Thyrotoxicosis (may be no other clinical signs)	Unusual
	Autonomic neuropathy (diabetes)	Rare
	Addison's disease	Rare
	Behçet's disease	Rare
	Hypoparathyroidism	Rare
Infiltrative gut diseases	Amyloidosis	Rare
	Intestinal vasculitis	Rare
	Mastocytosis	Rare
	Hypogammaglobulinaemia	Rare

Clinical features

History

- **Nature of diarrhoea**: watery, 'porridgy' and variable-consistency stool – as in 'Mechanisms of diarrhoea'; pale, fatty stools that are hard to flush away suggest steatorrhoea (pancreatic or small bowel cause).
- **Timing**: night-time diarrhoea is organic and excludes a diagnosis of IBS; morning diarrhoea suggests inflammatory bowel disease (IBD), IBS or alcohol misuse.
- **Associated features**:
  - Be alert to the 'red flag' or 'warning' features: rectal bleeding, weight loss, anaemia, nocturnal diarrhoea, and new onset in over 45-year-olds. Overt blood loss suggests a colonic cause.
  - Drug and surgical history (as per Box 3.1).
  - Systemic illness (diabetes, scleroderma, thyroid disease).
  - Family history (colorectal cancer, IBD, coeliac disease).

Rigid sigmoidoscopy is a useful part of the clinical assessment of the patient with diarrhoea – distal tumours, ulcerative colitis and infectious proctitis are readily evident, and biopsies can be taken. (NB: Microscopic colitis cannot be excluded by rectal biopsies alone.)

Investigation

- **Stool microscopy**: for *Giardia* (and other parasites or ova), although most labs use the more sensitive ELISA test for *Giardia*, *Cryptosporidium* and other parasites, which reduces the number of samples required from three to one. The presence of white blood cells and/or red blood cells on microscopy gives a clue as to whether there is an inflammatory cause or not.

- **Other stool tests**:
  - *Clostridium difficile* ELISA and toxin (if recent antibiotics, in the elderly or if other risk factors).
  - Culture (if suspect food poisoning with *Salmonella, Shigella, Campylobacter*).
  - Electron microscopy for viruses is rarely if ever needed.
  - Faecal calprotectin (a neutrophil-derived peptide) is used in some centres to distinguish inflammatory from other causes of diarrhoea. The problem with this is the possibility of false positive and negative results (positive and negative predictive value of around 70% for organic disease).

- **Blood tests**:
  - Haemoglobin: carcinoma, IBD, coeliac disease.
  - Mean corpuscular volume (MCV) elevated in coeliac disease (low folate), terminal ileal disease (low B_{12}), Crohn's, post-resection, alcohol misuse.
  - MCV reduced in carcinoma, IBD.
  - Serum potassium: classically low in VIPoma, but also in any severe diarrhoea (small bowel K^+ loss).
  - C-reactive protein (CRP) – preferred to erythrocyte sedimentation rate (ESR) – elevated in carcinoma (mild increase), IBD (greater increase) and infection (most elevated).
  - Thyroid function tests (TFTs).
  - Coeliac antibodies (see Chapter 14).

- **Endoscopy**:
  - Upper GI endoscopy and D2 biopsy: if suspect coeliac disease or *Giardia*.
  - Flexible sigmoidoscopy: if diarrhoea associated with fresh rectal bleeding.
  - Colonoscopy and ileoscopy with biopsies: largely reserved for patients with warning features or patients more than 45 years old.

- **Radiology**:
  - CT colonography: if patient unsuitable or unfit for colonoscopy.
  - Abdominal ultrasound or CT scan: if biliary or pancreatic disease suspected.
  - CT/MRI enterography: to exclude Crohn's disease, or intestinal lymphoma.

- **Further investigation**:
  - If above investigations do not reveal a cause, may need to consider admission for observation (food and stool chart) and 3-day stool weight estimation. If diarrhoea settles, or stool weight <200 g/day, treat as IBS or functional (laxative misuse); if stool weight >200 g/day, then further investigation is warranted.

  - Stool osmolality and volume after a 48-hour fast will identify secretory and osmotic causes of diarrhoea.
  - Laxative screen in suspected patients: this will need stool and serology samples.
  - Capsule enteroscopy: pick-up for diarrhoea is poor in CT/MRI enterography.
  - Lactose hydrogen breath test will identify hypolactasia, but it may be more practical to ask the patient to empirically follow a lactose-free diet and see how they respond.
  - Se-HCAT bile acid malabsorption test may be helpful, but an empirical trial of treatment with cholestyramine may be appropriate.

Treatment

Treatment is usually directed towards supportive care (maintaining fluid balance, treating pyrexia) and correcting the underlying cause. Symptomatic treatment may be undertaken with the following:

- Loperamide: acts on μ-opioid receptors in the myenteric plexus of the gut to reduce peristalsis and intestinal secretion; it does not cross into the CNS or cause dependence.
- Codeine: an opiate with analgesic and antidiarrhoeal properties; it can cross into the CNS and cause drowsiness and, in large doses, respiratory depression.
- Co-phenotrope: a combination drug of a synthetic opiate and atropine (anticholinergic), which reduces intestinal secretion and contraction; the anticholinergic effects mean that it is often poorly tolerated.

Prognosis

Worldwide, diarrhoea is an important cause of morbidity and mortality, particularly in children in developing countries. Around 760,000 children die each year because of diarrhoea. In the developed world diarrhoeal illnesses still cause significant morbidity and mortality, but most episodes are short and self-limiting. The prognosis of each of the common causes of diarrhoea is considered in the disease-specific chapters of this book.

Anal incontinence

This refers to involuntary passage of rectal content (gas or stool), and it is a source of major embarrassment to the sufferer.

Epidemiology

The symptom occurs more commonly with age, and on a weekly basis in 2% of community-dwelling over 70-year-olds.

Causes

Incontinence arises when there is disturbance of the:

- Anus,
- Rectum, or
- Coordination between anus and rectum.

In turn, this could be due to disorder of either structure or function of either organ. With regard to function, anal incontinence can be due to disturbed motor or sensory function. The overall possible pathophysiology is summarised in Figure 3.2, which also outlines the possible causes and relates these to the pathophysiology.

Clinical features

History

There are two forms of anal incontinence:

- **Urge incontinence** occurs when there is marked urgency to void the bowel, with incontinence occurring before the patient can get to a toilet.

- **Passive incontinence** is due to leaking of stool without perception of any urge.

History taking should also address the severity of the condition (need to wear pads, frequency of episodes, effects on lifestyle).

Investigation

- **Structure**: anal inspection, endoanal ultrasound (rarely pelvic CT or MR).
- **Function**: digital examination, anorectal manometry and sensory testing (rarely electromyogram, EMG).

Management

General

- Optimise stool consistency (antidiarrhoeal drugs – loperamide, codeine).
- Dietary advice (rationalise dietary fibre intake, avoid excess caffeine, alcohol).
- Review medications (if possible, discontinue any that cause diarrhoea).
- Anal sphincter exercises.

Specific

- Sphincter tear: surgical repair (when possible).
- Rectal prolapse or rectocoele: surgical repair.

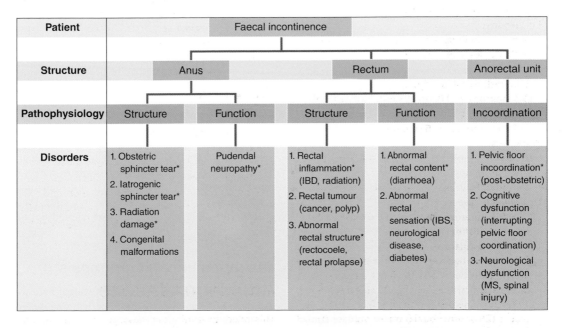

Patient	Faecal incontinence				
Structure	Anus		Rectum		Anorectal unit
Pathophysiology	Structure	Function	Structure	Function	Incoordination
Disorders	1. Obstetric sphincter tear* 2. Iatrogenic sphincter tear* 3. Radiation damage* 4. Congenital malformations	Pudendal neuropathy*	1. Rectal inflammation* (IBD, radiation) 2. Rectal tumour (cancer, polyp) 3. Abnormal rectal structure* (rectocoele, rectal prolapse)	1. Abnormal rectal content* (diarrhoea) 2. Abnormal rectal sensation (IBS, neurological disease, diabetes)	1. Pelvic floor incoordination* (post-obstetric) 2. Cognitive dysfunction (interrupting pelvic floor coordination) 3. Neurological dysfunction (MS, spinal injury)

Figure 3.2 Pathophysiology of faecal incontinence. The most common disorders are indicated with an asterisk. IBD, inflammatory bowel disease; IBS, irritable bowel syndrome; MS, multiple sclerosis.

- Disease causes of diarrhoea: specific medical treatment of each condition.
- Pelvic incoordination: biofeedback or sacral nerve stimulation (surgical procedure to electrically stimulate sacral nerves and hence improve sphincter function).

 ## Nerve stimulation modalities

Sacral nerve stimulation has been established as an effective therapy for severe faecal incontinence. It uses an electrode lead system connected to an implanted pulse generator to give chronic low-voltage stimulation of the sacral nerve root. It is by necessity invasive and expensive. Posterior tibial nerve stimulation has emerged as a less invasive alternative. Here, a fine-needle electrode is placed adjacent to the posterior tibial nerve to give the low-voltage stimulation. In a direct comparison study, the two techniques performed similarly over six months.

Prognosis

While faecal incontinence can have an enormous influence on quality of life, in itself it is a benign condition not associated with significant mortality.

Weight loss

Weight loss is a common cause for presentation to gastroenterology services. It should be remembered that there are 'physiological' reasons for weight loss, according to the simplistic formula:

Body weight = Food ingested − Exertion undertaken

In other words, reduced nutrient intake or excess exercise cause weight loss. Importantly, there are many non-GI causes of weight loss (Table 3.6).

Causes

See Table 3.6.

Epidemiology

In one study involuntary weight loss in the last six months occurred in 13% of the population.

Clinical features

History and investigation

Table 3.6 lists the conditions that should be considered in assessing weight loss. Particular attention should focus on the psychological and environmental

Table 3.6 Causes of weight loss.

Gastrointestinal	Oral disease GI malignancy Small bowel malabsorption Pancreatic disease Liver cirrhosis Inflammatory bowel disease (Crohn's > ulcerative colitis) Gut infestations (*Giardia*, small intestine bacterial overgrowth) Chronic intra-abdominal sepsis
Psychosocial	Eating disorders (anorexia > bulimia) Affective disorders Alcohol misuse (multifactorial) Chronic pain syndromes Starvation
Metabolic	Diabetes (type I especially) Hyperthyroidism Addison's disease Hypopituitarism Uraemia Chronic heart failure ('cardiac cachexia')
Chronic inflammatory diseases	Rheumatoid arthritis Connective tissue disorders Chronic obstructive pulmonary disease
Chronic infectious disease	Tuberculosis HIV/AIDS Abscesses
Malignancy anywhere	Especially common sites (lung, breast, cervix, prostate, lymphoma)

factors that may be influencing nutrient intake, and hence weight.

Body mass index (BMI) is used as a measure of weight that takes into account height. BMI is calculated as weight (in kg) divided by (height)^2 (in m^2). A value between 20 and 25 is normal, but sequential measurements showing a progressive reduction, even if they are within this normal range, should not be ignored.

Management and prognosis

The management and prognosis of weight loss are completely dependent on its underlying cause. In population studies weight loss is strongly associated with mortality. For this reason, it must be aggressively investigated and urgently managed.

Iron-deficiency anaemia

The physiology of the metabolism of iron is outlined in Box 3.3.

Epidemiology

Iron-deficiency anaemia (IDA) is a common problem: 30% of the world's population is affected and in the developed world, 5–12% of women and 1–5% of men have IDA. Until recently small bowel bleeding was a common cause of IDA that was very difficult to diagnose. Now patients have access to wireless capsule endoscopy and single-balloon enteroscopy for the detection and treatment of small bowel bleeding.

Causes

Gastrointestinal blood loss

Gastrointestinal (GI) blood loss is the leading cause of IDA in men and post-menopausal women. A bleeding lesion is identified in the GI tract in 50% of patients and rates of GI malignancy are 10–17% in men and post-menopausal women with IDA.

Malabsorption and deficient diets

Conditions affecting the absorption of iron, including coeliac disease, atrophic gastritis, severe Helicobacter pylori infestation, and duodenal bypass surgery for ulcer disease or obesity surgery, can cause iron-deficiency anaemia. IDA results from dietary deficiency alone only after adherence to a strict vegan diet for a period of two to three years.

Non-gastrointestinal blood loss

Blood loss from the airway or the urinary system can result in IDA, but is generally obvious. The exceptions to this are urothelial tumours, where asymptomatic blood loss can result in IDA. Rarely, chronic intravascular haemolysis results in IDA. These causes can be detected using dipstick urinalysis.

Clinical features

Patients often present with systemic symptoms of anaemia including malaise, exertional dyspnoea and even heart failure. History and examination should be aimed at detecting any evidence of blood loss or gastrointestinal disease. A careful dietary history is important to determine whether dietary iron intake is likely to be sufficient. A careful menstrual history must be taken in pre-menopausal women. Angular stomatitis and cheilosis, glossitis and koilonychias are non-specific findings that may be seen.

Investigation

The classic finding in IDA is a low haemoglobin and low mean corpuscular volume. In addition, the red cell distribution width (RDW) can be useful, with increasing RDW being equivalent to the anisocytosis seen on the blood film of a patient with IDA. While an increased serum total iron binding capacity, decreased serum transferrin and decreased serum iron are also typical, they are non-specific as to the cause of anaemia.

Serum ferritin is the single best laboratory marker of IDA that is readily available. Unfortunately, it is affected by age and inflammatory status. However, the likelihood ratio for IDA if the ferritin is above 100 mcg/l is very low, and conversely for a ferritin below 15 mcg/l is very high (Table 3.7). Thus, in the setting of anaemia, it is reasonable to consider a ferritin

Table 3.7 Likelihood ratio (LR) of iron-deficiency anaemia with different ferritin levels.

Serum ferritin	LR	95% CI
≥100 µg/l	0.08	0.07–0.09
45 < 100 µg/l	0.54	0.48–0.60
35 < 45 µg/l	1.83	1.47–2.19
25 < 35 µg/l	2.54	2.11–2.97
15 < 25 µg/l	8.83	7.22–10.44
≤ 15 µg/l	51.85	41.53–62.27

CI, confidence interval
Source: Guyatt GH, Oxman AD, Ali M, Willan A, McIlroy W, Patterson C Laboratory diagnosis of iron-deficiency anemia: an overview. J Gen Intern Med. 1992 7: 145–153. Adapted with permission of Springer Science + Business Media.

Box 3.3 Physiology of iron metabolism

Normal daily dietary intake of iron is approximately 15 mg. Gastric acid is essential to release iron from food and maintain it in the soluble ferrous (Fe^{2+}) form; this is why achlorhydria may cause iron deficiency. Ferrous iron is then absorbed through an active process in the duodenum and jejunum. Maximal absorption is between 2 and 4 mg/day, being at the upper figure when iron stores are low or there is chronic hypoxia. Absorbed iron can then be stored in the enterocytes as ferritin, or can be bound to the protein transferrin and circulated around the body.

below 100 mcg/l as the cut-off for further GI investigation. This means that patients with a ferritin in the >15 and <100 mcg/l range will have only an intermediate likelihood of true IDA, but this is somewhat offset by the fact that they are likely to be older and so at relatively increased risk of GI malignancy.

In patients with a ferritin between 15 and 100 mcg/l where the inflammatory markers are elevated, or there is known chronic inflammatory disease, soluble transferrin receptor levels can be helpful to distinguish between anaemia of chronic disease and IDA. Transferrin receptor is a carrier protein for transferrin. It is needed for the import of iron into the cell and is regulated in response to intracellular iron concentration. Low iron concentrations promote increased levels of transferrin receptor, to increase iron intake into the cell. Thus, serum transferrin concentration is usually elevated in patients with iron-deficiency anaemia.

Upper and lower gastrointestinal endoscopy

Upper and lower GI endoscopy is recommended in all men and post-menopausal women with IDA. In pre-menopausal women, if menstrual blood loss is significant, then gynaecological evaluation and management are likely to be the priority. However, GI evaluation is required in those with severe anaemia or anaemia refractory to iron therapy, GI symptoms, weight loss, those over 40 years of age, and where menstrual blood loss does not correlate with the severity of the IDA.

Although IDA is historically associated with lesions of the colon, upper GI tract lesions are also commonly found. Combined upper and lower GI endoscopy is therefore generally indicated.

Obscure gastrointestinal bleeding

In 5–10% of cases no cause for IDA is found at upper and lower GI endoscopy. In this setting repeat examination may be indicated, as missed lesions are not uncommon. A small bowel cause for IDA will be found in up to 75% with further investigation. Small bowel investigation should be offered to those with persistent or recurrent IDA.

Small bowel investigation

The options for small bowel investigation include radiological and radionucleotide studies, wireless capsule endoscopy (WCE), balloon enteroscopy and operatively assisted techniques. Operatively assisted enteroscopy is reserved for particular situations because of its cost and relative invasiveness. Radiological techniques may show larger lesions, but have low sensitivity for the full range of small bowel lesions and are generally not considered first-line investigations.

Wireless capsule endoscopy

Wireless capsure endoscopy (WCE) is the initial investigation technique recommended because of its superiority in terms of the length of bowel examined, the quality of the examination and the non-invasive

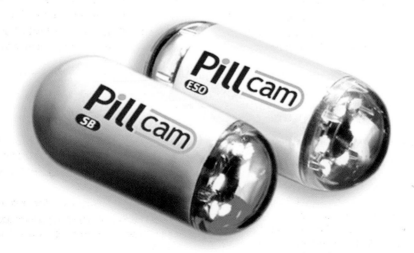

Figure 3.3 Wireless endoscopy capsule. Source: Kumar S. 2015. A GPU accelerated algorithm for blood detection in wireless capsule endoscopy images. Basel: Springer, Figure 1. Reproduced with permission of Springer Science + Business Media.

nature of the test. It has a sensitivity of 95% and a specificity of 86% for small bowel causes of IDA. A small capsule, just 11 mm in diameter, containing a light source, camera and radio-frequency emitter, is swallowed and a receiver worn on the belt for 8 hours to collect the images (Figure 3.3). The main risk is of the capsule becoming lodged in a small bowel stricture, requiring endoscopic or operative removal.

Balloon enteroscopy

Balloon enteroscopy (BE) gives a lower yield than WCE, but has the added benefit of allowing biopsy and therapeutic interventions, including coagulation of angiodysplasias, resection of superficial tumours and dilatation of strictures. It is seen as an adjunct to WCE, mainly for therapeutic use. BE uses a long, thin endoscope inside a shorter overtube, which has an inflatable balloon at its tip. The balloon is repeatedly inflated, withdrawn, deflated, advanced and inflated again. It thus grips the small bowel and pulls it back over the endoscope, allowing deep intubation of the small intestine. There are two types of BE, single and double balloon.

Management

Management is aimed at relieving the iron deficiency by giving oral iron or, if that is ineffective or intolerable, parenteral iron.

Prognosis

Because of its association with bleeding gastrointestinal lesions, iron deficiency can be caused by diseases with significant morbidity and mortality. The most concerning of these in a population sense is probably colorectal cancer. Once gastric and colonic neoplasia have been ruled out, fortunately the commonest causes of small bowel bleeding, in particular angiodysplasias, are benign.

 KEY POINTS

- In someone presenting with dysphagia, endoscopy is the first-choice investigation, except when a pharyngeal pouch is suspected, and it should generally be undertaken urgently.
- Vomiting, the violent expulsion of gastric and intestinal content, is distinct from regurgitation, and the list of possible diagnoses differs greatly between the two.
- To aid in diagnosis, primary constipation should be divided into those patients with a colon of normal diameter versus those with a dilated colon. Colonic transit studies can help to further define the diagnosis.

- Diarrhoea is usually the product of three basic mechanisms: osmotic diarrhoea, secretory diarrhoea and dysmotility diarrhoea. Defining the mechanisms involved helps to narrow the differential diagnosis.
- Gastrointestinal (GI) blood loss is the leading cause of iron-deficiency anaemia in men and post-menopausal women. A bleeding lesion is identified in the GI tract in 50% of patients and rates of GI malignancy are 10–17%.
- Serum ferritin is the single best laboratory marker of iron-deficiency anaemia that is readily available.

 SELF-ASSESSMENT QUESTION

(The answer to this question is given on p. 265)

A 66-year-old retired secretary has been taking warfarin for 15 years (for recurrent DVTs). She presents with a symptomatic anaemia (Hb 0.89 g/l), microcytosis (MCV 67 fl, normal range 76–100 fl) and hypochromia (MCH 20 pg/cell, normal range 26–34 pg/cell). She denies any abdominal pain, alteration of bowel habit, overt blood or weight loss. Examination reveals multiple telangiectasia on the lips and hands, but was otherwise entirely normal.

Regarding her anaemia, which of the following statements is most correct?

(a) Serum iron is likely to be more accurate than serum ferritin for detecting iron deficiency.

(b) The red cell distribution width in this patient is likely to be increased.

(c) Her anaemia is likely to be diet related.

(d) Given her age, it is best to perform gastroscopy first, followed by colonoscopy only if nothing is found.

(e) Radiological investigation of the small bowel is the next step after endoscopy.

4

Nutrition

Nutritional assessment is directed towards:

- Calorie–protein status.
- Specific mineral and vitamin status.

This information then guides a specific treatment approach. This chapter is designed to aid in understanding what happens to the individual in malnutrition, how to assess the effects of this and what interventions are available.

Nutritional physiology

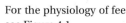

For the physiology of feeding, fasting and starvation, see Figure 4.1.

Glucose is essential to metabolism in the brain and renal medulla, and to red cell metabolism. Other organs mainly use fatty acids to produce energy. For this reason, under normal circumstances regulatory mechanisms maintain and control glucose levels in a tight range, both around the time of eating and between meals. Insulin is the main glucose-regulatory hormone. On eating, glucose is rapidly absorbed into the portal system, resulting in insulin secretion from the pancreas and a rise in insulin levels. Under the influence of insulin, the liver extracts a large percentage of that glucose and converts it to glycogen. Again under the influence of insulin, glucose reaching the periphery is taken up first into muscle and then into adipocytes.

Between meals glucose levels in the portal tract fall and the resultant decrease in insulin secretion prompts glycogenolysis, gluconeogenesis and lipolysis. Glycogenolysis occurs in the liver in order to maintain plasma glucose levels. At the same time, lipolysis is induced and fatty acids are released and become the major energy substrate for the body. Gluconeogenesis is induced in concert with glycogenolysis, converting glycerol, amino acids and fatty acids (via the citric acid cycle) to glucose.

Other hormones act on the regulatory mechanism, but their effect is limited compared to insulin, except in times of stress. These include glucagon, catecholamines and growth hormone. They have an anti-insulin effect, increasing glycogenolysis, gluconeogenesis and release of fatty acids and glycerol from adipose tissue, and amino acids from muscle.

Lipids enter the circulation as chylomicrons. These are large droplets of triglyceride emulsified by a surface monolayer of phospholipid and apolipoproteins. The apolipoproteins are transferred onto the chylomicrons from high-density lipoproteins (HDLs). When chylomicrons reach the peripheral capillaries of the heart and adipose tissue, lipoprotein lipase on the capillary endothelium binds them, and the triglycerides at the core of the chylomicron are rapidly hydrolysed to fatty acids, which are then taken up and utilised by peripheral tissues. HDL recycles the remaining surface phospholipids and apolipoproteins. Between meals chylomicrons disappear from the circulation and are replaced by very low-density lipoproteins (VLDLs), which are secreted by the liver. They are also bound and metabolised by lipoprotein lipase in peripheral capillaries.

Gastroenterology and Hepatology: Lecture Notes, Second Edition. Stephen Inns and Anton Emmanuel.
© 2017 John Wiley & Sons, Ltd. Published 2017 by John Wiley & Sons, Ltd.
Companion website: www.lecturenoteseries.com/gastroenterology

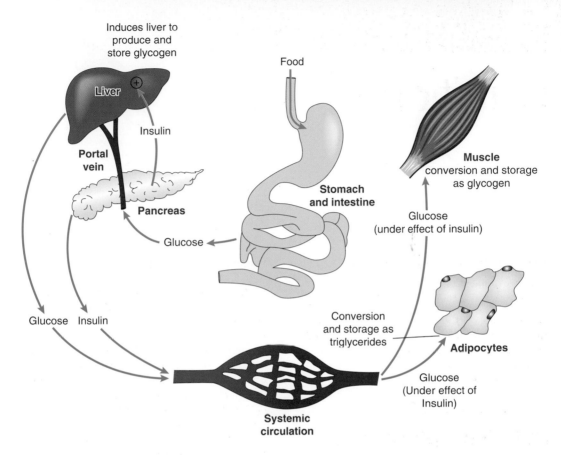

Figure 4.1a Feeding: An abundance of glucose triggers insulin release and its resultant storage as glycogen in the liver and muscle. Glucose is also converted to triglycerides in adipose tissue for storage when in excess.

Evaluation of nutritional status

About 30% of all patients in hospital are undernourished. A large number of these patients are undernourished when admitted to hospital, and in the majority of these undernutrition develops further while in hospital. Given that nutritional status contributes directly to morbidity and mortality in the majority of medical conditions, accurate and timely assessment of nutritional status and identification of patients needing nutritional input are essential. This assessment takes two forms:

- Nutritional screening, either in the community or at hospital admission.
- Nutritional assessment: a more detailed assessment performed by a nutrition expert and reserved for those patients identified by screening as being at nutritional risk.

Nutritional screening

Nutritional screening should be rapid and simple. It is conducted by admitting staff in the hospital or by the community healthcare team. All patients should be screened on admission to hospital. The aim is to stratify patients into nutritional risk groups and thus decide which patients should be referred on for further nutritional assessment and support, which can be managed using a nutrition plan as a part of the ordinary ward or home routine, and which are not at risk of malnutrition, but may need to be rescreened at specified intervals.

Nutritional assessment

The nutritional assessment is more detailed than screening and includes a full history, clinical examination (Table 4.1) and, where appropriate, laboratory investigations. An expert clinician, dietician or nutrition nurse conducts it. The assessment in turn leads

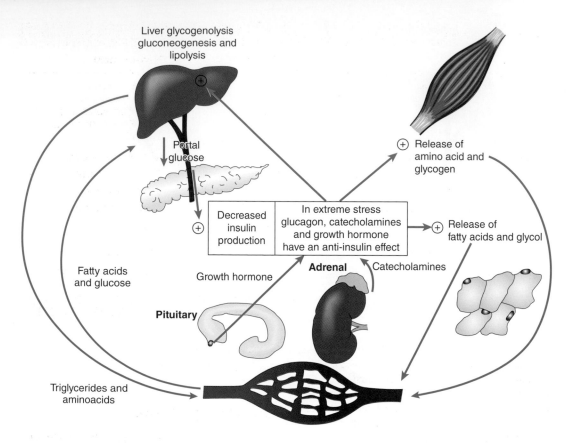

Figure 4.1b Fasting and starvation: When insulin levels in the portal tract fall, insulin secretion decreases and gluconeogenesis and glycogenolysis are induced. Fatty acids now become the major energy substrate for the body.

Table 4.1 Clinical manifestations of specific deficiency states.

Clinical	Deficiency	Measurement
Anorexia	Calories and protein	Subjective
Weight	Calories and protein	BMI <20 kg/m^2 Triceps skinfold thickness Mid-arm muscle circumference
Muscle wasting, oedema	Protein	Albumin <35 g/l Transferrin <2 g/l
Glossitis, cheilitis, stomatitis, koilonychias	Iron	Serum iron ↓ Serum ferritin ↓ Iron-binding capacity ↑
Weakness, proximal myopathy, tetany, paraesthesiae Chvostek and Trousseau signs	Calcium	Serum calcium ↓
Weakness, proximal myopathy, tetany, paraesthesiae	Magnesium	Serum magnesium ↓
Proximal myopathy	Phosphate	Serum phosphate ↓
Anorexia, diarrhoea, depression, anaemia, rash	Zinc	Serum zinc ↓
Night blindness, xerophthalmia	Vitamin A	Dark-adaptation time

(Continued)

Table 4.1 (Continued)

Clinical	Deficiency	Measurement
Bone pain, proximal myopathy	Vitamin D	Serum calcium ↓ Serum phosphate ↓ Alkaline phosphatase ↑ Bone X-ray, bone biopsy
Easy bruising	Vitamin K	INR >1.3
Peripheral neuropathy, psychosis, ophthalmoplegia	Vitamin B_1	Red cell transketolase
Stomatitis, anaemia, ataxia, mucosal fissures	Vitamin B_2	Red cell glutathione reductase
Diarrhoea, dermatitis, dementia	Nicotinamide	Urinary metabolites
Peripheral neuropathy, sideroblastic anaemia	Vitamin B_6	Aminotransferase activity
Peripheral neuropathy, macrocytic anaemia, subacute cord degeneration, vegans	Vitamin B_{12}	Serum B_{12}↓
Macrocytic anaemia, alcoholics	Folate	Serum folate ↓
Bleeding, periosteal haemorrhages, poor wound healing, gum hypertrophy	Vitamin C	White cell ascorbic acid

INR, international normalised ratio.

to a nutritional support plan. Following the initial assessment, nutritional and fluid status assessment is a continual process conducted by nursing, medical and dietetic staff, gauging the patient's ability to manage oral supplements, enteral feeding and/or parenteral feeding, with appropriate adjustments if requirements are not met.

Nutritional support

Nutritional support simply refers to the provision of nutrition above and beyond the normal diet and includes food fortification, oral nutritional supplementation (ONS), tube feeding and parenteral nutrition (PN); see Figure 4.2 and Box 4.1. It aims for increased intake of macro- and/or micronutrients. In certain circumstances a patient may receive one or a combination of modalities of support.

In general, the following principles are adhered to:

- High catabolic states need high calorie and nitrogen intake.
- Enteral feeding is preferred to parenteral feeding, and oral feeding is preferred to enteral feeding.
- A multidisciplinary team should determine nutritional needs and route of supplementation.

Five factors need consideration in deciding the replacement schedule:

- Calorie (fat and carbohydrate) requirement.
- Nitrogen (protein) balance.

- Minerals and vitamins.
- Fluid and electrolytes.
- Fibre.

Calorie replacement

Consideration of nutritional support is required when there has been >10% change in body weight, and depends on the specific illnesses surrounding the weight loss.

- General = highly catabolic states = 50 kcal/kg/24 h:
  - Intensive care, burns.
  - Chronic sepsis.
  - Following major surgery.
  - Malignancy.
- Gastrointestinal = intermediate catabolic states = 40 kcal/kg/24 h:
  - Intestinal fistula.
  - Short bowel syndrome.
  - Acute pancreatitis.
  - Crohn's disease.
- Prolonged inadequate dietary intake = low catabolic states = 30 kcal/kg/24 h:
  - Dysphagia post-cerebrovascular accident (CVA).
  - Neurological illness.

Protein replacement

In a healthy individual the protein requirement is 0.12 g nitrogen/kg body weight/day (1 g nitrogen per 6.25 g protein on average). Patients with protein malnutrition, inflammatory or infective disease and other

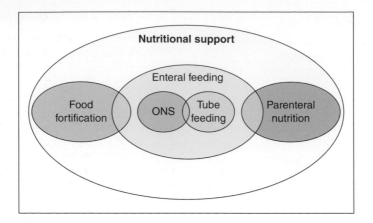

Figure 4.2 Range of options for nutritional support. ONS: oral nutritional supplementation

---

Box 4.1 Methods of delivery of nutritional replacement

Oral
- A variety of nutritional supplements are available
- Amount required is judged according to actual oral intake

Nasogastric feeding
- Appropriate for patients needing up to 4 weeks of feeding
- If there is gastric emptying delay, nasojejunal tubes may be used

Gastrostomy feeding
- Percutaneous endoscopic gastrostomy (PEG) tubes used if >4 weeks of feeding needed
- Jejunostomy extensions can be placed if there is gastric emptying delay or risk of aspiration with gastric feeding
- Home PEG feeding with small domestic feeding pumps is feasible

Parenteral feeding
- Careful balance of nitrogen and electrolytes is required
- Tunnelled central venous lines are preferred to peripheral lines (due to risk of sepsis and clotting)
- Home parenteral nutrition is needed for some patients with intestinal failure

---

catabolic conditions (e.g. surgery, burns) will have greater requirements. In the severely unwell, aiming for a positive nitrogen balance is often not possible or advisable, as nitrogen losses actually increase with increasing nitrogen intake, and high nitrogen intakes lead to a metabolic burden. Generally, in unwell patients, provision of 0.20 (0.17–0.25) g nitrogen/kg body weight/day should be sufficient.

Mineral, vitamin and trace element replacement

Protein energy malnutrition particularly predisposes to deficiencies of micronutrients and these should be corrected. For ONS and tube feeds the vitamin and trace element content is regulated. As these recommendations are based on a daily intake of 2000 kcal, advice from a dietician should be sought about the most appropriate enteral feeds and micronutrient supplements to use for an individual patient.

Fluid and electrolyte replacement

Usually between 1.5 and 3.0 l of fluid are given to adults receiving enteral or parenteral nutrition (PN). In general, 30–35 ml/kg body weight/day of fluid is required, with additional requirements for those with fever and losses of other body fluids. Electrolyte requirements vary greatly and should be tailored to the individual by monitoring serum, and in some circumstances urinary electrolytes. In general, 1–1.5 mmol/kg/day of sodium, chloride and potassium and 0.3–0.7 mmol/kg/day of phosphate are appropriate. In standard enteral and parenteral regimens, daily intakes of sodium are 80–100 mmol, potassium 60–150 mmol and phosphate 15–40 mmol. Daily weighing, fluid intake charts, serum biochemistry and daily examination of the patient (for dehydration, oedema etc.) are necessary for monitoring.

Fibre replacement

Soluble fibres have a prebiotic effect (i.e. they stimulate growth of beneficial bifidobacteria and lactobacilli) and on fermentation provide short-chain fatty acids, which are essential to the metabolism of the cells lining the colon. Less soluble fibre acts as a bulking agent, increasing stool output and frequency, and reducing colonic transit time. Patients receiving enteral nutrition may benefit from feeds containing a mix of insoluble and soluble fibres, particularly if long-term tube feeding is their sole source of nutrition, in order to maintain gut integrity, function and flora. For those receiving PN, it is acknowledged that to maintain gut integrity and function, where possible and appropriate, some feeding into the gut should be maintained.

Parenteral nutrition

Indications

It is clear that in patients with complete, irreversible intestinal failure, PN support is life saving. However, the use of PN in other clinical situations, often short term, is more controversial. Although meta-analyses have not shown improvements in clinical outcome with PN overall, they have shown improvements in complication rates among malnourished patients. In general, PN should only be considered when partial or complete intestinal failure has occurred and oral nutrition or enteral tube feeding (ETF) is not possible or has failed.

Administration

The GI tract should be utilised as much as possible in order to maintain gut hormone secretion, enzyme production, mucosal absorptive capacity and resistance to bacterial translocation. When a patient is on PN, they should be reassessed regularly with the aim of transferring to oral feeding or ETF.

Access is via a dedicated feeding line. This can be either a peripheral feeding line or central venous catheter. Peripheral lines give ease of venous access, but peripheral veins cannot tolerate high infusion rates or high osmolarity solutions, such as lipid-free solutions.

Complications

Complications can be divided into line-related complications and metabolic complications.

Line-related complications

Early line-related complications include local haematoma, arterial puncture and pneumothorax. Catheter-related sepsis remains the most serious complication of PN. Meticulous line care is vital and patients with suspected line sepsis should have their PN stopped temporarily and blood cultures taken peripherally and from all catheter lumens. Generally, lines should be removed and replaced after 24 hours of appropriate antibiotics. However, it is reasonable to attempt sterilisation of a long-term tunnelled line. Central vein thrombosis is relatively common; however, it is usually not clinically evident.

Metabolic complications

The risk of refeeding syndrome is high and all patients who are to receive PN must be carefully assessed and managed with this in mind. Hyperglycaemia is common and is largely due to the insulin resistance associated with severe disease. In the setting of critical illness, benefits have been seen with aggressive management of even minimal hyperglycaemia with the use of intensive insulin therapy.

Abnormal liver-function tests (LFTs) are common, but usually relate to the underlying disease, sepsis and drugs rather than to the PN itself. Steatosis may results from overadministration of glucose and lipid, and is due to the resultant hyperinsulinaemia, lipogenesis and hepatocyte fat deposition. In those receiving long-term PN there is a risk of cholestasis. The exact aetiology of this is unknown, but may relate to increased lithogenicity of bile with interruption of enterohepatic bile acid circulation, reduced gallbladder motility and biliary sludge because of no oral intake, bacterial overgrowth and nutrient deficiencies, including choline, taurine and carnitine. Long-term PN also places the patient at risk of metabolic bone disease and micronutrient deficiencies, particularly in the setting of ongoing intestinal loss.

Enteral nutrition

Oral nutritional supplements

The oral route of nutrition should always be preferred. ONS provides macronutrients and micronutrients, usually in a liquid form. Polymeric feeds contain protein, carbohydrate and fat, together with electrolytes, minerals, trace elements and vitamins. These are much more palatable than elemental feeds, which contain protein as amino acids and generally have low fat content, often providing the fat as medium-chain triglycerides.

The main indication for ONS is the presence of disease-related malnutrition, which may occur in many patient groups, including those with cancer, the elderly, surgical patients and others with severe acute or chronic diseases. Other indications include preoperative preparation of a malnourished patient, inflammatory bowel disease, short bowel syndrome, intractable malabsorption (which can include patients with a range of GI, including pancreatic, and liver diseases), post-total gastrectomy, dysphagia, bowel fistulae and dialysis (continuous ambulatory peritoneal dialysis, haemodialysis). Provision of ONS tends not to suppress food intake substantially and so total nutritional intake can be significantly improved.

Enteral tube feeding

ETF should be considered if supplements are insufficient to ensure an adequate intake and recovery, or where oral intake is unsafe and contraindicated. The conditions in which tube feeding should be a part of routine care include:

- Protein-energy malnutrition (>10% weight loss) with little or no oral intake for 5 days.
- <50% of the required oral nutrient intake for the previous 7–10 days.
- Severe dysphagia or swallowing-related difficulties, e.g. head injury, strokes, motor neurone disease.
- Major, full-thickness burns.
- Massive small bowel resection.
- Low-output enterocutaneous fistulae.

ETF is provided by two main routes in the majority of patients: via nasogastric tube (NGT) or percutaneous endoscopic gastrostomy (PEG). Generally administration is via a pump and sterile administration set, delivering continuous infusions of feed over many hours. Sometimes boluses of feed are given with gastric but not jejunal tube feeding.

As inpatients, on the whole, tend to be fed for short periods of time, nasogastric feeding using a fine-bore feeding tube (polyurethane) is appropriate, at least initially, in most patients. Tubes should be placed by a trained health professional and correct positioning should be checked, by X-ray initially, to ensure that there is no malpositioning into the lungs or elsewhere. Some authorities recommend checking tube position by aspirating stomach contents prior to every feeding episode (checking for pH 5 or less using pH indicator paper). Secure fixing of the tube to the nose and face is essential. Where ETF will be longer term,

PEG is the most common route used. For patients at increased risk of regurgitation of feed and/or pulmonary aspiration, gastric atony or gastroparesis, post-pyloric feeding into the duodenum or jejunum should be considered.

PEG tube insertion is an invasive procedure requiring careful patient selection and informed consent from the patient and family. Patients should have a recent platelet count, haemoglobin and coagulation screen available. Where possible, antiplatelet drugs and anticoagulants should be stopped prior to the procedure. Antibiotics are administered before the procedure to reduce the risk of tube-related infection.

Physiology of starvation

During starvation the body utilises liver glycogen stores as well as gluconeogenesis to form glucose (see Figure 4.1). Gluconeogenesis is glucose synthesis using the breakdown products of lipid and protein. During this process adipose tissue releases large quantities of fatty acids and glycerol, and muscle releases amino acids. With the depletion of glycogen stores, ketone bodies (produced as a by-product of gluconeogenesis) and free fatty acids replace glucose as a major energy source. The result is the catabolism of adipose tissue and muscle, with a resultant loss of lean body mass.

With refeeding there is a shift from fat back to carbohydrate metabolism. The resultant glucose load triggers insulin release, which in turn increases the cellular uptake of glucose, phosphate, potassium, magnesium and water, and promotes protein synthesis. It is these nutrient, electrolyte and fluid fluxes that can produce the refeeding syndrome (see the next section).

The refeeding syndrome

The refeeding syndrome can be defined as a syndrome consisting of metabolic disturbances that occur as a result of reinstitution of nutrition to patients who are starved or severely malnourished. At-risk patients include the following:

- Those with kwashiorkor or marasmus, anorexia nervosa, or other causes of chronic malnutrition (e.g. from carcinoma or in the elderly).
- Chronic alcoholics.
- After prolonged fasting (e.g. hunger strikers).

- Following a duodenal switch operation for obesity.
- Oncology patients receiving prolonged chemotherapy.
- Postoperative patients.

Body–fluid fluxes can result in cardiac failure, dehydration or fluid overload, hypotension, prerenal failure and sudden death. The major metabolic disturbances, their pathological basis and treatment are summarised in Table 4.2.

Refeeding syndrome must be considered in any patient who is to receive nutrition, be it oral, enteral or parenteral, after a period of starvation or reduced nutritional intake. Electrolyte disorders must be corrected and the patient made fluid replete prior to beginning refeeding. At-risk patients must be monitored closely, in particular their vital functions, fluid balance and plasma electrolytes, including magnesium and phosphate. Hypophosphataemia is common not only in refeeding syndrome, being present in 2% of hospital admissions.

Intestinal failure

Intestinal failure (IF) results from loss of absorption due to obstruction, dysmotility, surgical resection, congenital defect or disease, and is characterised by the inability to maintain protein energy, fluid, electrolyte or micronutrient balance. IF can be divided into three types:

- **Type 1**: self-limiting intestinal failure as occurs following abdominal surgery.
- **Type 2**: intestinal failure in severely ill patients with major resections of the bowel and septic, metabolic and nutritional complications.
- **Type 3**: chronic IF requiring long-term nutritional support.

Short bowel syndrome (SBS) is IF resulting from the loss of small intestinal absorptive capacity for anatomical reasons. The normal length of the small intestine ranges from 260 to 800 cm and a patient with <200 cm of viable bowel is at risk of SBS, although methods for measuring residual bowel are inaccurate, making assessment of this risk difficult. Dependence on PN may result when the small intestine is shorter than 100 cm in the absence of an intact and functional colon, or 60 cm in the presence of a completely functional colon. Following shortening, the intestine adapts by increasing villous diameter and height, which, in addition to some slight lengthening of the small bowel, increases the absorptive surface. As this process evolves over years, especially in children, some patients may go from being PN dependent to PN independent with time.

The vast majority of cases of IF are related to acquired SBS and result from the surgical resection of bowel, related to recurrent Crohn's disease, vascular events such as a mesenteric arterial embolism or venous thrombosis, volvulus, trauma, tumour resection or congenital abnormalities in children. Functional IF results when malabsorption occurs despite intact bowel length. Causes include chronic intestinal pseudo-obstruction syndrome, refractory sprue, radiation enteritis and congenital villous atrophy.

Management of Type 2 intestinal failure

Management of the severely ill patient following major resections of the bowel, and the often-resultant complications, is of the utmost importance to prevent further surgical intervention, and reduce the associated high morbidity, mortality and risk of progression to Type 3 IF. Management of these patients requires a skilled multidisciplinary team combining dieticians, pharmacists, biochemists, enterostomal therapists, nurses, microbiologists, radiologists, pain specialists, surgeons and physicians. Experts in this area recommend a temporal sequence in managing the various facets of intestinal failure in these patients and have coined the term 'Sepsis–Nutrition–Anatomy–Plan' or the 'SNAP' approach. Here attention is first paid to managing sepsis, in particular draining intra-abdominal collections; then the patient's nutritional status is carefully assessed and rectified; following this the intra-abdominal anatomy is clearly delineated in order to guide further management; finally, a long-term plan for the restoration of intestinal continuity is instituted, often involving medical management of six months to a year prior to any further attempt at surgical intervention.

Medical therapy

Medical therapy for IF consists of providing adequate nutrition of macro- and micro-nutrients, sufficient fluids, and correcting and preventing acid–base disturbances. In some patients this may require supplementary enteral nutrition and management of electrolyte and fluid losses: orally using salt solutions, or by subcutaneous or intravenous administration. A proportion of patients will be PN dependent and for them home PN (HPN) is often possible, following a period of hospital management and training.

HPN is associated with a significant risk of complications, however, including liver and biliary complications,

Table 4.2 Nutrient deficiencies in refeeding syndrome: Their consequences and management.

Nutrient/electrolyte disturbance	Normal physiology	Consequences of disturbance	Treatment
Hypophosphataemia	Body phosphate 500–800 g 80% in bony skeleton and 20% soft tissues and muscle Major intracellular anion Transcellular movement results from carbohydrate or lipid ingestion and acid–base alterations Intake about 1 g/day: • 80% absorbed in the jejunum • Found in protein-rich food, cereals and nuts Output: • 90% renal • 10% GI loss Important intracellular buffer Structural role as a component of phospholipids, nucleoproteins and nucleic acids Central role in cellular metabolic pathways, including glycolysis and oxidative phosphorylation Essential in 2,3-diphosphoglycerate	Skeletal muscle weakness and myopathy Cardiomyopathy Seizures, perturbed mental state and paraesthesia Prolonged hypophosphataemia osteomalacia Rhabdomyolysis Thrombocytopenia, impaired clotting processes Reduced leucocyte phagocytosis and chemotaxis Haemolysis Erythrocyte 2,3-diphosphoglycerate depletion, resulting in a leftward shift in haemoglobin–oxygen dissociation curve (i.e. haemoglobin has a greater affinity for oxygen)	Severe hypophosphataemia rare, most cases are clinically insignificant Treatment only if plasma phosphate concentration <0.30 mmol/l or symptomatic Intravenous phosphate replacement with the Vannatta regimen: • 9 mmol of monobasic potassium phosphate in half-normal saline continuous intravenous infusion over 12 h • Not with hypercalcaemia (risk of metastatic calcification) or hyperkalaemia • Plasma phosphate, calcium, magnesium and potassium monitored closely • Infusion stopped once plasma phosphate >0.30 mmol/l

Hypomagnesaemia	Mandatory for optimal cell function
	Cofactor to many enzymes
	Found mainly in bone and muscle
	Largely absorbed in the upper small intestine
	70% of dietary magnesium eliminated in faeces
	Major excretory route is through the kidneys
		Hypomagnesaemia, defined as <0.5 mmol/l or if symptomatic
		Mechanism likely multifactorial:
		• Intracellular flux with carbohydrate feeding
		• Poor dietary intake
		• Pre-existing poor magnesium
		Severe hypomagnesaemia:
		• Cardiac arrhythmias • Paraesthesia
		• Torsade de pointes • Tetany
		   • Seizures
		• Abdominal discomfort • Irritability
		   • Confusion
		• Anorexia • Weakness
		• Tremor • Ataxia
			Can be corrected by oral magnesium but salts poorly absorbed and lead to GI upset
			Intravenous replacement:
			• Magnesium sulphate (50% solution containing 2.1 mmol/ml)
			• 24 mmol of magnesium sulphate over 6 h
			• Close monitoring of plasma magnesium
			May facilitate treatment of refractory hypokalaemia
			Plasma calcium concentration also should be checked

Thiamine deficiency (vitamin B1)	Carbohydrate refeeding causes increased cellular thiamine utilisation	Wernicke's encephalopathy: ocular disturbance, confusion, ataxia and coma, Korsakov's syndrome: short-term memory loss and confabulation	50–250 mg thiamine should be given at least 30 min before refeeding is instigated More thiamine might be necessary until the patient is stabilised NB: Some preparations associated with anaphylaxis Oral thiamine can be given as 100 mg tablets once daily
Hypokalaemia	Regulated by the kidney distal nephron Increased by aldosterone, alkalosis Essential for maintaining cell-membrane action potential	Clinical manifestations rare unless severe (<3.0 mmol/l): • Cardiac: arrhythmias, hypotension and cardiac arrest • Gastrointestinal: ileus and constipation • Neuromuscular dysfunction: weakness, paralysis, paraesthesia, confusion, rhabdomyolysis and respiratory depression • Potentiation of digitalis toxicity • Glucose intolerance • Metabolic alkalosis • Worsening of hepatic encephalopathy	Cautious intravenous potassium administration Ideally, the rate should not exceed 20 mmol/h and should not be >40 mmol/l in the intravenous infusion mixture Close monitoring of plasma potassium is important Electrocardiographic monitoring preferable

GI, gastrointestinal.

catheter-related infections, catheter occlusion and metabolic bone disease, including osteomalacia and osteopenia. Long-term users accrue a 10–15% yearly chance of dying from a therapy complication. While HPN is clearly life saving when required, it is associated with a reduced quality of life compared to patients with SBS who do not require HPN, similar to that experienced by patients with chronic renal failure treated by dialysis.

Surgery and intestinal transplantation

Non-transplant surgical treatment for IF includes approaches that increase nutrient and fluid absorption by either slowing intestinal transit or increasing intestinal surface area. Particularly important is the restoration of intestinal continuity, such as reanastomosis of the small intestine with the colon, since it can be performed with a relatively low morbidity and mortality, and often with a good probability of discontinuation of PN therapy because of improved fluid absorption.

Intestinal transplantation is rarely performed, the number limited by its risk. Three-year patient survival after isolated intestinal transplantation is approximately 70%, which is not comparable with the 90% three-year survival in at-home, stable, PN-treated patients. Hence imminent liver failure is currently the most appropriate indication, followed by patients failing PN therapy (<20% 1-year survival).

Post-transplant complications include:

- Postoperative haemorrhage.
- Vascular leaks.
- Obstruction.
- Biliary leaks or obstruction.
- Allograft rejection (frequent and may result in graft loss, being most common in the early postoperative period).
- Infection, which is the leading cause of morbidity and mortality and is a result of the relatively high levels of immunosuppression required and the technically difficult nature of the surgery and aftercare.
- Epstein-Barr virus (EBV) and post-transplant lymphoproliferative (PTLD) disorder, which are a concern and are more common than in solid-organ transplants.
- Graft-versus-host disease (GVHD), which is on the whole mild and self-limiting.

 KEY POINTS

- Nutrional management is aimed at the accurate assessment and adequate and safe treatment of calorie–protein and specific mineral and vitamin deficiencies.
- 30% of all patients in hospital are undernourished, so accurate and timely assessment of nutritional status and identification of patients needing nutritional input is essential.
- Nutritional support simply refers to the provision of nutrition above and beyond the normal diet and includes food fortification, oral nutritional supplementation (ONS), tube feeding and parenteral nutrition (PN).
  - ○ The oral route of nutrition should always be preferred.
  - ○ Enteral tube feeding should be considered if supplements are insufficient to ensure an

  adequate intake and recovery, or where oral intake is unsafe and contraindicated.
  - ○ In general, PN should only be considered when partial or complete intestinal failure has occurred and oral nutrition or enteral tube feeding is not possible or has failed.
- The refeeding syndrome is a potentially life-threatening syndrome consisting of metabolic disturbances that occur as a result of reinstitution of nutrition to patients who are starved or severely malnourished.
- Intestinal failure (IF) results from loss of absorption due to obstruction, dysmotility, surgical resection, congenital defect or disease, and can be divided into three types depending on chronicity.

SELF-ASSESSMENT QUESTION

(The answer to this question is given on p. 265)

A 15-year-old girl is admitted to the medical ward by her psychiatrist because her eating disorder has led to marked undernutrition. Her BMI is 16 kg/m² and she has disturbed vital signs in the form of a heart rate of 42 beats per minute, postural hypotension and core body temperature of 36.5 °Celsius.

Regarding the treatment of this patient, which of the following statements is most correct?

(a) Her low mood and poor decision making relate to her pre-existing psychiatric disorder and not her nutritional status.

(b) Vitamin A deficiency could lead to nerve and bone marrow abnormalities.

(c) If thiamine levels are normal, no supplementation should be given.

(d) On refeeding she must be carefully monitored for hypoglycaemia, hypokalaemia, hypophosphataemia and hypomagnesaemia.

(e) Tube feeding is preferred over oral nutrition in this situation.

5

Gastrointestinal infections

Oral infections

Candidiasis

Candida albicans is a mouth commensal that may proliferate in immunocompromised patients (newborns, those with AIDS, diabetes, patients receiving cytotoxics) or those taking antibiotics. The diagnosis is usually obvious from the appearance of small white clumps adherent to the mucosa. Dysphagia or painful swallowing raises the possibility of oesophageal involvement. Oral candidiasis is treated with nystatin or amphotericin (which can also be used prophylactically in at-risk patients). Resistant candidiasis, and oesophageal involvement, may require fluconazole.

Vincent's angina

Borrelia vincenti may invade the mucosa in immunocompromised patients or those with appalling oral hygiene. Deep, sloughing ulcers cause severe pain and halitosis; systemic features (fever and malaise) are frequent. Local anaesthetic mouthwashes or oral antibiotics may be needed, depending on severity.

Parotitis

Viral (mumps) or bacterial infections (postoperative) of the parotid glands cause parotid swelling and pain. Oral antibiotics may help, but surgical drainage is required if there is abscess formation. The differential for parotid swelling includes:

- Salivary gland stones.
- Sjögren's syndrome.
- Sarcoidosis.
- Tumours (mostly benign adenoma, rarely mucoepidermoid tumours or cancers).

Oesophageal infections

Oesophageal candidiasis is a common observation at upper GI endoscopy. Less frequent are viral infections, of which herpes simplex is the most important. The features of these are shown in Table 5.1.

Helicobacter pylori infection

Epidemiology

Infection with *Helicobacter* is extremely common throughout the world, especially in the developing world. In north European and North American populations, about one-third of adults are infected, whereas in south and east Europe, South America and Asia, the prevalence of *H. pylori* is often higher than 50%. *H. pylori* remains highly prevalent in immigrants coming from countries with a high prevalence of the infection. Low socioeconomic conditions in childhood are the most important risk factors for *H. pylori* infection.

Gastroenterology and Hepatology: Lecture Notes, Second Edition. Stephen Inns and Anton Emmanuel.
© 2017 John Wiley & Sons, Ltd. Published 2017 by John Wiley & Sons, Ltd.
Companion website: www.lecturenoteseries.com/gastroenterology

Table 5.1 Features of oesophageal infections.

	Candida	Herpes simplex
At-risk groups	Immunocompromised, elderly, antibiotic use	Immunocompromised
Spread	Downwards from mouth	Contagious (other herpes lesions)
Symptoms	Odynophagia, dysphagia	Odynophagia, dysphagia, joint pain
Endoscopic appearance	Creamy plaques, mucosa normal	Mucosal ulceration ± vesicles
Treatment	Fluconazole or amphotericin	Acyclovir
Prognosis	Recurrent, even if correct immune system	Can be eradicated, especially if correct immunocompromise

Table 5.2 Disorders associated with *Helicobacter pylori* infection.

Strong association	Uncertain association
Gastritis (chronic and acute)	NSAID-related ulcer
Peptic ulcer (gastric and duodenal)	Gastro-oesophageal reflux disease
Menetrier's disease	Functional dyspepsia
Cancer of the stomach	
MALT lymphoma	

NSAID, non-steroidal anti-inflammatory drug.

Clinical features

While usually asymptomatic, *H. pylori* infection is associated with certain disorders (Table 5.2). It interacts with host factors (age, genetic susceptibility) and environmental factors (smoking, drugs) to result in either:

- Antral gastritis (predisposes to duodenal ulcer), or
- Pan-gastritis (predisposes to gastric carcinoma).

Gastric ulcers are associated with both antral and pan-gastritis.

Investigation

This can be through means that are invasive (endoscopic, shaded in Table 5.3) or non-invasive (breath, stool or blood test, unshaded in Table 5.3).

The principle underlying the urea breath test and Campylobacter-like organism (CLO) test is that *H. pylori* produces the enzyme urease, which can cleave urea to ammonia and CO_2. In the breath test, ^{13}C or ^{14}C is included in a test meal and can be detected by mass spectrometer (^{13}C) or radiation count (^{14}C). In the CLO test, the biopsies are incubated with urea substrate and a colour pH indicator: ammonia production turns the indicator pink.

Management

First-line treatment is one week of 'triple therapy', namely a proton pump inhibitor (PPI) and two antibiotics (out of amoxycillin, clarithromycin and metronidazole).

Second-line treatment involves quadruple therapy, including bismuth-containing preparations, or triple therapy incorporating tetracycline. However, in most circumstances treatment failure is due to poor compliance.

Prognosis

Helicobacter is an important cause of gastric cancer worldwide. Around 780,000 cases of non-cardia gastric cancer per year are thought to be attributable to *H. pylori*. This represents 6.2% of the 12.7 million total cancer cases that occur worldwide each year. For this reason, it is important that eradication is confirmed following treatment, usually with a stool antigen test six weeks after completion of therapy.

Table 5.3 Diagnostic methods to detect *Helicobacter pylori*.

	Serology (IgG)	Urea breath test	Faecal antigen test	Urease (CLO) test	Histology	Bacterial culture
Advantages	Specific Quick Useful for screening	Specific and sensitive	Specific and sensitive Cheap	Specific Quick Cheap	Specific and sensitive	'Gold standard' Can test antibiotic sensitivity
Disadvantages	No use to test eradication (IgG antibodies persist for months or years after eradication) False negatives in older people	Need to stop PPIs, antibiotics 4 weeks Requires radiation or mass spectrometer Slow	Need to stop PPIs, antibiotics 4 weeks	Insensitive Need to stop PPIs, antibiotics 4 weeks	Slow Need to stop PPIs, antibiotics 4 weeks	Slow Insensitive Need to stop PPIs, antibiotics 4 weeks

CLO, Campylobacter-like organism; IgG, immunoglobin G; PPI, proton pump inhibitor.

Acute gastroenteritis

Infection in the GI tract usually results in diarrhoea, abdominal pain and occasionally vomiting. Since spontaneous resolution usually occurs in <4 days, investigation for the specific organism is only required in:

- Elderly patients, especially those in institutions.
- Immunocompromised patients.
- Symptoms >5 days.
- Epidemics.

Epidemiology

The frequency of infection and the infectious agent vary widely between age groups and countries, but worldwide infectious gastroenteritis is an important cause of morbidity and mortality, particularly among infants in developing countries. In the developed world the majority of food-borne infections are of viral aetiology and of those the commonest are the *noroviridae*.

Causes

See Table 5.4.

Clinical features

- **History of ingesting suspicious food**:
  - Incubation 1–6 h: *Bacillus cereus, Staphylococcus aureus.*

Table 5.4 Infectious causes of acute diarrhoea.

Virus	Norovirus* Rotavirus*
Bacteria	Salmonella Shigella Escherichia coli Campylobacter Yersinia Clostridium perfringens
Bacterial toxins	E. coli Shigella Clostridium difficile Staphylococcus aureus Clostridium botulinum Vibrio cholera Bacillus cereus
Protozoa	Giardia lamblia Cryptosporidium Cyclospora

* Commonest causes.

  - Incubation 8–18 h: *Shigella, E. coli, Campylobacter, Clostridium perfringens.*
  - Incubation 12–36 h: *Salmonella, Clostridium botulinum.*
- **Diarrhoea** – all organisms cause diarrhoea, bloody in *Shigella*, enterotoxic *E. coli, Campylobacter.*
- **Abdominal pain**, *especially in Campylobacter.*
- **Vomiting**, especially in *Bacillus cereus* and *Staphylococcus aureus.*
- **Systemic features**, especially in *Shigella, Campylobacter, and Yersinia.*

Investigations

- Stool culture and microscopy: for cysts and trophozoites.
- Serology for toxins:
  - *C. difficile*.
  - *E. coli*.
  - *Shigella*.
  - *Campylobacter*.
- Sigmoidoscopy and biopsy only indicated if symptoms persist >2 weeks.
- Joint X-rays and aspiration if joint is swollen and there is fever and leucocytosis.

Management

- **General supportive treatment**:
  - Resuscitation: oral rehydration solution is preferred to IV rehydration, if patient is not vomiting.
  - Meticulous hand hygiene.
  - Antidiarrhoeals (loperamide) should be avoided in most cases, especially in children (when fatal paralytic ileus may occur).
  - Antiemetics may be used more liberally.
  - Food poisoning is a notifiable disease.
- **Specific treatment**:
  - Viruses:
    - Typically self-limiting within 5 days, but may be fatal in elderly and immunocompromised – especially norovirus.
    - Epidemics occur in hospitals and institutions – through uncooked food and hand-to-hand transmission.
    - Supportive treatment only is needed.
  - *Salmonella*:
    - Antibiotic therapy is avoided, as it prolongs gallbladder carriage of the organism.
    - Ciprofloxacin is the first-choice antibiotic, trimethoprim being the alternative.
    - Asymptomatic carriers need no specific management other than advice about good hand hygiene.
  - *Shigella*:
    - If antibiotics are needed, ciprofloxacin is preferred.
  - *E. coli*:
    - Occurs in outbreaks, usually from infected meat.
    - Ciprofloxacin is the first-choice antibiotic, but increases the risk of developing haemolytic uraemic syndrome (due to toxin release).
  - *Campylobacter*:
    - If symptoms persist, ciprofloxacin or erythromycin may be used.

- *Yersinia*:
  - Diagnosis requires stool culture or elevated antibodies on serology.
  - Tetracycline for 2 weeks is the first-choice antibiotic.
- *C. difficile*:
  - This is a Gram-positive anaerobe that is found everywhere, with 2% of the population being asymptomatic carriers.
  - In hospitals the spores are resistant to most disinfectants.
  - Spectrum of infection occurs, from:
    Asymptomatic carriage, to
    Isolated diarrhoea, to
    Pseudo-membranous colitis (based on endoscopic appearance of a grey 'membrane' overlying colonic mucosa), to
    Death.
  - Risk factors:
    Antibiotics: high risk – cephalosporins, clindamycin; medium risk – penicillins, co-trimoxazole, macrolides; low-risk – metronidazole, vancomycin, metronidazole, ciprofloxacin, aminoglycosides.
    Old age or immunocompromised.
    Concomitant chemotherapy or proton pump inhibitor (PPI).
  - Diagnosis: *C. difficile* toxins A (95%) and B (5%); in many laboratories a screening test for the presence of *C. difficile*, such as a glutamate dehydrogenase enzyme immunoassay, is performed first.
  - Management:
    Stop causative antibiotic and *avoid* antidiarrhoeals.
    Careful nursing and hand hygiene.
    Oral metronidazole for 7–10 days.
    Oral (*not* IV) vancomycin for 14–28 days.
    Role of probiotics and faecal bacteriotherapy are under investigation for this common hospital condition.
  - Prognosis: 30% mortality in hospital patients.
- *Listeria monocytogenes*:
  - Usually ingested in unpasteurised products.
  - Caution required in those who are immunocompromised and in pregnant women, where there is significant mortality and risk to the foetus.
- *Giardia*:
  - Chronic infection is a significant potential problem.
  - Course of metronidazole or single-dose tinidazole will usually eradicate the protozoa.

○ *Cryptosporidium*:
  – Supportive treatment only is needed as it is self-limiting.
  – Immunocompromised may require azithromycin.
○ *Cyclospora*:
  – Common cause of chronic diarrhoea in returning travellers.
  – Responds to a course of co-trimoxazole.

Prognosis

The vast majority of episodes of acute gastroenteritis resolve spontaneously. Complications of acute gastroenteritis occur rarely, but those listed here are classic.

- **Chronic diarrhoea**:
  ○ Post-infectious IBS (see Chapter 15).
  ○ Persistent infection (immunosuppressed, *Giardia*).
  ○ Secondary hypolactasia (especially in children, Asian origin).
- **Reactive arthritis**:
  ○ May follow *Salmonella* or *Shigella*.
- **Reiter's syndrome** (asymmetrical polyarthritis, conjunctivitis, orogenital mucosal ulceration):
  ○ May follow *Yersinia* or *Campylobacter*.
- **Erythema nodosum**:
  ○ May follow *Yersinia* or *Campylobacter*.
- **Toxic megacolon**:
  ○ Especially with *Clostridium difficile*, *Yersinia*, *Campylobacter*, *E. coli*.
  ○ More often relates to undiagnosed ulcerative colitis complicated by infection.
- **Asymptomatic carrier state** (*Salmonella*).

Intestinal tuberculosis

Mycobacterium tuberculosis or *bovis* may cause intestinal infection by:

- Ingestion of infected milk.
- Blood-borne spread from the lung.
- Rarely, direct spread from adjacent organs.

Epidemiology

While not uncommon in the developing world, intestinal tuberculosis (TB) is a rarity in the developed world and tends to affect the immigrant population (sub-Saharan Africa, South-East Asia), often many years after arriving in the host country. The malnourished, immunocompromised and institutionalised are also at particular risk.

Clinical features

- **Ileocaecal disease** (commonest):
  ○ Diarrhoea, abdominal pain, weight loss and systemic ill health.
  ○ Rarely, presentation is with an acute abdomen (TB appendicitis, obstruction or perforation).
  ○ An abdominal mass is often present.
- **TB adenitis**:
  ○ Mimics appendicitis.
- **TB peritonitis**:
  ○ Weight loss, systemic ill health and ascites (diagnosis is established by staining and culture of paracentesed ascites).

Investigations

The main differential diagnosis is with Crohn's disease and *Yersinia* infection and differentiation can be difficult.

- Standard TB investigations are often unhelpful: two-thirds of patients will have a normal chest X-ray, and Mantoux testing is poorly sensitive for current infection.
- Tissue diagnosis is required, and also helps with determining drug sensitivity:
  ○ Ascites: exudate with increased lymphocytes, supported by Ziehl–Nielsen staining and culture of acid-fast bacilli.
  ○ Peritoneal biopsy, with Abrams' needle or at laparoscopy.
- Abdominal CT or contrast follow-through often reveals features indistinguishable from Crohn's disease (small bowel thickening, intra-abdominal lymphadenopathy, peritoneal reaction).
- Colonoscopy is also indistinguishable from Crohn's disease, but does allow for biopsies to be taken.

Management

- Triple therapy (rifampicin, isoniazid and pyrazinamide) for 2 months followed by dual therapy (rifampicin, isoniazid) for 4 months.
- Ethambutol may be needed if resistance is suspected.
- Monitoring response: symptoms, weight, erythrocyte sedimentation rate (ESR), C-reactive protein (CRP), haemoglobin (Hb).
- Monitoring adverse events: liver enzymes.
- Surgery is indicated for:
  ○ Obstruction.
  ○ Complications (perforation, haemorrhage).
  ○ Large abdominal mass (poor antimicrobial penetrance).
- TB is a notifiable disease.

Miscellaneous gut infections

Amoebiasis

- Mostly in immigrant populations, after ingestion of contaminated water or food containing *Entamoeba histolytica*.
- Classically it occurs in patients receiving a course of corticosteroids.
- Usually asymptomatic, but a pancolitis occurs in 10% of those infected, and very rarely a fatal toxic megacolon may occur.
- Rarely, perianal manifestations and fistulisation may occur, resembling Crohn's disease.
- **Diagnosis**:
  ○ *Entamoeba histolytica* antigen in stool *and* serum; this is preferred to microscopy of warm stool to look for the amoeba. Biopsies may show the flask-shaped mucosal ulceration and trophozoites.
  ○ One-quarter of patients may develop an amoebic liver abscess (especially men); the risk is of rupture into the peritoneum or pleural cavity.
  ○ Diagnosis of liver abscess requires imaging (ultrasound or CT) with drainage revealing thick brown ('anchovy sauce') fluid.
- **Management**: metronidazole for 5 days followed by paromomycin to eradicate luminal parasites. Three sequential clear stool samples confirm eradication.

Typhoid and paratyphoid

- Mostly in returning travellers, caused by *Salmonella typhi* or *paratyphi*.
- Symptoms are usually systemic and non-specific (milder in paratyphoid).
- Classic triad is bradycardia, 'rose-spot' rash and constipation (later diarrhoea).
- Hepatosplenomegaly and a leucopaenia are often present.
- Small bowel haemorrhage or perforation occurs in 10%; encephalopathy in 5%.
- **Diagnosis**: usually depends on bone marrow culture (blood culture is only positive in the early stages, when the diagnosis is usually not suspected).
- **Management**: ciprofloxacin or chloramphenicol to eradicate the bacterium, and prednisolone for encephalopathy.

Parasite worm infections

- Roundworm, hookworm, threadworm, whipworm and tapeworm are consumed either by eating contaminated uncooked meat or through the faeco-oral route.
- Infections are usually asymptomatic, but may cause low-grade abdominal distension and nausea. A low-grade anaemia is common with all. Tapeworms are the most likely to give more dramatic symptoms (fever, enterocolitis, cyst formation in brain or muscle, weight loss). There may be pruritus ani or visible worms in the faeces.
- **Diagnosis** is suggested by an eosinophilia, but requires faecal examination for confirmation. Sellotape applied to the anal margin will on examination reveal threadworm, especially common in children.
- **Treatment**: tapeworm requires niclosamide as a stat dose, and the other infections will respond to 3 days of mebendazole or levamisole.

Anal infections

Anal warts

Human papilloma virus (HPV) is the commonest sexually transmitted virus, and is highly contagious. The warts are frequently multiple, with a characteristic cauliflower appearance, and may extend to the dentate line.

Treatment is usually with a topical antiviral (such as podophyllin, podofilox or imiquimod). Alternatively, destructive local therapies such as laser, cryotherapy or electrocoagulation may be considered. Surgery is reserved for large clusters of lesions or when there is extension into the rectum.

Chlamydia

This is the commonest sexually transmitted disease in the developed world, affecting women slightly more often than men. Urethral discharge and dysuria precede a shallow ulcer on the penis before the characteristic groin lymphadenopathy occurs. In rare late stages, inflammation of the rectum may occur. Diagnosis is based on antibody and complement fixation testing, only occasionally needing histology. Treatment is with azithromycin, doxycycline or co-trimoxazole.

Syphilis, gonorrhoea and herpes simplex

These sexually transmitted infections occur most frequently in those practising anoreceptive intercourse. Treatment is along standard lines.

Gut symptoms in HIV infection

Any part of the GI tract may be affected in patients with HIV infection; opportunistic gut infections should raise the suspicion of AIDS in these patients. Any of the preceding infections may occur, but specific symptom patterns suggest specific opportunistic infections:

- **Oral ulceration**: herpes simplex, *Candida*, *Neisseria gonorrhoea*, syphilis.
- **Dysphagia**: cytomegalovirus (CMV; see next section), *Candida*.

- **Abdominal pain**: TB, CMV in the gallbladder (intestinal lymphoma, Kaposi's sarcoma).
- **Diarrhoea**: TB, *Giardia*, *Cryptosporidium*, *Cyclospora*, *Chlamydia*, CMV and herpes simplex.
- **Rectal stricture**: *Chlamydia*, lymphogranuloma venereum.
- **Rectal bleeding**: lymphogranuloma venereum, syphilis (anal cancer, Kaposi's sarcoma).

Cytomegalovirus

CMV can invade the mucosa of any region of the gut, causing the symptoms already discussed. Histology is diagnostic, showing *multiple* intranuclear inclusion bodies. CMV infection of the colon can occur in any immunocompromised patient, not just those with AIDS; specifically also in patients with a flare-up of ulcerative colitis who have received immunosuppression (prednisolone, azathioprine). Since viraemia is fatal, aggressive treatment may be needed, with intravenous ganciclovir or foscarnet.

 KEY POINTS

- Many chronic gastrointestinal infections are more common in the developing world and in migrants from those countries. Infections include intestinal tuberculosis, *Helicobacter pylori* and parasitic infestations.
- Travellers are at risk of acute diarrhoea – often from enterotoxigenic *Escherichia coli* – and chronic infection – from amoebiasis, typhoid and paratyphoid.

- Sexually transmitted infections can affect the gut, particularly in those who have anoreceptive intercourse and in association with HIV.
- Tuberculosis can be very difficult to distinguish from Crohn's disease and a high index of suspicion must be held, particularly where patients have emigrated from areas of high endemicity.

 SELF-ASSESSMENT QUESTION

(The answer to this question is given on p. 266)

An 83-year-old woman presented with a 3-day history of worsening diarrhoea starting 5 days after discharge from hospital (she had been admitted for pneumonia). Her bowels were opening 10–15 times by day and night, passing watery stool without blood. On examination, she had a temperature of 37.8 °C with a pulse of 96 beats/min and a blood pressure of 110/58 mmHg. Her chest was clear, and her abdomen was soft but diffusely tender.

Regarding the investigation and management of her condition, which of the following statements is most correct?

(a) She should proceed directly to colonoscopy to rule out colonic carcinoma.

(b) Demonstrating the presence of *C. difficile* is insufficient to confirm the diagnosis of *C. difficile*–related diarrhoea.

(c) The absence of bloody diarrhoea makes infection with *C. difficile* much less likely than with *Campylobacter*.

(d) Given her profuse diarrhoea and evidence of dehydration, she should be given loperamide to slow the diarrhoea.

(e) IV vancomycin is indicated to cover the most likely pathogens in her situation.

Gastrointestinal investigations

Structural tests

Radiology

Plain X-rays

- Erect chest X-ray: free air under the diaphragm = perforation.
- Abdominal X-ray:
  - Dilated bowel loops and fluid level = obstruction or ileus.
  - Calcification:
    - Chronic pancreatitis.
    - Gallstones (only 10% radio-opaque).

Contrast studies

The principle is to provide radio-opaque contrast using an insoluble salt (such as barium sulphate) or water-soluble medium (gastrograffin); the mucosal images can be enhanced by the double-contrast technique (with co-inflation of gas and contrast). These are real-time studies, so as well as showing mucosal detail, they also give *some* information about gut motility.

Contrast swallow

- **Indications**:
  - Dysphagia (where upper GI endoscopy may be dangerous due to pharyngeal pouch).
  - Suspected dysmotility (where upper GI endoscopy is unhelpful).
  - Size of hiatus hernia (if not quantified at upper GI endoscopy).
  - (Other – heartburn, chest pain.)
- **Limitations**:
  - Upper GI endoscopy shows better mucosal detail and allows biopsy.
  - Aspiration risk.

Contrast meal (usually barium)

- **Indications**:
  - Epigastric pain with 'normal' upper GI endoscopy; possible linitis plastic.
  - Vomiting with 'normal' upper GI endoscopy; possible gastric outlet obstruction or dysmotility.
  - Suspected perforation (water-soluble medium).
- **Limitations**:
  - Upper GI endoscopy shows better mucosal detail and allows biopsy.
  - Poor at detecting early cancer.
  - Essentially replaced by endoscopy in current practice.

Contrast follow-through

- **Indications**:
  - Crohn's disease: suspected or to quantify extent.
  - Diarrhoea or abdominal pain with normal endoscopy and histology.
  - Suspected small bowel obstruction.
  - (Anaemia – superseded by capsule endoscopy.)
- **Limitations**:
  - Ionising radiation exposure.
  - Expertise dependent.
  - In most centres currently reserved for particular situations and CT or MRI enterography is the main modality for small bowel imaging; capsule

Gastroenterology and Hepatology: Lecture Notes, Second Edition. Stephen Inns and Anton Emmanuel.
© 2017 John Wiley & Sons, Ltd. Published 2017 by John Wiley & Sons, Ltd.
Companion website: www.lecturenoteseries.com/gastroenterology
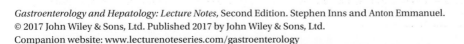

endoscopy for anaemia or where clinic suspicion is high but radiology negative.

Contrast enema

- **Indications**:
  - ∘ Altered bowel habit.
  - ∘ Suspected diverticulosis where colonoscopy may be difficult or dangerous.
  - ∘ Suspected megacolon (where lower GI endoscopy can give false negatives).
  - ∘ (Anaemia or rectal bleeding.)
- **Limitations**:
  - ∘ Uncomfortable for patient.
  - ∘ Does not visualise rectal mucosa well (especially if patient is unable to retain contrast due to incontinence).
  - ∘ Ionising radiation exposure.
  - ∘ Compared to colonoscopy, poor mucosal definition, cannot biopsy lesions and same bowel preparation required.
  - ∘ Very rarely used in modern practice.

Ultrasound

- **Indications**:
  - ∘ Abdominal masses: tumour, abscess, cyst.
  - ∘ Organomegaly.
  - ∘ Jaundice.
  - ∘ Gallstones.
  - ∘ Biliary tract dilatation.
  - ∘ Ascites.
  - ∘ Guided procedures (liver biopsy, cyst aspiration, stent insertion).
- **Limitations**:
  - ∘ Low sensitivity for lesions <5 mm.
  - ∘ Poor views if obstructed (gas) or obese.
  - ∘ Expertise dependent.
  - ∘ Poor for imaging retroperitoneal structures.

CT scanning

Oral contrast helps mucosal definition; intravenous contrast shows vascular lesions.

- **Indications**:
  - ∘ Tumour staging (colorectal, gastric, etc.).
  - ∘ Crohn's disease.
  - ∘ Pancreatic disease.
  - ∘ Bile duct stones (better than ultrasound).
  - ∘ Hepatic tumour staging.
  - ∘ Guided procedures (cyst aspiration, stent insertion).
  - ∘ CT colonography (non-invasive colonic imaging, but requires full bowel prep, and may miss lesions <1 cm).

- **Limitations**:
  - ∘ Ionising radiation exposure.
  - ∘ May 'under-stage' tumours.
  - ∘ Expertise dependent.

MRI scanning

- **Indications**:
  - ∘ Tumour staging (especially oesophagogastric).
  - ∘ Crohn's disease (small bowel and perianal).
  - ∘ Suspected neuroendocrine tumours.
  - ∘ Suspected chronic pancreatitis (secretin-stimulated MR).
  - ∘ Hepatic tumour staging.
  - ∘ MR cholangiopancreatography (MRCP).
- **Limitations**:
  - ∘ Expertise dependent.
  - ∘ Claustrophobic for some patients.
  - ∘ Time consuming.
  - ∘ Not feasible if metal prostheses in situ.

Mesenteric angiography

- **Indications**:
  - ∘ GI haemorrhage with normal upper and lower GI endoscopy.
  - ∘ Suspected arterio-venous malformation.
  - ∘ Suspected mesenteric ischaemia.
- **Limitations**:
  - ∘ Contrast-induced nephropathy.
  - ∘ Requires sufficiently brisk bleeding to document source.

Endoscopy

Video-endoscopy enables passage of flexible instruments into the upper and lower extremes of the gut, allowing both direct visualisation of the mucosa and biopsy or procedural interventions.

Upper GI endoscopy

Performed under sedation with intravenous benzodiazepine, or local anaesthetic throat spray only. Should be avoided if perforation is suspected; also caution following recent myocardial infarction or if suspected atlanto-axial subluxation (e.g. rheumatoid arthritis).

- **Indications – diagnostic**:
  - ∘ Abdominal pain.
  - ∘ Haematemesis or melaena.
  - ∘ Dysphagia.
  - ∘ Weight loss.
  - ∘ Iron-deficiency anaemia (necessitates distal duodenal biopsy).
  - ∘ Vomiting.

- Biopsy of upper GI tract following radiology procedure.
- Gastric ulcer follow-up.
- Balloon enteroscopy: an invasive technique allowing visualisation of distal duodenum and jejunum in cases of suspected bleeding or pain of intestinal origin.
- **Indications – therapeutic**:
  - Endoscopic treatment of oesophageal varices.
  - Dilatation of stricture.
  - Insertion of stent to palliate strictures.
  - Placement of PEG tube.
- **Complications**:
  - Perforation (0.1%).
  - Over-sedation resulting in respiratory depression (0.01%).
  - Aspiration pneumonia (avoidable with good nursing assistance and pharyngeal suctioning).

Flexible sigmoidoscopy

Performed (often without sedation) following enema; only the left colon and rectum are examined.
- **Indications**:
  - Fresh rectal bleeding.
  - Quantify activity in known ulcerative colitis patient.
- **Complications** of perforation and haemorrhage are extremely rare.

Colonoscopy

Performed after full bowel preparation and with conscious sedation; the entire colon and if possible the terminal ileum are examined.
- **Indications – diagnostic**:
  - Altered bowel habit (constipation or diarrhoea).
  - Rectal bleeding.
  - Iron-deficiency anaemia.
  - Suspected inflammatory bowel disease.
  - Follow-up of abnormal barium enema.
  - Colorectal cancer screening.
  - Surveillance:
    - Post-colectomy for cancer.
    - For adenoma.
    - For inflammatory bowel disease.
- **Indications – therapeutic**:
  - Polypectomy.
  - Argon or laser photocoagulation of vascular lesion.
  - Dilatation or stent insertion.
- **Complications**:
  - Incomplete examination (10%), depending on expertise.

- Perforation (0.5% therapeutic procedures, 0.1% diagnostic ones).
- Haemorrhage (twice the perforation rate).
- Cardiorespiratory depression if over-sedated.
- Infective endocarditis (avoidable with prophylactic antibiotics in at-risk patients, i.e. those with previous endocarditis or prophylactic heart valves).

Endoscopic retrograde cholangiopancreatography

ERCP is performed after minimum four hours fasting and with conscious sedation or general anaesthetic (GA). A specialised side-viewing endoscope is used to visualise the ampulla of Vater in the duodenum and instruments including catheters, sphincterotomy devices, stone-extraction devices and stents can be inserted into the pancreatic or bile duct. Fluoroscopy is used to image contrast injected into the biliary and pancreatic duct systems (Figure 6.1).
- **Indications – diagnostic**:
  - Biliary pain or cholestatic liver tests when ultrasound and magnetic resonance cholangiopancreatography (MRCP) have failed to show a cause.
  - With the advent of MRCP the role for diagnostic ERCP has virtually disappeared.
- **Indications – therapeutic**:
  - Removal of biliary stones.
  - Dilatation or stenting of biliary stricture (biliary tumour or extrinsic compression).
  - Endoscopic sphincterotomy for sphincter dysfunction.
- **Complications**:
  - Failed examination (10%), depending on expertise.
  - Perforation (less than 1%).
  - Haemorrhage following sphincterotomy.
  - Cardiorespiratory depression if over-sedated.
  - Cholangitis if complete drainage is not achieved.
  - Pancreatitis is the most feared complication, ~5% in most series. Higher risk if young, previous post-ERCP pancreatitis, female, cannulation of pancreatic duct, sphincter of Oddi dysfunction.

Endoscopic ultrasound

Performed with specialised endoscopes, bearing a revolving ultrasonic probe at the tip of the scope.

- **Indications**:
  - Staging of cancers of oesophagus, rectum and pancreas.
  - Drainage of pancreatic pseudocysts.

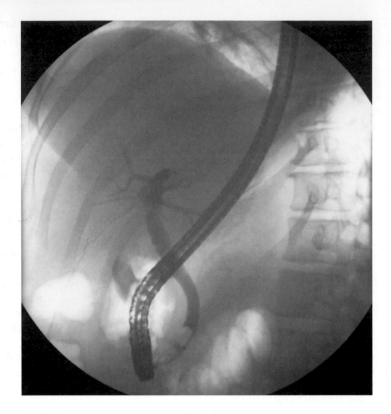

Figure 6.1 Normal endoscopic retrograde cholangiopancreatography (the lucency at the distal end of the bile duct is an inflated balloon).

○ Lymph node biopsy.
○ Assessment of anal sphincters in faecal incontinence.

Video-capsule enteroscopy

Allows visualisation of distal small bowel by a swallowed disposable video capsule.
- **Indications**:
  ○ Obscure GI bleeding.
  ○ Recurrent anaemia.
  ○ Where the clinical suspicion for small bowel disease (e.g. Crohn's disease) is high but radiology is negative.
- **Limitations**:
  ○ Caution required if strictures are suspected, as the capsule can then obstruct.
  ○ Expense.

Radioisotope studies

Meckel's scan

- Technetium (^{99m}Tc) is selectively taken up by parietal cells.

- Thus, intravenous infusion of labelled ^{99m}Tc allows localisation of ectopic tissue in a **Meckel's diverticulum**.

Labelled white cell scan

- Patient's own leucocytes are extracted and radiolabelled before being reintroduced.
- Thus, they migrate to sites of infection or inflammation (Crohn's disease), which can now be localised.

Labelled red cell scan

- Patient's own erythrocytes are extracted and radiolabelled before being reintroduced.
- Thus, they can be seen as they are extravasated from the gut.

Bile acid absorption test

- Radiolabelled bile acid substrate is consumed orally, and should be absorbed and stored as ^{75}SeHCAT.
- Test allows quantification of the amount that is retained after 7 days, with anything <5% retention being abnormal.

Physiological tests

Gut hormone analysis

Performed to assess secretory diarrhoea or suspected Zollinger–Ellison syndrome. Requires cessation of proton pump inhibitor for 2 weeks. Results are of the fasting levels of:

- Gastrin.
- Glucagon.
- Vasoactive intestinal polypeptide (VIP).
- Pancreatic polypeptide.
- Somatostatin.
- Calcitonin.

Breath tests

These depend on the following simple principle:

Substrate + Physiological or Pathological host factor
$\rightarrow$ Physiological metabolite(s) + Gas by-product

For each test, the principle is exploited to measure a lack or excess of the host factor. The methodology for each test is that the substrate is given and gas samples are collected regularly for 120 min.

Lactose hydrogen breath test

To diagnose hypolactasia ('lactose intolerance').
- Substrate = lactose.
- Host factor = brush border lactase levels (physiological).
- Physiological metabolites = glucose and galactose.
- Gas by-products = nil:
  - In hypolactasia, the lactose is not digested and so enters the colon, where it is metabolised by bacteria-releasing hydrogen.
  - Positive result is an elevated breath hydrogen sooner than 120 min (i.e. when lactose substrate has reached the colon).

Glucose (or lactulose) hydrogen breath test

To diagnose small intestine bacterial overgrowth.
- Substrate = glucose (or lactulose).
- Host factor = bacteria present in small intestine (pathological).
- Physiological metabolite = energy.
- Gas by-product = hydrogen:
  - In bacterial overgrowth, the flora in the small intestine digests the glucose-releasing hydrogen.
  - Positive result is an elevated breath hydrogen sooner than 60 min (i.e. well before substrate has reached colonic flora).

^{14}C-xylose carbon dioxide breath test

To diagnose small intestine bacterial overgrowth.
- Substrate = ^{14}C-xylose.
- Host factor = bacteria present in small intestine (pathological).
- Physiological metabolite = energy.
- Gas by-product = carbon dioxide:
  - In bacterial overgrowth, the flora in the small intestine digests the xylose-releasing $^{14}CO_2$.
  - Positive result is an elevated breath $^{14}CO_2$ sooner than 60 min (i.e. well before substrate has reached colonic flora).

^{14}C-triolein carbon dioxide breath test

To diagnose fat malabsorption.
- Substrate = ^{14}C-triolein (a triglyceride).
- Host factor = lipase enzymes (physiological).
- Physiological metabolite = oleic acid.
- Gas by-product = carbon dioxide:
  - In fat malabsorption, there is less hydrolysis of the triolein substrate, hence less oleic acid produced, hence less $^{14}CO_2$.
  - Positive result is a reduced breath $^{14}CO_2$ sooner than 60 min (i.e. well before substrate has reached colonic flora).

^{14}C- or ^{13}C-urea carbon dioxide breath test

To identify the presence of *Helicobacter pylori* (especially to confirm eradication in those who have been treated but have persistent or recurrent symptoms).
- Substrate = ^{14}C- or ^{13}C-urea.
- Host factor = *Helicobacter pylori* (pathological).
- Physiological metabolite = ammonium.
- Gas by-product = carbon dioxide:
  - In *Helicobacter pylori* infection there is increased cleavage of urea by the bacteria (which possess the enzyme urease) and hence an increase of CO_2.
  - Positive result is an elevated breath $^{14}CO_2$ or $^{13}CO_2$ at 20 min.

Mucosal inflammation tests

Intestine permeability studies

- **Principle**: the normal small bowel absorbs mono-, not di-, saccharides. Once absorbed they are excreted in the urine. An increase in permeability allows both mono- and di-saccharides to be absorbed.
- **Method**: oral lactulose and rhamnose are ingested, before accurate urinary measurement of the sugars, expressed as a ratio.
- **Results**: increased permeability in Crohn's disease and coeliac disease.

Faecal calprotectin

- **Principle**: calprotectin is a peptide expressed by colonic neutrophils.
- **Method**: faecal estimation of concentration of calprotectin.
- **Results**: increased levels in colonic inflammation, infections and cancers.

Oesophageal physiology

Stationary manometry

A transnasal catheter is passed into the oesophagus and gives information (see Figure 6.2) about:

- Contractions in the body of the oesophagus.
- Function and pressure of the lower oesophageal sphincter (LOS).

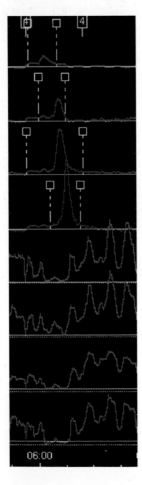

Figure 6.2 Stationary oesophageal manometry trace showing normal peristalsis in upper four graphs and relaxation of lower oesophageal sphincter in lower four graphs. Each horizontal division represents 5 s.

High-resolution manometry is the current state of the art and involves recording of intraluminal pressure using a large array of closely spaced pressure sensors (Figure 6.3).

LOS, lower oesophageal sphincter; UOS, upper oesophageal sphincter.

- **Indications**:
  - Suspected achalasia: manometry is the diagnostic test, showing:
    - Absence of peristalsis in body of oesophagus (mandatory).
    - Non-relaxation of the LOS (often).
    - Elevated LOS pressure (occasional).
    - Elevated pressures in body of oesophagus (occasional).
  - Suspected other oesophageal dysmotility (though ambulatory studies may be needed).
  - Prior to proposed antireflux surgery (to exclude dysmotility prior to surgery).

Ambulatory manometry

A transnasal catheter is placed in the oesophagus for a 24-hour period, measuring contraction patterns while the patient continues normal activities.

- **Indication**: Chest pain where coronary artery disease has been excluded (to exclude oesophageal spasm).

Ambulatory pH studies

A transnasal pH catheter is placed in the oesophagus for 24–48 hours, or alternatively a wireless pH probe is clipped into the oesophagus, allowing:

- Quantification of degree of acid exposure.
- Timing of symptom episodes with objective episodes of reflux into the oesophagus.
- **Indications**:
  - Suspected gastro-oesophageal reflux where endoscopy shows no oesophagitis (to confirm whether there is objective acid reflux).
  - Refractory gastro-oesophageal reflux (to confirm adequacy of acid suppression).
  - Prior to proposed antireflux surgery (to confirm pathological degree of acid reflux).

Recent advances include ambulatory impedance studies, which allow quantification not only of acid reflux but also of non-acid reflux episodes, and the addition of multiple sensors to the catheter, allowing simultaneous measurement of fluid movement through the whole oesophagus.

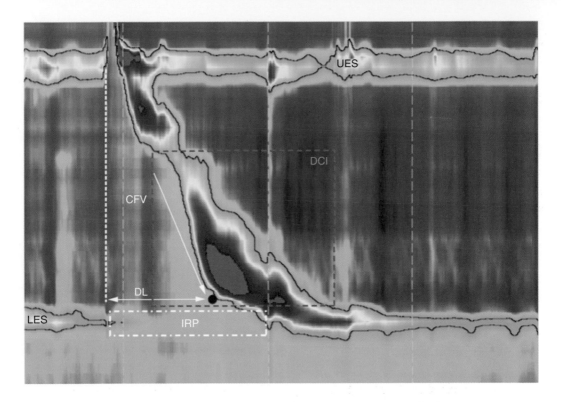

Figure 6.3 High-resolution oesophageal manometry: normal water swallow. The two bands of high pressure correspond to the UOS and LOS. The UOS relaxes at the start of the swallow, and the LOS relaxes as the contraction front traverses the oesophageal body (x-axis: distance from LOS to UES, y-axis: time, the intraoesophageal pressure is represented by colours [red: higher, green: lower, blue: background pressure]). Source: Zerbib F, Omari T. Oesophageal dysphagia: manifestations and diagnosis. Nat Rev Gastroenterol Hepatol. 2015;12: 322–331. doi:10.1038/nrgastro.2014.195. Reproduced with permission of Nature Publishing Group.

Gastric emptying

In suspected gastroparesis, endoscopy and contrast studies are often normal (with the exception of possibly showing persistence of gastric content despite an adequate period of fasting). The rate of gastric emptying can be accurately quantified using a *radio-isotope-labelled meal*, with different labels on the solid (technetium) and liquid (indium) phase of the test meal. Normal emptying is for 50% of the solid phase to be empty by 90 min.

Whole gut transit

Oroanal transit time in health is highly variable, but approximates to between 20 and 40 hours, the majority of that time being spent in the colon. This rate of transit can be assessed by undertaking an abdominal X-ray on day 5 after three sets of distinct *radio-opaque markers ('shapes study')* have been ingested on days 1, 2 and 3 (see Figure 3.1). Persistence of excessive numbers of any one of the sets of markers indicates slow transit, and is a valuable test in patients with chronic constipation.

Anorectal physiology

This term refers to a battery of tests undertaken to investigate anorectal function in a laboratory setting. They are complementary to a focused history of bowel function and imaging studies (most commonly endo-anal ultrasound or proctography). Measures are obtained of:

- Anal sphincter pressure.
- Rectal sensitivity and compliance.
- Anorectal reflexes.
- **Indications**:
  ◦ Faecal incontinence.
  ◦ Suspected Hirschsprung's disease (see Chapter 16).
  ◦ Prior to ileoanal pouch surgery (to confirm sphincter competence).

KEY POINTS

- Contrast studies have essentially been replaced by endoscopy in current practice.
- Capsule endoscopy allows mucosal visualisation of the small bowel for anaemia or where clinical suspicion for mucosal disease is high but radiology negative.
- With the advent of MRCP, the role for diagnostic ERCP has virtually disappeared.
- Endoscopic ultrasound allows operators to overcome the limitations of transabdominal ultrasound, namely the distance from the area of interest to the probe and any gas in the way.

- High-resolution manometry is the current state of the art and involves recording of intraluminal pressure using a large array of closely spaced pressure sensors.
- Wireless oesophageal pH studies have improved the acceptability and tolerability of ambulatory pH telemetry.
- Recent advances in oesophageal pH studies include ambulatory impedance studies, which allow quantification not only of acid reflux but also of non-acid reflux episodes.

SELF-ASSESSMENT QUESTION

(The answer to this question is given on p. 266)
A 62-year-old man presents with intermittent rectal bleeding. The blood is mixed in with the stool. He has lost no weight and his bowel habit has not changed significantly. He is not anaemic. There is no significant family history of gastrointestinal disease.

Regarding the investigation of his complaint, which of the following statements is most correct?

(a) The risk of perforation due to diagnostic colonoscopy is less than 1 in 1000 procedures.

(b) The risk of haemorrhage with polypectomy is less than 1 in 500 procedures.

(c) Barium enema is the standard first-line test for rectal bleeding.

(d) CT colonography has equal sensitivity and specificity to colonoscopy for colonic lesions less than 1 cm.

(e) Antibiotics should be routinely administered at colonoscopy to avoid infective endocarditis.

Part II

Gastrointestinal Emergencies

7

Acute gastrointestinal bleeding

Acute upper gastrointestinal bleeding

The **clinical features** of gastrointestinal bleeding are blood loss and shock. Observing the pattern of blood loss can help to localise bleeding to an extent, and carefully stratifying risk based on haemodynamic compromise and other patient factors is crucial to appropriate management. **Haematemesis** (vomiting blood) occurs when the bleeding source is proximal to the jejunum, and **melaena** (tarry stool) usually occurs when blood loss is proximal to the caecum. Gastrointestinal bleeding is a common cause of inpatient mortality, but the outcome very much depends on the expertise available – 5% in the best centres and 20% in others. The aims of management are to:

- Resuscitate the patient.
- Arrest the bleeding.
- Prevent or promptly recognise rebleeding.

Causes and epidemiology (in order of occurrence)

- Peptic ulcer (duodenal > gastric).
- Gastric erosions/gastritis.
- Mallory–Weiss tear.
- Gastro-oesophageal varices (~5% of acute bleeds, but 80% of mortality).
- Duodenitis.
- Oesophagitis.
- Tumours (gastric > oesophageal).
- Gastric antral vascular ectasia (GAVE).

- Dieulafoy lesions.
- Hereditary haemorrhagic telangiectasia.
- Aorto-enteric fistula.
- Clotting defect.

Investigation and management – general

- Assess initial Rockall score to predict mortality risk (Table 7.1).
- Initial resuscitation.
- Intravenous access.
- Give colloid (preferred to crystalloid) if hypotensive or tachycardic.
- If Rockall shock score 2, insert central venous catheter and urinary catheter and get a surgical consultation.
- Keep nil by mouth (until endoscopy).
- **Initial investigations**:
  - Check bloods for FBC, renal and liver function, and clotting status.
  - If major blood loss, cross-match blood; if not, group and save blood.
  - Arterial blood gases, chest X-ray and electrocardiogram (ECG) if cardiorespiratory disease present.
  - Upper GI endoscopy: best performed on a daytime list, but emergency procedure indicated if there is:
    - High likelihood of variceal bleed (history of or stigmata of chronic liver disease).
    - Rebleeding of a hospital patient.
    - Bleeding after endoscopy.
    - High chance of acute surgery.

Gastroenterology and Hepatology: Lecture Notes, Second Edition. Stephen Inns and Anton Emmanuel.
© 2017 John Wiley & Sons, Ltd. Published 2017 by John Wiley & Sons, Ltd.
Companion website: www.lecturenoteseries.com/gastroenterology

Table 7.1 Rockall score – initial.

Criterion		Score
Age	<59	0
	60–79	1
	>80	2
Shock	None	0
	Pulse >/=100 and SBP >/= 100	1
	SBP < 100	2
Comorbidity	None	0
	Cardiac/lung /major	2
	Renal/liver/cancer	3
Total		0–7

SBP, systolic blood pressure.

Table 7.2 Rockall score – post-endoscopy.

Criterion		Score
Endoscopic diagnosis	Normal, Mallory–Weiss tear	0
	Any other lesion	1
	Upper GI cancer	2
Stigma of recent bleed	None, black spots	0
	Clot, visible vessel, blood in stomach	2
Post-endoscopy sub total		0–4
Total	Add initial score	0–11

GI, gastrointestinal.

- Endoscopic intervention is preferred to surgery for peptic ulcer (thermocoagulation, adrenaline injection, vessel clip) and for varices (see Chapter 20).
- Endoscopy also permits check of *Helicobacter pylori* status in peptic ulcer patients.
- Assess post-endoscopy Rockall score to predict risk (Table 7.2).

Investigation and management – specific

Oesophagogastric varices

See Chapter 20.

Peptic ulcers

See also Chapter 13.

- High-dose intravenous omeprazole or pantoprazole (proton pump inhibitor, PPI) in high-risk bleeding (halves chance of rebleeding).
- Whether oral or lower-dose PPI might be effective is not yet clear.
- Tranexamic acid (an antifibrinolytic) may help reduce bleeding, but the evidence for a mortality benefit is still not available.
- Monitor for rebleeding:
  ○ Rise in heart rate (most sensitive indicator).
  ○ Fall in venous pressure or urine output.
  ○ Overt haematemesis (more sensitive than melaena).
- Liaise with surgical team especially if:
  ○ High-volume transfusion (>5 units RBC) required.
  ○ There is continued bleeding, or rebleeding, despite endoscopy.
  ○ A spurting vessel was seen at endoscopy.

Mallory–Weiss tears

- Typical feature is that bleeding is not seen in the initial vomitus.
- Acid suppression not required (>90% heal spontaneously).
- Continued bleeding may, rarely, warrant endoscopic therapy.

Gastric erosions

- Usually related to a combination of NSAIDs, alcohol and stress.
- Treatment is with a PPI for 2–4 weeks.

Aorto-enteric fistula

- Consider in any patient who has had aortic graft surgery and presents with GI blood loss.
- Diagnosis is best made by abdominal CT.
- Management requires surgery rather than endoscopy.

No source of bleeding found

- Most often due to a common lesion missed at upper GI endoscopy, so careful re-examination by an expert is warranted, especially if there is continued bleeding.
- Rarely, other lesions may be the cause:
  ○ Dieulafoy lesion that has healed by time of endoscopy.
  ○ Distal duodenal bleeding (NSAID, Zollinger–Ellison peptic ulcers).
  ○ Meckel's diverticulum.

Prognosis

Prognosis is largely determined by the degree of shock at presentation, the risk of rebleeding and patient factors such as comorbidity. Some causes of bleeding do carry a higher morbidity and mortality risk, particularly variceal bleeding (50% 3-year mortality) and bleeding from malignancies (95% 3-year mortality).

Acute lower gastrointestinal bleeding

This is distinct from melaena in that blood loss is either red–brown or fresh and bright. Causes are almost invariably due to a colonic or anal source of blood loss; a more useful classification is according to frequency of particular lesions occurring.

Causes (in approximate order of frequency)

- Haemorrhoids: these are so common that they may occur synchronously with other causes.
- Anal fissure.
- Colorectal polyps.
- Colorectal cancer.
- Ulcerative colitis > Crohn's colitis.
- Rectal prolapse.
- Diverticular disease.
- Angiodysplasia.
- Ischaemic colitis.
- Solitary rectal ulcer syndrome with/without rectal prolapse.
- Vasculitis.
- Small intestinal disease (lymphoma, diverticula).

Management

- Initial resuscitation.
- Initial investigation.
- Check bloods for FBC, renal and liver function, clotting status.
- If major blood loss, cross-match blood; if not, group and save blood.
- Prompt lower GI endoscopy:
  - Colonoscopy if altered bleeding.
  - Flexible sigmoidoscopy if fresh rectal bleeding.
  - Upper GI endoscopy is only required if there is major circulatory collapse (when the source may be a rapidly bleeding upper GI lesion causing the presentation).
- Mesenteric angiography is only needed if there is continued heavy bleeding (loss of >1 g Hb/4 h).
- If there is recurrent bleeding and no source has been identified:
  1. Repeat colonoscopy by an expert; *if nil found, go to 2.*
  2. Consider an upper GI source: gastroscopy or push enteroscopy may be indicated; *if nil found, go to 3.*
  3. Video-capsule enteroscopy; *if nil found, consider 4 or 5.*
  4. CT angiography; *or*
  5. Scintigraphic red cell scan.
- In most cases, spontaneous cessation of bleeding occurs. However:
  - If blood loss continues from an identified source, consideration of surgical resection is reasonable.
  - If blood loss continues from an unidentified source, laparotomy with on-table colonoscopy/enteroscopy.

 KEY POINTS

- Observing the pattern of blood loss can help to localise bleeding.
- Carefully stratifying risk based on haemodynamic compromise and other patient factors is crucial. A scoring system such as the pre-endoscopic Rockall's score can assist with this.
- Haematemesis (vomiting blood) occurs when the bleeding source is proximal to the jejunum, and melaena (tarry stool) usually occurs when blood loss is proximal to the caecum.

- Ongoing obscure upper GI bleeding is most often due to a common lesion missed at upper GI endoscopy, so careful re-examination by an expert is warranted.
- Continued obscure lower GI bleeding despite negative colonoscopy requires further investigation of the small bowel.

SELF-ASSESSMENT QUESTION

(The answer to this question is given on p. 266)

A 67-year-old man presents with black tarry stool and postural dizziness for the last day. On arrival his heart rate is 96 beats/min and his blood pressure lying is 98/52. He has been taking voltaren for mechanical back pain for the last 2 weeks. There is no history of, or risk factors for, liver disease.

Regarding the management of his condition, which of the following statements is most correct?

(a) The presence of melaena suggests that the source is proximal to the pylorus.

(b) The mortality associated with this situation is low and unpredictable.

(c) Immediate gastroscopy and cessation of bleeding are the priority in his treatment.

(d) Tranexamic acid has not been shown to reduce mortality in acute upper GI bleeding.

(e) Proton pump inhibitors may help to prevent peptic ulcer bleeding, but have no place in acute upper GI bleeding.

8

Acute upper and lower gastrointestinal emergencies

Gastrointestinal emergencies account for a significant proportion of acute presentations to the A&E department – both to surgeons and physicians. The potential presentations are listed anatomically in this section. Presentations with isolated acute abdominal pain are covered in Chapter 3.

Acute total dysphagia

Sudden complete dysphagia for solids and liquids is a medical emergency requiring instant relief of obstruction. The commonest cause is bolus food impaction on a pre-existing lesion (cancer, benign stricture, web). The dangers relate to the risk of aspiration pneumonia, and the extreme distress to the patient from not being able to swallow even their saliva.

Causes and epidemiology

Very little epidemiological data regarding the prevalence and pathogenesis of acute total dysphagia is available. However, acute dysphagia is not an uncommon cause for urgent endoscopy in most endoscopy centres. The underlying causes include eosinophilic oesophagitis, reflux oesophagitis with Stricturing, oesophageal malignancy and stricturing from past surgery or radiotherapy.

Clinical features

Patients generally present with a clear history of having swallowed a bolus of food that was less well chewed or harder than usual, followed by a sense of a foreign body in the oesophagus and often the inability to swallow anything, including saliva. There may be cough resulting from aspiration and, on rare occasions, laryngeal spasm and resultant stridor.

Investigation and management

- Reassurance.
- Rehydration.
- Endoscopic removal of obstruction.
- Endoscopic dilatation of stricture if appropriate; if not, an enteral feeding tube should be placed if oral nutrition will not be safe.
- Treat aspiration pneumonia if appropriate.
- Give advice about avoiding dysphagia:
  ○ Good dentition and careful mastication.
  ○ Avoid fibrous foods.
  ○ Plentiful drinks, especially carbonated.
  ○ Proton pump inhibitor (PPI) if stricture present.

Prognosis

The vast majority of obstructions can be dealt with safely by endoscopy. There is, however, an associated risk of perforation or haemorrhage, and this is higher

Gastroenterology and Hepatology: Lecture Notes, Second Edition. Stephen Inns and Anton Emmanuel.
© 2017 John Wiley & Sons, Ltd. Published 2017 by John Wiley & Sons, Ltd.
Companion website: www.lecturenoteseries.com/gastroenterology

than that for a diagnostic procedure. The main determinant of morbidity and mortality is the underlying pathology. Eosinophilic oesophagitis is one of the commoner reasons for food bolus impaction, but survival is excellent; the converse is true for oesophageal malignancy.

Oesophageal rupture

Causes and epidemiology

This is a very rare consequence of oesophageal trauma and is known eponymously as Boerhaave's syndrome when it results from vigorous vomiting. In order of frequency, causes are:

- Endoscopy or other instrumentation (usually small tears).
- Chest trauma.
- Forceful severe vomiting (usually large tears).

Clinical features

Sudden severe chest pain after an obvious provoking cause. The differential includes myocardial infarction, dissecting aneurysm, acute pancreatitis and gastrointestinal perforation.

Investigations

Investigations are therefore driven towards confirming the condition, excluding the differential diagnosis (in parenthesis in the following), identifying the site of perforation and identifying complications:

- ECG and cardiac enzymes (MI).
- Erect chest X-ray (dissecting aneurysm, perforated viscus, pneumothorax) will also show surgical and mediastinal emphysema, and possibly a pleural effusion as a complication of the rupture.
- CT scan chest and abdomen (dissecting aneurysm, perforated viscus).
- Serum amylase (acute pancreatitis >> perforated viscus).
- Gastrograffin swallow: to confirm location.

Management

- Analgesia (potent).
- Intravenous fluids and keep nil by mouth.
- Urgent surgical opinion.

Large tears (based on gastrograffin swallow) and spontaneous ruptures

- Intravenous antibiotics (metronidazole and broad-spectrum agent).
- *Early* surgical repair.
- Enteral nutrition (via jejunal feeding tube).

Small tears

- Conservative management (and operate if fever or pneumothorax develops).
- If rupture complicates oesophageal malignancy, a cuffed oesophageal tube can be placed to palliate.

Prognosis

The mortality of oesophageal perforation depends largely on the size of the tear and the timeliness and success of surgery. In Boerhaave's syndrome the untreated mortality is essentially 100%, and even with treatment there is still a mortality rate of around 25%.

Acute diarrhoea

The epidemiology, causes, presentation and prognosis of acute diarrhoea are detailed in Chapter 5. This section serves only as a primer for management in the acute setting.

Management
Fluid replacement

- Oral replacement is sufficient in most cases.
- Isotonic fluid is required to replace diarrhoeal losses (which are isotonic themselves).
- Glucose is required to drive mucosal absorption of the ions in this isotonic fluid.
- This combination of isotonic fluid and glucose is found in oral rehydration solutions (ORSs).
- A few figures:
  - Adults lose 1 l of fluid for every 24 h with moderate diarrhoea (6–8 stools/day).
  - Typically 200 ml of isotonic fluid is lost with each stool.
  - One sachet of commercial oral rehydration solution provides 200 ml of isotonic fluid.
  - Fluid replacement of diarrhoea as described needs to *supplement* the minimum 1.5 l of liquid that an adult needs per day.

Antibiotic therapy

- Antimicrobials are not usually indicated since acute infections typically last only 1–3 days (in addition to the risks of antibiotic-related diarrhoea and emerging antibiotic resistance).
- Antibiotics are indicated only in certain patient groups (see Chapter 5).
- Antibiotics are also indicated in epidemic diarrhoea, in order to control the spread of infection.

Antidiarrhoeal therapy

Antidiarrhoeal agents are best avoided, as they may prolong carriage of the organism, and as such they are absolutely contraindicated in cases of bloody diarrhoea (where an enteroinvasive organism may be causative). They may trigger intussusception or ileus in children.

Gut obstruction and ileus

Epidemiology and causes

Obstruction of the passage of intestinal contents can be caused by mechanical obstruction or by paralysis of the normal motility of the gut. Both are common

causes of inpatient care, affecting 20% of patients admitted to hospital for abdominal pain. While the gut can be affected at any level, the majority (over 80%) of episodes involve the small bowel. The causes are listed in Table 8.1.

Clinical features

History

The history of the symptoms preceding intestinal obstruction gives invaluable clues as to the location and cause (Table 8.1). In the patient with a past history of laparotomy and sudden onset of central abdominal pain and vomiting, adhesional obstruction of the small bowel is most likely. Patients with obstruction within a hernia may give a history of a pre-existing hernia, usually inguinal or incisional. More chronic progressive presentations suggest an inflammatory or malignant cause of obstruction.

Proximal obstruction is associated with marked vomiting and pain, but not usually abdominal distension. More distal small bowel lesions tend to result in more abdominal distension and less vomiting. Marked unexplainable weight loss suggests a malignant process or a chronic inflammatory disease such as Crohn's disease. Generally, pain caused by small

Table 8.1 Causes of gut obstruction.

Mechanism	Site	Examples
Mechanical	Extrinsic	Intestinal hernia* Adhesions* Volvulus (sigmoid >> caecal >> gastric)
	Mural	Malignancy (carcinoma >> lymphoma > carcinoid)* Diverticular disease Stricturing Crohn's disease NSAID-induced strictures Radiation enterocolitis Intestinal tuberculosis
	Luminal	Foreign body Bezoar (food bolus) Intussusception Gallstone ileus
Paralytic ('ileus')	Multiple sites	Postoperative* Chronic intestinal pseudo-obstruction Intestinal ischaemia
	Retro-peritoneal	Pancreatitis Tumours (sarcoma) Retro-peritoneal fibrosis
	Metabolic	Hypokalaemia Diabetic ketoacidosis Acute renal failure

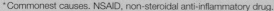

*Commonest causes. NSAID, non-steroidal anti-inflammatory drug.

intestinal obstruction is felt in the central abdomen. It may be colicky in nature, waxing and waning over periods of minutes. Severe localised unremitting pain is suggestive of strangulated obstruction.

Colonic lesions on the left side may be associated with rectal bleeding or a change in the stool calibre. There may be difficulty with evacuation but, if the lesion allows passage of fluid stool only, there may be pseudo-diarrhoea. Pain from colonic obstruction tends to be felt periumbilically and in the hypogastrium.

Examination

On general observation the patient may be in obvious pain and/or vomiting. The nutritional status should be assessed. The abdomen, including the inguinal regions, must be carefully examined for the presence of hernias. Tenderness may be generalised and will not necessarily aid localisation of the lesion. Bowel sounds may be high pitched where an overactive small bowel attempts to push luminal substrate through a narrow opening. They may be absent in established obstruction. Peritonism occurs where the viscus has perforated. Rectal examination must always be performed in order to rule out palpable rectal lesions, establish whether there is stool in the rectum and detect left-sided colonic bleeding.

Management – general

- **Initial resuscitation**:
  - Intravenous access.
  - Give crystalloid, including potassium.
  - Insert nasogastric suction tube.
  - Keep nil by mouth (until endoscopy).
- **Initial investigations**:
  - Plain abdominal X-ray (Figure 8.1), supine and erect; look for:
    - Gas distribution: valvulae conniventes (traverse the full width of the small intestine) or haustra (partially traverse the width of the colon).
    - Fluid levels.
    - Luminal dilatation.
    - Mucosal oedema.
  - Erect chest X-ray: look for air under the diaphragm.
  - Check bloods:
    - For FBC: increased white cell count suggests strangulation.
    - Renal and liver function: hypokalaemia and increased urea are found in ileus.
  - Abdominal CT scan: this is the most useful examination to determine site and cause of obstruction.

(a)

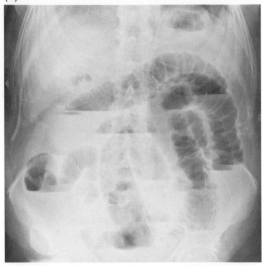

(b)

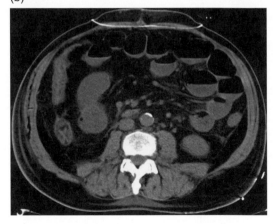

Figure 8.1 Imaging in diagnosis of acute GI obstruction in a patient with small bowel obstruction. (a) Plain abdominal radiograph. (b) Computer tomography. Source: Hucl T. Acute GI obstruction. Best Pract Res Cl Ga. 2013;27: 691–707, Fig 1. Reproduced with permission of Elsevier.

- Arterial blood gases: severe vomiting causes metabolic alkalosis.
- If there is strangulation (fever, rebound tenderness and increased white count), then surgery is required.
- Monitor:
  - Hydration status (venous pressure, signs of hydration).
  - Nasogastric aspirate volume.
  - Urine output.
  - Electrolyte status.

Management – specific (Table 8.2)

- **Paralytic ileus:**
  - Stop provoking drugs (anticholinergics) and minimise opiate analgesia.
  - Give crystalloid, including potassium.
  - Meticulous attention to hydration and serum potassium.
  - Consider domperidone, metoclopramide or erythromycin (prokinetics).
  - Consider parenteral nutrition if prolonged.
- **Intussusception:**
  - Diagnosis is often established by ultrasound.
  - Barium or gastrograffin meal may be therapeutic in reducing intussusception.
- **Meckel's diverticulum:** treat surgically if that is the cause.
- **Volvulus:**

  - Sigmoid: deflating the gut (flatus tube or colonoscopy) is preferable to surgery.
  - Caecal: recurrence is frequent, so surgery is advised.
  - Gastric: surgery to reduce the volvulus and repair diaphragmatic hiatus that allows the gastric volvulus.

Prognosis

The prognosis obviously depends largely on the underlying cause and access to appropriate therapy. Most cases of postoperative ileus resolve spontaneously and without complication, but malignant causes of obstruction are associated with poor outcomes. Where strangulation and resultant ischaemia occur, the outcome is very poor without emergent surgery.

Foreign bodies

In the case of swallowed foreign bodies, the priority is to safeguard the airway. If the object is impacted in the pharynx, or is likely to become so on attempted removal, then an ENT surgeon should be available. Once past the pylorus, spontaneous anal passage is the norm, though rarely perforation at the ileocaecal

valve may occur. Severe pain and fever should raise the concern of perforation.

Causes and epidemiology

Foreign body ingestion is common in small children but does occur in adults, either inadvertently when food is inadequately chewed or purposefully, often in the setting of psychiatric disease. Little data exists regarding the true prevalence of ingested foreign bodies, but in one US study 4% of parents reported the swallowing of a coin by their child – the commonest object swallowed by children.

Investigation and management

- Reassure the patient.
- Perform chest and abdominal X-rays to confirm nature and quantity of ingested item (normal X-rays do not exclude the diagnosis).
  - Sharp items and batteries:
    - If within the oesophagus or stomach, remove at endoscopy (an overtube is needed to protect the pharynx on extubation).
    - If past the pylorus, commence watchful waiting.
  - Blunt items and coins: watchful waiting, as most will spontaneously pass.
  - Smuggled drug packets:
    - Surgical removal is preferred to endoscopic (due to risk of rupture).
    - Monitor for risks of overdose in case of rupture.
  - Rectal foreign bodies:
    - Usually need surgical removal at examination under anaesthetic.
    - Treat the patient with dignity.
    - Consider psychiatric referral as appropriate.

Prognosis

Outcome depends on the nature of the object and access to appropriate interventions. Most swallowed objects pass spontaneously. However, foreign bodies are a common problem and deaths do occur: one US study estimated the death rate associated with ingested foreign bodies to be as high as 0.5 per 100,000 head of population per year.

Table 8.2 Symptoms, investigation and management of gut obstruction according to site of obstruction.

Site of obstruction	Common causes	Typical symptoms	Diagnosis	Management options
Oesophagus	Malignancy	Progressive difficulty swallowing, particularly 'hard' foods	Upper GI endoscopy	Dependent on stage and grade (see Chapter 28) Palliation: • Endoluminal stent • Radiotherapy laser therapy Curative: • Surgery • Radiotherapy
	Peptic stricture	Frequently past history of reflux symptoms Slowly progressive dysphagia to solids	Upper GI endoscopy	Endoscopic dilatation followed by PPI long term
	Food bolus obstruction Foreign body	Sudden onset of pain and dysphagia Unable to swallow saliva	Plain X-ray if foreign body Upper GI endoscopy	Endoscopic removal Rule out underlying lesion in food bolus obstruction
Stomach	Pyloric stenosis (related to peptic ulcer disease in adults)	Slowly progressive	Upper GI endoscopy	Surgical pyloroplasty Endoscopic dilatation
	Gastric cancer	Progressive postprandial vomiting and upper abdominal bloating Cachexia	Upper GI endoscopy	
	Gastroparesis	Intermittent nausea and vomiting Association with diabetes mellitus	Scintigraphic meal to estimate gastric emptying half time Upper GI endoscopy shows no outlet obstruction but may show large gastric residue	Careful diabetic control Prokinetics (gastric pacing)
Duodenum	Pancreatic cancer	Progressive pain, nausea and vomiting Cachexia	CT abdomen Upper GI endoscopy ERCP	Curative: • Whipple's procedure Palliative: • Endoluminal stent • Surgical bypass
Jejunum and ileum	Benign extrinsic obstruction • Adhesions • Hernia	Sudden onset of pain, nausea and vomiting Abdominal distension depending on site	Small bowel radiology, particularly enteroclysis	Surgical management

	Clinical features	Investigations	Management
Crohn's stricture	Diarrhoea Malabsorption Relapsing and remitting symptoms	Small bowel radiology • Enteroclysis • MRI • Ultrasound Colonoscopy and ileoscopy Enteroscopy Capsule endoscopy (risk of capsule retention)	Medical therapy of Crohn's disease Surgical resection or stricturoplasty Endoscopic dilatation of ileocaecal valve and terminal ileal strictures
Small bowel carcinoma and lymphoma	Progressive nausea, vomiting and bloating	Small bowel radiology CT abdomen	Surgical resection with or without chemotherapy
Meckel's diverticulum	History of occult GI bleeding in some	Small bowel radiology Meckel's scan	Surgical resection
Colon and rectum			
Colorectal carcinoma	Rectal bleeding and change in stool form with left-sided lesions Cachexia	Colonoscopy CT colonography Barium enema	Surgical excision with or without chemotherapy Endoluminal stenting or ostomy formation for palliation
Benign stricture • Diverticular • Crohn's disease		Colonoscopy CT colonography Barium enema	Medical therapy of Crohn's disease Surgical resection Endoscopic dilatation in Crohn's disease
Extrinsic compression • Uterine cancer • Ovarian carcinoma • Lymphoma		CT abdomen Colonoscopy Barium enema	Surgical or other treatment of underlying lesion Endoluminal stenting for palliation
Sigmoid volvulus	Constipation, abdominal distension	Plain X-ray or gastrograffin enema	Flatus tube, endoscopic deflation or surgical resection
Foreign body insertion		Plain X-ray Rigid or flexible sigmoidoscopy	Per anal or surgical extraction

CT, computed tomography; ERCP, endoscopic retrograde cholangiopancreatography; GI, gastrointestinal; MRI, magnetic resonance imaging; PPI, proton pump inhibitor.

KEY POINTS

- Sudden complete dysphagia for solids and liquids is a medical emergency requiring instant relief of obstruction, usually by endoscopy.

- Boerhaave's syndrome is oesophageal rupture as the catastrophic and very rare consequence of vigorous vomiting. Even with treatment there is a mortality rate of around 25%.

- Most cases of acute diarrhoea require only oral rehydration solutions (ORSs). Antimicrobials are not usually indicated and antidiarrhoeal therapy is best avoided.

- Gut obstruction and ileus are common causes of inpatient care, affecting 20% of patients admitted to hospital for abdominal pain. The majority (over 80%) of episodes involve the small bowel.

 SELF-ASSESSMENT QUESTION

(The answer to this question is given on p. 266)

A 52-year-old man with known Crohn's disease presents with acute, severe, retrosternal pain after copious and vigorous vomiting. Four hours ago he started taking polyethylene glycol preparation for a planned colonoscopy to assess the activity of his inflammatory bowel disease. He started vomiting approximately 15 minutes after the second litre of fluid.

Regarding his presentation, which of the following statements is most correct?

(a) Urgent endoscopy is indicated to determine the cause of his pain.

(b) The pattern of symptoms suggests that he has a colonic stricture as a result of his Crohn's disease.

(c) Use of an antiemetic and further preparation is indicated to ensure that he is ready for his colonoscopy.

(d) In this situation the mortality risk is very low as long as appropriate treatment is instigated early.

(e) A plain erect chest X-ray is the first investigation of choice.

9

Acute liver failure

Acute failure of liver synthetic and metabolic function in the presence of encephalopathy, and the absence of pre-existing liver disease, defines acute liver failure (ALF). This entity presents the clinician with a particular set of diagnostic and management problems, often requiring the input of a specialist liver service.

The most common causes of death in ALF are:

- Cerebral oedema.
- Infection.
- Multiorgan failure.

The aim of management is to avoid these complications and allow the liver to regenerate. Acute liver transplantation remains the only definitive therapy when supportive care fails.

Epidemiology and causes

ALF is rare, with only about 2000 cases per year reported in the US. However, it makes up 6% of the liver failure–related deaths in the same population. The prevalent underlying causes vary between countries: paracetamol overdose is the commonest cause in the US, Europe and the UK, as are idiosyncratic drug reactions. In developing countries hepatitis delta virus superinfection is more common because of high rates of chronic hepatitis B virus infection. Where hepatitis E virus is endemic, there is a high incidence of hepatic failure in women who are pregnant.

Pathophysiology

Systemic inflammatory response syndrome and infection

ALF is haemodynamically characterised by a hyperdynamic circulation with high cardiac output and low systemic vascular resistance. The pathophysiological mechanisms underlying these haemodynamic disturbances are unclear, but increased nitric oxide production and cyclic guanosine monophosphate (cGMP) have been demonstrated during the later stages of the disease.

These changes can occur in the absence of microbiologically confirmed infection.

More than 80% of ALF patients do develop infection, mostly pulmonary. Patients with ALF are functionally immunosuppressed (related to Kupffer cell and polymorph dysfunction, as well as reduction of fibronectin, opsonins, chemoattractants and components of the complement system). Hence, fever and leucocytosis may not occur in the face of sepsis. The majority of pathogens are Gram-positive organisms, usually staphylococci. Fungal infections, occurring in about a third of patients, are difficult to detect and are associated with a grim prognosis.

Gastroenterology and Hepatology: Lecture Notes, Second Edition. Stephen Inns and Anton Emmanuel.
© 2017 John Wiley & Sons, Ltd. Published 2017 by John Wiley & Sons, Ltd.
Companion website: www.lecturenoteseries.com/gastroenterology

Hepatic encephalopathy and raised intracranial pressure

Hepatic encephalopathy and raised intracranial pressure (ICP) progress hand in hand. Initially encephalopathy develops without raised ICP, but as it progresses to grade 3–4 there is a high risk of increased ICP developing (Table 9.1). The pathogenic mechanisms centre on failure of the liver to clear mainly nitrogenous waste from the bloodstream. Worsening encephalopathy is associated with worsening prognosis (see Table 9.2).

Raised ICP can lead to brainstem herniation, which is the commonest cause of death. Putative mechanisms include:

- Accumulation of osmolytes (such as glutamine) in brain cells, and hence uptake of water into the cells.
- Cerebral blood flow changes: initial decrease due to loss of the autoregulatory mechanisms to maintain perfusion pressure, and then later increase due to inappropriate vasodilation.
- Disruption of the blood–brain barrier with leakage of plasma into the cerebrospinal fluid.

Coagulopathy

Due to the liver's role in the production of coagulation factors, inhibitors of coagulation and components of the fibrinolytic system, as well as the clearance of activated clotting factors, disturbance of its function

Table 9.1 Grading of hepatic encephalopathy.

Grade	Level of consciousness	Personality and intellect	Neurological signs	Electroencephalogram abnormalities
0	Normal	Normal	None	None
Subclinical	Normal	Normal	Abnormalities only on psychometric testing	None
1	Day/night sleep reversal Restlessness	Forgetfulness Mild confusion Agitation Irritability	Tremor Apraxia Incoordination Impaired handwriting	Triphasic waves (5 Hz)
2	Lethargy Slowed responses	Disorientation to time Loss of inhibition Inappropriate behaviour	Asterixis Dysarthria Ataxia Hypoactive reflexes	Triphasic waves (5 Hz)
3	Somnolence Confusion	Disorientation to place Aggressive behaviour	Asterixis Muscular rigidity Babinski signs Hyperactive reflexes	Triphasic waves (5 Hz)
4	Coma	None	Decerebration	Delta/slow wave activity

Table 9.2 King's College criteria of poor prognosis in acute liver failure.

	Criterion	Paracetamol-induced ALF	Non-paracetamol-induced ALF
		Either $pH < 7.3$ or all of 1, 2 and 3	Either INR >6.5 or 3 of the following 5
1	INR	>6.5	>3.5
2	Creatinine	>300 µmol/l (>3.4 mg/dl)	>300 µmol/l (>3.4 mg/dl)
3	Encephalopathy	Grade 3 or 4	
4	Patient age		<11 or >40
5	Days from jaundice to coma		>7 days
6	Drug toxicity		present

ALF, acute liver failure; INR, international normalised ratio.

results in a complex coagulopathy characterised by factor deficiency and intravascular coagulation. The prothrombin time (PT) is widely used to assess coagulation and is a useful guide to prognosis.

Renal, electrolyte and metabolic disturbance

Renal impairment is common; 70–80% of those who have cerebral oedema require some form of extracorporeal renal replacement. The aetiology of renal dysfunction is a combination of:

- Effects of liver cell failure itself (hepatorenal syndrome).
- Acute tubular necrosis (related to sepsis, endotoxaemia, bleeding or hypotension).

Because paracetamol has a direct effect on the renal tubule, renal failure is particularly common in the setting of overdose with this agent.

Serum creatinine is the preferred indicator of renal function, as urea synthesis by the liver will be decreased. **Hypokalaemia** develops as a result of renal losses and can be compounded iatrogenically if potassium is not adequately replaced. **Hypophosphataemia**, **hypocalcaemia** and **hypomagnesaemia** also commonly develop. **Hyponatraemia** is usually seen only in the latter stages of disease. **Acidosis** commonly develops because of:

- Inadequate tissue perfusion causing lactic acidosis.
- Respiratory depression or pulmonary complications causing respiratory acidosis.

Acidosis occurs particularly in paracetamol overdose, and is a determinant of prognosis.

Hypoglycaemia occurs in 40% of patients and is due to failure of gluconeogenesis and raised insulin levels because of reduced hepatic uptake. Neuroglycopaenia can contribute to reduced consciousness.

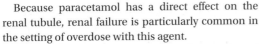

Clinical features

History

Obtaining an accurate history can be very difficult when faced with an encephalopathic patient. Appropriate third-party information must be obtained, both to guide diagnostic thinking and to decide on the appropriateness of possible liver transplantation:

- Onset and duration of the disease.
- Propensity for, or known, pre-existing liver disease (focusing on alcohol and drug consumption, both prescription and illicit).

- Patient's social context.
- Premorbid function and social support networks.

The time between onset of the first symptoms of illness and hepatic encephalopathy divides the illness into hyperacute (within 7 days), acute (between 8 and 28 days) and subacute (>28 days) subgroups.

In the hyperacute subgroup, the prognosis is better than for those with acute or subacute disease.

The features prior to onset of jaundice are non-specific, including nausea and malaise. Vomiting is common but abdominal pain rare. Jaundice *precedes* the onset of hepatic encephalopathy. Coma may then develop rapidly within a few days.

Rarer pathogens should be sought if there is no drug or alcohol history, including plant substances, and potential infectious exposures. It is important to recall the time delay of 2–3 days between paracetamol overdose and liver damage.

Worldwide, viral infection and, in the developed world, paracetamol overdose and idiosyncratic drug reactions are by far the commonest causes (Box 9.1). However, the list of possible differential diagnoses is long and when an alternative diagnosis seems likely, historical features should guide investigation. In up to 15% of cases no cause will be found.

Examination

Differentiation of ALF from acute or chronic disease is aided by careful observation for the stigmata of chronic liver disease, in particular the presence of a hard liver, marked splenomegaly and spider naevi.

Investigations

Prognostic tests (Table 9.2)

The first task for the clinician is to select those patients with ALF most likely to require transfer to a specialist liver unit. Once they are under the care of a transplant unit, criteria have been defined that allow the selection of candidates appropriate for transplantation:

- **A**rterial blood gas measurement (especially in paracetamol overdose).
- **B**ilirubin.
- **C**oagulation studies.
- Thrombocytopaenia (secondary to **d**isseminated intravascular coagulation).

Additional tests

- While the transaminases are of little prognostic value, a low albumin indicates poor prognosis.

Box 9.1 Causes of acute liver failure

Viral
- HAV and HBV typically
- HDV, HEV, HSV, CMV, EBV, HVZ, paramyxovirus, adenovirus, haemorrhagic fever viruses (HCV rarely causes ALF)

Drugs and toxins (these lists are necessarily incomplete)
- Dose-dependent: acetaminophen, CCl4, yellow phosphorus, *Amanita phalloides, Bacillus cereus toxin*, sulphonamides, tetracycline, Ecstasy (methyldioxymethamphetamine), herbal remedies
- Idiosyncratic: halothane, INH, rifampicin, valproic acid, NSAIDs, disulphiram

Vascular
- Right heart failure
- Budd–Chiari syndrome
- Veno-occlusive disease
- Shock liver (ischaemic hepatitis)
- Heatstroke

Metabolic
- Acute fatty liver of pregnancy
- Wilson's disease
- Reye's syndrome
- Galactosaemia
- Hereditary fructose intolerance
- Tyrosinaemia

Miscellaneous
- Malignant infiltration (liver metastases, lymphoma)
- Autoimmune hepatitis, sepsis

Indeterminate
- Includes primary graft non-function in liver transplanted patients

ALF, acute liver failure; CCl₄, carbon tetrachloride; CMV, cytomegalovirus; EBV, Epstein–Barr virus; HAV, hepatitis A virus; HBV, hepatitis B virus; HCV, hepatitis C virus; HDV, hepatitis D virus; HEV, hepatitis E virus; HSV, herpes simplex virus; HVZ, herpes varicella zoster virus; INH, isoniazid; NSAIDs, non-steroidal anti-inflammatory drugs.

- Paracetamol levels may have decreased by the time a patient presents with fulminant hepatic failure (FHF), but it is helpful to document this.
- Serum IgM anti-A antibodies diagnose acute hepatitis A.
- Hepatitis B surface antigen may have already been cleared and hepatitis B surface antibody will not yet have appeared, so the hepatitis B IgM core antibody is necessary for diagnosis. It is very useful to store serum at an early stage, as further virological studies might be needed later on. In patients found to be positive for hepatitis B, serum anti-delta should be checked.

- Anti-hepatitis C (HCV) virus antibodies should be checked, but are unlikely to be positive this early in the disease. Diagnosis of acute HCV requires polymerase chain reaction (PCR) for HCV RNA.
- Hepatitis E serology (the virus is prevalent both in the UK and in foreign travellers).
- Pregnancy testing must be performed in women of childbearing potential.
- In patients with risk factors for thromboembolism or vasculopathy, assessment of the liver vasculature using ultrasound Doppler and echocardiography can be helpful.
- Ultrasound of the liver will outline liver architecture and show infiltrating lesions.
- In young patients, rare metabolic and autoimmune disease should be considered. The diagnosis of Wilson's disease is difficult as serum caeruloplasmin is unreliable; in this setting an increased serum-free (unbound) copper may be more reliable than any other study results. An autoimmune hepatitis screen should be sent.

Management

Management is supportive (in an intensive care bed with strict monitoring of vital signs and fluid balance), allowing time for the liver to regenerate. This requires careful attention to the complications of liver failure and aggressive treatment of these as they develop. A proton pump inhibitor or H₂ antagonist is given to prevent gastroduodenal bleeding. Enteral nutrition, or in less severe cases oral caloric supplementation, should be given. Patients in whom transplant is appropriate should be sent to a specialist centre for comprehensive assessment. Artificial liver support may be available in some centres.

Hepatic encephalopathy and cerebral oedema
Grade 1–2 encephalopathy

- Sedation should be avoided as this may worsen confusion.
- Patients should not receive a high-protein diet, although there is debate regarding the benefit of low-protein diets.
- Phosphate enemas and lactulose should be administered so that the patient has two semi-soft bowel motions per day.

Grade 3–4 encephalopathy

- Patients generally require sedation and mechanical ventilation (risk of concomitant cerebral oedema is high).
- Hyperthermia, hypercapnoea, hypoglycaemia and hyperglycaemia must be avoided.
- Specific therapies for raised ICP include mannitol (mainstay of treatment), barbiturates (used less commonly than previously), hypothermia (experimental), hypertonic normal saline, vasopressors, and hepatectomy and liver transplantation.

Renal, metabolic and electrolyte disturbances

- Hypoglycaemia is treated with 100 ml 50% glucose intravenously if the blood sugar falls below 3 mmol/l, followed by an infusion of 5% or 10% dextrose. The blood glucose should be checked at least hourly. Further 50% glucose is given if it falls again.
- Iatrogenic hypokalaemia must be carefully monitored for and replaced.
- Hypocalcaemia, hyponatraemia, hypophosphataemia and hypomagnesaemia are common and require adequate replacement.
- Adequate volume repletion and the avoidance of nephrotoxins are central to the maintenance of renal function. Renal replacement therapy should be undertaken early in established renal failure. Continuous, rather than intermittent, treatment is preferred.

Infection

Regular culture screens should be carried out, including daily sputum and urine culture. Line sites must be carefully monitored. Antibiotics are indicated in patients with any clinical suggestion of infection.

The rationale for the use of prophylactic antibiotics is based on the very high risk of infection in ALF and evidence that systemic inflammatory response is important in the pathogenesis of increased ICP in ALF. Attempts to reduce infection with prophylactic antibiotics are successful, but serious resistance problems emerge in up to 10% of patients.

Prophylactic antifungals should be considered early because of diagnostic difficulties and the high mortality associated with systemic fungal sepsis.

Circulatory and respiratory dysfunction

The circulatory disturbance of ALF is characterised by vasodilatation and increased cardiac output. Hypotension may respond to volume repletion, but many patients will require vasopressor therapy directed by invasive haemodynamic monitoring. The preferred drug for vasopressor support is noradrenaline.

Adrenal dysfunction contributes to refractory hypotension, but supraphysiological doses of corticosteroids, while reducing norepinephrine requirements, do not improve survival.

The main mechanism of lung injury is adult respiratory distress syndrome with or without pulmonary sepsis. Sepsis, haemorrhage, pleural effusions, atelectasis and intrapulmonary shunts can also contribute to respiratory difficulty. Pulmonary sepsis should be aggressively sought and treated.

Coagulopathy

Patients should routinely receive intravenous vitamin K. Because the prothrombin time is an important prognostic variable, infusion of fresh frozen plasma is advocated only for control of bleeding or at the time of invasive procedures. Thrombocytopaenia, with or without disseminated intravascular coagulation, correlates much more closely with the risk of clinical bleeding than INR, and should be monitored closely.

Bioartificial liver support and liver transplantation

A variety of extracorporeal liver-support devices, such as haemodialysis, haemofiltration, charcoal haemoperfusion, plasmapheresis and exchange transfusions, have been advocated and essentially serve as toxin filters. More recently bio-artificial livers using cell-based therapies have been developed. Despite promising case reports and small series, no controlled study has shown a long-term survival benefit. These techniques seem to be better at 'bridging' patients to transplantation than at improving transplant-free survival.

Liver transplantation (see Chapter 21), although never subjected to a prospective controlled trial, is considered the only proven therapy. Before the era of liver transplantation less than half of the patients with ALF survived. Nowadays, liver transplantation for ALF offers an overall survival of 65–80%. However, the outcome remains worse than in those transplanted for chronic liver disease.

Living donor liver transplantation is now established in some centres and is being increasingly used due to the scarcity of deceased donor organs. Auxiliary liver transplantation, where a partial liver graft is transplanted while leaving part of the native liver in situ, has been used for patients in whom there is anticipation of recovery of normal liver function. Total hepatectomy with portocaval shunting is a temporising measure that may be employed as a method of stabilising a critical patient until a donor liver becomes available.

KEY POINTS

- While ALF is rare, it still makes up 6% of liver failure–related deaths.
- Paracetamol overdose is the commonest cause of ALF in the developed world.
- In developing countries hepatitis delta virus superinfection and hepatitis E virus in women who are pregnant are more common.
- Patients with ALF are functionally immunosuppressed and may not show the classic signs of sepsis.
- Raised intracranial pressure can lead to brainstem herniation, which is the commonest cause of death in patients with ALF.
- Bioartificial liver-support techniques exist, but are best at 'bridging' patients to transplantation.

SELF-ASSESSMENT QUESTION

(The answer to this question is given on p. 266)

A 21-year-old woman with a history of depression and previous self-harm is brought in admitting to an overdose of 60 g of paracetamol 24 h earlier. She is started on an infusion of N-acetylcysteine, but by 48 h after ingestion her arterial pH is 7.2, INR is 6.6, creatinine 347 micromol/L, white cell count is normal. She is afebrile but is confused and disoriented, with asterixis evident on examination.

Regarding her further treatment, which statement is most correct?

(a) Her pH alone means that she is at high risk and should be considered for transfer to a specialist liver unit.

(b) Her INR alone means that she is at high risk and should be considered for transfer to a specialist liver unit.

(c) She should be transferred to a centre with extracorporeal liver support, as this has been shown to reduce mortality and prevent transplantation in paracetamol-induced acute liver failure.

(d) The commonest cause of death in this situation is renal failure.

(e) Infection is unlikely in this situation, particularly given the absence of fever and leucocytosis.

Pancreatobiliary emergencies

Acute pancreatitis

Acute inflammation of the pancreas can arise from a variety of insults, and frequently involves peripancreatic tissues and at times remote organ systems. It is potentially lethal and appears to be increasing in incidence. The diagnosis is based on characteristic abdominal pain and nausea, combined with elevated serum levels of pancreatic enzymes. To ensure best management, the diagnosis must be considered early, the disease severity assessed to guide decision making and adequate fluid resuscitation instituted immediately.

Epidemiology

This is a common emergency condition, with incidence rates up to 80 in 100,000 per year. There has been an apparent increase in the incidence of acute pancreatitis in the past 40 years. This may be due to improved diagnostic capability during this period, but may also reflect a true increase due to a greater prevalence of risk factors such as higher alcohol consumption. The mortality in patients with acute pancreatitis is approximately 5%. About half of deaths occur within the first two weeks of illness, generally attributed to organ failure.

Causes

In acute pancreatitis the pathological process involves inflammation, oedema and necrosis of pancreatic tissue, as well as inflammation and injury of extrapancreatic organs. Although alcohol abuse and gallstone disease cause 70–80% of acute pancreatitis, a range of other insults can lead to the same end result. The exact mechanisms by which these factors initiate acute pancreatitis are presently unknown. In the case of gallstones or microlithiasis (sludge), increased ductal pressure is probably involved. With prolonged alcohol intake (>100g/day for >3–5 years), protein plugs may form in small pancreatic ductules. Obstruction by these protein plugs may cause premature activation of pancreatic enzymes. An alcohol binge in such patients can trigger pancreatitis by activating pancreatic enzymes.

Pancreatobiliary anatomy and mechanical causes

Because of the association of the pancreatic duct with the bile duct, obstruction can occur when biliary material impacts in the common segment of the common bile and pancreatic duct (Figure 10.1). This is more likely to occur when biliary sludge and small debris are involved. For similar reasons, dysfunction of the sphincter of Oddi, with very high sphincter pressures, may lead to pancreatitis. One of the complications of endoscopic retrograde cholangiopancreatography (ERCP) is acute pancreatitis, occurring at a rate of up to 15% following complex ERCP. Other types of trauma and pancreatic and periampullary tumours can also precipitate pancreatitis. Finally, a rare cause of pancreatitis may be pancreas divisum, where there is failure of the dorsal and ventral ducts to fuse in the embryo so that most of the pancreatic juice flows through the minor pancreatic duct and papilla (Figure 10.1). A comprehensive list of causes is in Table 10.1.

Gastroenterology and Hepatology: Lecture Notes, Second Edition. Stephen Inns and Anton Emmanuel.
© 2017 John Wiley & Sons, Ltd. Published 2017 by John Wiley & Sons, Ltd.
Companion website: www.lecturenoteseries.com/gastroenterology

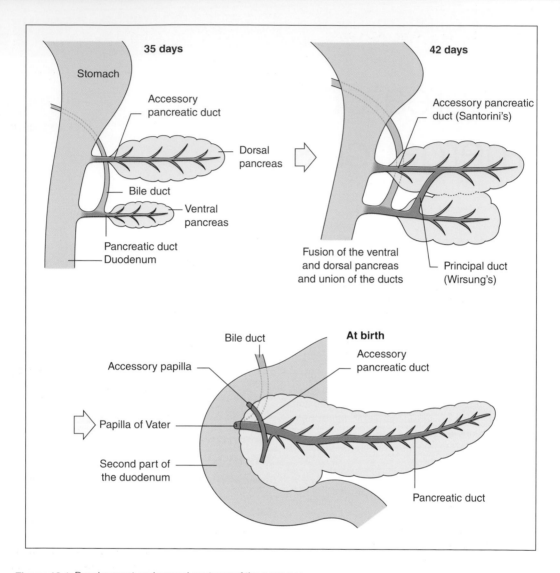

Figure 10.1 Development and normal anatomy of the pancreas.

Clinical features

Complications

Systemic inflammatory response syndrome

With inflammation of the pancreas comes activation of pancreatic enzymes (including trypsin, phospholipase A_2 and elastase) within the gland itself. These enzymes in turn damage tissue, activating complement and the inflammatory cascade, thus producing cytokines. Inflammatory products that enter the systemic circulation produce a systemic inflammatory response. This can result in acute respiratory distress syndrome, cardiovascular failure and renal failure. The systemic effects are mainly mediated through an increase in capillary permeability and decrease in vascular tone.

Other complications

The result of acute pancreatitis is effectively a chemical burn, as activated enzymes and cytokines enter the peritoneal cavity, resulting in capillary leakage of pancreatic fluid.

- **Pseudocysts**: in about 40% of patients, collections of pancreatic fluid and tissue debris form around the pancreas. In half the cases these collections

Table 10.1 Causes of acute pancreatitis.

Cause	Example
Drugs	α-methyldopa 5-aminosalicylate ACE inhibitors Azathioprine Cimetidine Cytosine arabinoside Dexamethasone Ethinylestradiol Frusemide Isoniazid Mercaptopurine Metronidazole Norethindrone Pentamadine Procainamide Stilbogluconate Sulphamethazole Sulphamethoxazole Sulindac Tetracycline Trimethoprim
Infectious	Coxsackie B virus, cytomegalovirus, mumps
Inherited	Multiple known gene mutations, including a small percentage of cystic fibrosis patients
Mechanical/ structural	Gallstones, ERCP, trauma, pancreatic or periampullary cancer, choledochal cyst, sphincter of Oddi stenosis, pancreas divisum
Metabolic	Hypertriglyceridaemia, hypercalcaemia (including hyperparathyroidism)
Toxins	Alcohol, methanol
Other	Pregnancy, postrenal transplant, ischaemia from hypotension or atheroembolism, tropical pancreatitis

ACE, angiotensin-converting enzyme; ERCP, endoscopic retrograde cholangiopancreatography.

resolve spontaneously; in the remainder either infection sets in or the collections become surrounded by a fibrous (not epithelial) lined capsule and are called pseudocysts. These pseudocysts may themselves become infected, haemorrhage or rupture.

- **Metabolic complications** of pancreatitis include:
  - Hypocalcaemia (a drop in serum calcium is usually due to concomitant hypoalbuminaemia; however, ionised calcium may fall due to intraperitoneal saponification).
  - Hypomagnesaemia.
  - Hyperglycaemia.
- **Haematological complications** in the form of disseminated intravascular coagulopathy may occur.
- **Infectious complications** may complicate severe pancreatitis, where there is necrosis and haemorrhage of the gland. Enteric bacteria may infect the necrotic tissue after 5–7 days. In addition, pancreatic pseudocysts may become infected.

History

The main symptom of acute pancreatitis is **abdominal pain** that is usually epigastric in location. It typically increases in severity over a few hours before reaching a plateau that may last for several days. The pain radiates through to the back in about 50% of patients. Sitting up and leaning forward may reduce pain, but coughing, vigorous movement and deep breathing may accentuate it.

Nausea and vomiting are common. Gallstone pancreatitis may be more sudden in onset, whereas that associated with alcoholism may come on more slowly. Pain beyond about a week is likely to result from the development of local complications.

Examination

Observation reveals an acutely ill and sweaty patient who is tachycardic and tachypnoeic. Blood pressure (BP) may be transiently high or low, with significant postural hypotension. Temperature may be normal or even subnormal at first but may increase to 37.7–38.3 °C within a few hours. Level of consciousness may be reduced. Respiratory examination may reveal basal crackles consistent with atelectasis.

Abdominal signs may vary from mild tenderness to generalised peritonitis. Blue–grey discoloration of the flanks, due to exudation of fluid stained by pancreatic necrosis into the subcutaneous tissue, is known as Grey–Turner's sign. Similar discoloration in the periumbilical area is known as Cullen's sign. In about 20% of patients there will be upper abdominal distension caused by gastric distension or displacement of the stomach by a pancreatic inflammatory mass. Pancreatic duct disruption may cause ascites (pancreatic ascites). Bowel sounds may be hypoactive.

Investigation

The diagnosis of acute pancreatitis is made in the presence of typical **clinical features** together with a high plasma concentration of **pancreatic enzymes**. Serum amylase analysis is the most widely available test. However, concentrations decline quickly over 2–3 days. In addition, hyperamylasaemia is found in several non-pancreatic diseases and its specificity for acute pancreatitis is around 88%. Diagnosis should therefore not rely on arbitrary limits of values three or four times greater than normal. Lipase has a superior sensitivity and specificity for acute pancreatitis.

Following a thorough history and physical examination, all patients should have:

- Serum amylase (and if available lipase).
- FBC.
- Electrolytes and renal function.
- Coagulation screening.
- Liver enzymes.
- Serum lactate.
- Calcium, magnesium.
- Glucose.
- Arterial blood gases and pH.
- Biliary ultrasonography.

Any abnormalities should be monitored and tests repeated within 48 hours to allow further risk stratification.

Follow-up investigations, during the recovery phase, should include fasting plasma lipids and calcium, as both may be secondarily reduced during the acute episode. Convalescent viral antibody titres and repeat biliary ultrasonography are warranted if the cause is not obvious. Further investigations are indicated by the clinical situation.

For **recurrent idiopathic acute pancreatitis**, exclusion of the following is essential:

- Pancreatic cancer.
- Microlithiasis.
- Chronic pancreatitis.
- Pancreas divisum.

This is undertaken by:

- Ultrasonography: considered the investigation of first choice because of its ability to show gallstones and dilated bile ducts. Its weakness is in detecting stones within the lower and common bile duct.
- CT: mainly indicated for the detection and staging of the complications of acute severe pancreatitis, especially pancreatic necrosis.
- Endoscopic ultrasonography: perhaps the most sensitive modality for detecting biliary causes and may guide the use of ERCP.
- ERCP: may be needed to detect microlithiasis or provide sphincter of Oddi manometry; its main role in acute pancreatitis currently is the treatment of biliary causes.
- MRI: like CT, can identify gallstones or a tumour, as well as local complications. MRI may also identify early duct disruption that is not seen on CT.

Management

- Aggressive fluid resuscitation is the central aspect of management of acute pancreatitis.
- Treatment of pain usually requires opiate analgesia; while morphine is generally avoided because of concerns that it might exacerbate pancreatitis by increasing sphincter of Oddi tone, no definitive human study supports this.
- Early risk stratification guides allocation to critical care and nutritional support.

Risk stratification

In assessing the patient with acute pancreatitis, stratification of the severity of an episode is essential as it guides appropriate allocation of critical care beds, ERCP, CT scanning and nutritional support. The severity of acute pancreatitis is defined by the presence or absence of organ failure, local complications or both, and can be assessed using specific scoring systems. The best known of these is the Ranson criteria, completed 48 hours after onset of the episode (Box 10.1).

Elevated C-reactive protein levels at 24–48 hours after onset are also useful in predicting severity. In

Box 10.1 Ranson's prognostic signs help predict the prognosis of acute pancreatitis

Five of Ranson's signs can be documented at admission:
- Age >55 years
- Serum glucose >11.1 mmol/l (>200 mg/dl)
- Serum LDH >350 IU/l
- AST >250 U
- WBC count >16,000/µl

The rest are determined within 48 hours of admission:
- Hct decrease >10%
- BUN increase >1.78 mmol/l (>5 mg/dl)
- Serum Ca <2 mmol/l (>8 mg/dl)
- PaO_2 <60 mmHg (<7.98 kPa)
- Base deficit >4 mmol/l (>4 mEq/l))
- Estimated fluid sequestration >6 l

Mortality increases with the number of positive signs:
- <3 signs positive, the mortality rate is <5%
- 3–4 signs positive, the mortality rate is 15–20%

addition there are markers of severity not included in standard scoring systems that should be considered:

- Obesity (a BMI of >30) is associated with a two- to threefold increase in the risk of a severe clinical course.
- A haematocrit >44% is a clear risk factor for pancreatic necrosis, although it is a poor predictor of the severity of disease.
- Several clinical findings, including thirst, poor urine output, progressive tachycardia, tachypnoea, hypoxaemia, agitation, confusion, a rising haematocrit level and a lack of improvement in symptoms within the first 48 hours, are warning signs of impending severe disease.

Nutritional support

Early enteral nutrition should be the goal for all patients with acute pancreatitis. Nutritional support is essential for all patients with severe disease. Enteral nutrition is superior to parenteral in terms of cost, safety and risk of septic complications. In severe pancreatitis, the nasojejunal route of feeding is usually recommended. However, a clear benefit of this over nasogastric feeding has not been shown. Serum glucose concentrations should be monitored and in the critically ill patient should be maintained at or below 6.1 mmol/l by the use of intensive insulin treatment.

Gallstones

ERCP and sphincterotomy within 72 hours of disease onset are indicated for patients with acute severe gallstone pancreatitis. In patients with mild gallstone pancreatitis, it is important to prevent recurrence. A cholecystectomy with intraoperative cholangiography should be undertaken as soon after recovery as possible; if the patient is not fit for cholecystectomy, then ERCP and sphincterotomy are sufficient.

Other treatment modalities

Antibiotic prophylaxis is effective in preventing infection of necrotic pancreatic tissue. However, it is also associated with the development of antibiotic resistance and is reserved for patients with pancreatic necrosis proven on CT. Antibiotics should be used early when infection is suspected. Initial therapy is with agents active against enteric organisms.

If patients have >30% necrosis on CT scanning, then further investigation to detect infected necrotic tissue is indicated. Positive bacteriology from samples gained by fine-needle aspiration of pancreatic or peripancreatic necrotic tissue, or the presence of retroperitoneal gas on CT, is an indication for necrostomy. The standard techniques for necrostomy are surgical; however, radiological and endoscopic techniques have been trialled.

Prognosis

The mortality from acute pancreatitis is 5–10% and relates mostly to multiorgan failure early in the disease, and septic complications of pancreatic necrosis late in the disease. As already explained, scoring systems are helpful in stratifying those at greatest risk so that they can be offered more intensive therapy. New strategies using genetic, transcriptomic and proteomic profiling and also functional imaging looking for specific disease patterns are under investigation and may offer more accurate methods for stratifying disease severity earlier in the course of the disease.

Acute cholangitis

Epidemiology

Acute cholangitis presents as a complication of about 1% of cases of cholelithiasis. Male and female, median age 50–60 years.

Causes

Acute bacterial cholangitis develops when bacterial infection complicates obstruction within the biliary tract. Partial obstruction imparts increased risk compared to complete obstruction. Infection is generally thought to occur through direct extension of bacteria from the duodenum. Haematogenous spread through the portal venous system could be another route. Bacterial colonisation of the bile duct alone generally does *not* result in cholangitis.

Causes of acute bacterial cholangitis:

- Choledocholithiasis or sludge.
- Biliary strictures.
- Choledochal cysts, choledochocoele, Caroli's disease.
- Stenosis of the papilla of Vater.
- Parasitic infections.
- Iatrogenic (e.g. post-ERCP).

Clinical features

The classic presentation is with Charcot's triad:

- Fever.
- Right upper quadrant (RUQ) pain (may be absent in the elderly).
- Jaundice.

In severe cases, mental confusion and hypotension may also be present (Reynold's pentad). In these cases, urgent biliary decompression is needed.

Investigations

- **Bloods**: all patients should have serum biochemistry, FBC and a clotting screen performed. In the early stage there may be a pronounced and disproportionate increase of aminotransferases (ALT, AST). This may cause confusion with viral hepatitis, since in the early stage bile ducts are often not (yet) dilated on ultrasound.
- **Transabdominal ultrasound** is the first step in detecting bile-duct (as well as associated gallbladder) stones. However, the distal bile duct may be difficult to visualise because of air-containing intestinal loops in front of it. While the specificity of ultrasound in stone detection is almost 100%, the sensitivity in detecting bile-duct stones is rather low (27–49%). The finding of bile-duct dilatation is invaluable, as it indicates the presence of posthepatic obstruction.
- **MRCP** is more sensitive than transabdominal ultrasound (overall >90%) in detecting bile-duct stones. However, its sensitivity is lower in cases with small stones and/or very dilated bile ducts.

- **Endoscopic ultrasonography** allows excellent visualisation of the bile duct, including the distal part that may be difficult to see on conventional ultrasound. It has a high sensitivity to detecting bile-duct stones.
- **ERCP** is considered the gold standard investigation. The disadvantages are its invasiveness and risk of complications (morbidity 3%, mortality 0.2% for diagnostic ERCP). A great advantage is the possibility of proceeding to therapeutic ERCP with papillotomy, stone extraction and/or nasobiliary drainage or stenting.

Differential diagnosis

- Gallbladder:
  - Acute cholecystitis.
  - Mirizzi's syndrome.
- Intra-abdominal:
  - Acute appendicitis.
  - Perforated duodenal ulcer.
  - Hepatic abscess.
  - Acute hepatitis.

Management

While 80–90% of cholangitis patients respond satisfactorily to initial conservative therapy with broad-spectrum antibiotics and adequate intravenous hydration, it is wise to perform ERCP in all patients as early as possible: immediately in septic patients, otherwise within 24 hours.

Choice of antibiotics is influenced by patient characteristics (e.g. antibiotic hypersensitivity, renal function, hearing loss, severity of disease, previous instrumentation of the bile ducts) and results of biliary (if taken) and blood cultures.

Endoscopic therapy for acute gallstone cholangitis is superior to surgical treatment. Percutaneous transhepatic drainage or surgery should be considered when ERCP is impossible or has failed in expert hands. If there are significant coagulation disturbances, large and multiple stones or an unstable patient, nasobiliary drain placement or biliary stents are preferred as the initial treatment. Stone removal can then be performed at a later stage, after recovery from the acute episode. Elective cholecystectomy should be performed in the majority of cases.

Prognosis

The sepsis produced by acute cholangitis can be extreme and the mortality as high as 5%. Mortality is greater in the elderly and those with comorbid disease, including cirrhosis, malignancy, liver abscess, hypoalbuminaemia or coagulopathy. In patients with severe cholangitis (Reynold's pentad) the mortality is as high as 50%.

KEY POINTS

- 80% of cases of acute pancreatitis are caused by alcohol or gallstone obstruction, but a long list of other possible causes must be considered.

- Pancreatitis effectively results in a 'chemical burn' to the peritoneum, and morbidity and mortality relate to the resultant systemic inflammatory response and later development of necrosis and sepsis.

- Clinical scoring systems allow the stratification of risk in acute pancreatitis, and molecular techniques are being developed that may further refine these tools.

- Acute cholangitis largely results from partial biliary obstruction and resultant stasis and sepsis.

- The classic clinical presentation of cholangitis is Charcot's triad (fever, right upper quadrant pain and jaundice).

- Early ERCP (<72 hours in severe gallstone pancreatitis and <24 hours in cholangitis with sepsis) is an important therapeutic tool.

- Elective cholecystectomy is warranted in the majority of patients post-cholangitis.

 SELF-ASSESSMENT QUESTION

(The answer to this question is given on p. 267)

A 56-year-old man is admitted urgently with severe central abdominal pain radiating through to the back. Initial lab results show serum amylase 600, WCC 16, Hb 15, ALT 72, AST 89, ALP 180, bilirubin 39, INR 1.2, glucose 14, LDH 755.

Regarding this man's condition, which of the following statements is most true?

(a) A high BMI is protective in acute pancreatitis.

(b) Ranson's criteria can be used to predict mortality at admission.

(c) Amylase is only 88% specific for acute pancreatitis and elevation to greater than 4 times the upper limit of normal cannot be considered diagnostic.

(d) Lipase is less sensitive and specific than amylase for the diagnosis of acute pancreatitis.

(e) Opiates must be avoided in acute pancreatitis because they increase sphincter of Oddi tone.

Part III

Regional Gastroenterology

11

Oral cavity

The oral cavity is the first portion of the digestive system: it receives food, commences digestion by mechanically breaking up the solid food into smaller particles and then combines these with saliva.

Oral ulcers

Aphthous ulcers are the commonest cause of oral ulceration. These are painful, superficial breaches of the mucosa of the lips, tongue, gums or buccal membranes. They are recurrent in up to a third of the normal population, but if other systemic features are present, then alternative causes need to be considered (Box 11.1).

Usually just antiseptic mouthwashes will suffice to allow spontaneous healing, but topical salicylates or steroids can induce rapid healing. Rare patients with severe, recurrent ulcers need oral steroids.

Oral cancer

Squamous cell carcinoma is increasing in incidence, and is aetiologically related to:

- Smoking or tobacco chewing.
- Alcohol excess.
- Malnutrition.
- Betel nut chewing (in Asian populations).

It may present as a lump, or an ulcerated lesion or a white patch in the mouth ('leukoplakia'). Cervical lymphadenopathy is usually a sign of late presentation. Radical radiotherapy is often undertaken, and is preferable to surgical resection, which often needs extensive dissection.

Oral manifestations of inflammatory bowel disease

Crohn's disease

- 0.5% of Crohn's patients show oral features.
- Usually young males, often co-existing with anal Crohn's.
- Usually multifocal, firm painless lumps (unless ulcerated, see Box 11.1).
- Diagnosis confirmed by biopsy.
- Usually self-limiting, may need topical steroid.

Ulcerative colitis

- Rarer than oral Crohn's.
- Usually male, any age.
- Usually multifocal, shallow, pustular lesions.
- Usually responds to treatment of colonic disease.
- Occasionally needs topical steroid or dapsone.

Gastroenterology and Hepatology: Lecture Notes, Second Edition. Stephen Inns and Anton Emmanuel.
© 2017 John Wiley & Sons, Ltd. Published 2017 by John Wiley & Sons, Ltd.
Companion website: www.lecturenoteseries.com/gastroenterology

Box 11.1 Causes of oral ulceration

Idiopathic aphthous ulcers

GI disease
- Coeliac disease
- Crohn's disease

Infection
- Herpes simplex
- Vincent's angina
- Candidiasis

Systemic disease
- Systemic lupus erythematosus (SLE)
- Behçet's disease
- Pemphigus
- Pemphigoid

Drugs
- Stevens–Johnson syndrome

Neoplasia
- Oral cancers
- Leukaemia

Dental enamel erosion

This can arise from GI causes:

- Gastro-oesophageal reflux disease.
- Chronic alcoholism (recurrent vomiting, neglect and malnutrition).
- Recurrent vomiting in bulimia.

Hereditary haemorrhagic telangiectasia

Four forms of this autosomal dominant disorder are described. All are characterised by:

- Mucosal and skin telangiectasia.
- Arteriovenous malformations (AVMs) in the internal organs.

Gardner syndrome

An autosomal dominant (chromosome 5) disorder of intestinal polyposis (with high rates of developing into cancer). Head and neck features are prominent:

- Unerupted teeth.
- Jaw osteomas.
- Jaw enostoses (growths on internal surface of bone cortex).
- Epidermoid cysts on head and neck.

Peutz–Jegher's syndrome

An autosomal dominant (chromosome 19) disorder of benign hamartomatous intestinal polyps and hyperpigmented macules on the lips and oral mucosa. Patients are at increased risk of all cancers, particularly GI and pancreatic, so once this is diagnosed screening is mandatory.

KEY POINTS

- Aphthous ulcers are recurrent in up to a third of the normal population, but if other systemic features are present, then alternative causes need to be considered.
- Oral squamous cell carcinoma is increasing in incidence.
- Hereditary haemorrhagic telangiectasia is often suspected when telangiectasia is seen in the oral mucosa.

- Gardner syndrome, a disorder of intestinal polyposis, is also associated with prominent head and neck features.
- Peutz–Jegher's syndrome, a condition characterised by hamartomatous intestinal polyps, also demonstrates hyperpigmented macules on the lips and oral mucosa and is associated with a 15-fold increase in the risk of developing intestinal cancer.

Oesophagus

Gastro-oesophageal reflux disease (GORD)

Epidemiology

Gastro-oesophageal reflux (GOR) is one of the most prevalent symptoms, with 10–20% of the population in the developed world experiencing at least weekly heartburn. Given the high prevalence of GOR symptoms, it should only be considered a disease when frequent symptoms or complications occur. Around 20% of patients undergoing endoscopy for upper GI symptoms are found to have reflux oesophagitis.

Causes

In health, GOR episodes occur throughout the day, especially after meals. However, these do not usually cause symptoms due to the following antireflux mechanisms:

- Lower oesophageal sphincter (LOS) pressure: the tone produced by the combination of smooth circular muscle at the distal oesophagus and striated muscle of adjacent diaphragm. The LOS resists the pressure gradient from abdomen to thorax that predisposes towards reflux. The LOS normally relaxes to allow food into the stomach, and also does so several times a day to allow swallowed air out of the stomach – these are called *transient LOS relaxations (TLOSRs)*.

- Angle of Hiss: the oblique angle between the cardia and oesophagus, which provides an anatomical barrier (Figure 12.1a).
- Oesophageal clearance: any material refluxed into the oesophagus is normally rapidly cleared back into the stomach by oesophageal contractions.

Impairment of any of these defences may result in reflux symptoms:

- **Hiatus hernia** herniation of the stomach into the thorax. Although present in 30% of over 50-year-olds, it is usually asymptomatic. There are two forms: sliding (much commoner) and rolling (Figure 12.1b). A hiatus hernia causes reflux by reducing LOS pressure, increasing TLOSRs and straightening out the angle of Hiss. A very rare complication of a hiatus hernia is development of **gastric volvulus**, when the stomach twists on itself causing severe pain and dysphagia; diagnosis is by chest X-ray showing a thoracic air bubble, and management is by nasogastric tube decompression followed by surgical referral.
- **Gastroparesis** – any condition that delays gastric emptying (pregnancy, binge drinking, poorly controlled diabetes) can increase gastric volume and hence the pressure gradient encouraging reflux. TLOSRs are also prolonged in gastroparesis. This is why eating large, calorie-rich meals (especially before lying flat) promotes reflux.
- **Increased intra-abdominal pressure**: pregnancy, obesity and chronic cough all increase the pro-reflux pressure gradient, hence weight loss may help GOR symptoms.

Gastroenterology and Hepatology: Lecture Notes, Second Edition. Stephen Inns and Anton Emmanuel.
© 2017 John Wiley & Sons, Ltd. Published 2017 by John Wiley & Sons, Ltd.
Companion website: www.lecturenoteseries.com/gastroenterology

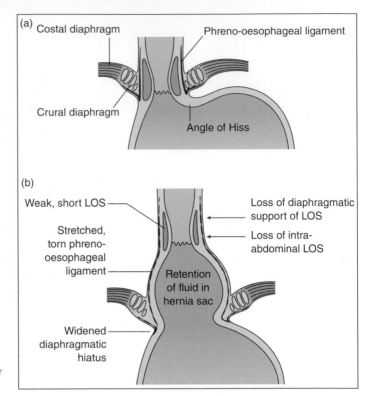

Figure 12.1 (a) Normal distal oesophagus and proximal stomach; (b) Distal oesophagus and proximal stomach with hiatus hernia (LOS, lower oesophageal sphincter).

- **Unhealthy lifestyle** smoking, eating fat- and calorie-rich foods and binge drinking reduce LOS pressure and increase TLOSRs. These factors, and regular use of NSAIDs, also increase gastric acid production, resulting in more acid being available to cause reflux.

Clinical features

See Table 12.1.

Investigations

Investigations are indicated in middle-aged or elderly patients with alarm symptoms present. Endoscopy is the first-line investigation (to exclude other conditions causing similar symptoms).

 24-hour (or longer) pH measurement is helpful if surgery is being considered or the exact diagnosis is unknown. NB: There is poor correlation between endoscopic change, degree of acid reflux (on pH testing) and burden of symptoms.

Clinicopathological manifestations

- **Oesophagitis**: defined as endoscopic change ranging from minor erythema to frank ulceration and stricturing (classified as Los Angeles grades A to D, respectively). Anaemia from oesophagitis is rare

Table 12.1 Clinical features of gastro-oesophageal reflux.

Heartburn	} Related to bending,
Fluid/food regurgitation	} straining and tight clothing
Waterbrash (= reflex salivation in response to oesophageal acid)	
Nocturnal cough (due to gastric fluid refluxing to the larynx when lying flat)	
Chest pain (secondary to acid-related oesophageal muscle spasm)	
Dysphagia or odynophagia (= painful or difficult swallowing), rare in uncomplicated GORD	

and if present, another cause of anaemia should be sought.
- **Oesophageal stricture** (Box 12.1): this typically complicates severe and chronic oesophagitis and results in narrowing of the distal oesophagus following repeated peptic ulceration and scarring. It presents as dysphagia and requires treatment by endoscopic dilatation. At this time, biopsies may help to exclude malignancy. Following dilatation, long-term proton pump inhibitors (PPIs) are

(nausea, dysphagia, chest pain) and may result in 'buried islands' of Barrett's mucosa under the epithelium.
- Endoscopic mucosal resection can be used to excise Barrett's mucosa, but carries a significant risk of perforation and structuring is common. It is generally used in patients already found to have dysplasia.
- Antireflux surgery does not stop the progression of Barrett's oesophagus.
  - Surveillance frequency depends on the severity of dysplasia, but the value of this surveillance remains controversial.
  - When high-grade dysplasia is observed, oesophagectomy may be considered in patients fit enough for such surgery, since 40% will be found to have a cancer present at resection. Endoscopic mucosal resection or radioablative therapy of localised lesions has become mainstream therapy, especially in those not fit for surgery.

indicated (both as secondary prevention and to minimise reflux symptoms after dilatation).
- **Barrett's oesophagus**:
  - Also known as columnar-lined oesophagus, this is an endoscopic or pathological diagnosis defined as metaplasia of distal oesophageal mucosa from squamous to columnar epithelium. It is thought to arise as an adaptive response to chronic acid exposure.
  - Typically asymptomatic.
  - Its importance lies in the fact that it is a premalignant condition, predisposing to the development of oesophageal adenocarcinoma. This is a cancer that is rapidly increasing in incidence. However, it is important to remember that the actual rate of developing cancer is low, incidence figures being 1 in 200 patient years. Particularly at risk are:
    - White males.
    - Over 50-year-olds.
    - The obese.
    - Smokers (though not alcohol misusers).
  - Diagnosis is based on mucosal appearances and histology; multiple biopsies should be taken to look for **intestinal metaplasia** (a histological precursor of malignancy).
  - There are a range of management options:
    - Acid-suppressive therapy does not induce regression of Barrett's oesophagus.
    - Endoscopic ablation through photodynamic therapy or radiofrequency ablation is effective, but is associated with significant local side-effects

Management

Conservative

- **Lifestyle modification** strategies (weight loss, smoking cessation, avoiding fatty meals prior to bedtime, elevation of the bed head) are usually complied with poorly.
- **Antacids** provide effective symptom relief for 40% of patients and may be needed several times a day.

Medical

- **H$_2$ receptor antagonists** are as effective as antacids and need be taken less frequently.
- **PPIs** achieve symptom relief in the overwhelming majority of patients, and are especially effective when symptoms are severe. Unlike other medical agents, they also heal oesophagitic mucosa. The newer PPIs are licensed for 'on-demand' use to relieve symptoms. Some patients need long-term treatment, in which case the lowest effective dose should be used. According to patient preference – and for the rare patient who does not respond to PPIs – consideration of more interventional treatments (see subsequent sections) may be needed.

Endoscopic

- **Endoscopic fundoplication** is an experimental technique for patients with significant symptoms in the context of a small or no hiatus hernia.

Surgical

- **Laparoscopic or open fundoplication** is the more established – and more invasive – method to treat refractory reflux symptoms. It is suitable for patients with large hiatus hernias. However, it is not curative (>60% of patients need to restart PPIs) and it does not prevent Barrett's cancers. It may be more cost-effective than maintenance PPI use, but only after 8 years. Adverse effects are seen in up to 15% of patients:
  - Dysphagia.
  - Excess flatulence.
  - 'Gas-bloat' syndrome (inability to belch).

Prognosis

The majority, around 80%, of people with GORD relapse once medication is discontinued, so GORD can be considered a chronic condition. However, the vast majority suffer no long-term complication of this and, as already outlined, progression to adenocarcinoma is rare.

Caustic oesophagitis

Corrosive ingestion

Deliberate self-harm through ingestion of bleach or battery acid causes acute oropharyngeal and oesophageal ulceration, and stricture formation in the chronic situation. Management is with analgesia, antiemetics and keeping the patient nil by mouth. Acutely, oesophageal perforation is the major risk, and endoscopy should be avoided. If dysphagia develops later on, endoscopic dilatation of any strictures may be performed, but is hazardous.

Drug-induced oesophagitis

NSAIDs, potassium supplements and bisphosphonates may cause oesophageal ulceration, especially if the tablets get stuck above an oesophageal stricture. Liquid or parenteral preparations should be considered in patients with known strictures.

Oesophageal motility disorders

Manometry is pivotal to the diagnosis of oesophageal motility disorders, and the advent of high-resolution manometry has allowed the accurate quantitation of certain features of normal and abnormal oesophageal physiology (see Chapter 6).

Achalasia

Achalasia is a progressive, debilitating disorder of oesophageal function that is characterised by:

- Failure of propagation of peristalsis in the body of the oesophagus.
- Progressive dilatation of the body of the oesophagus.
- Failure of relaxation of the LOS.
- High-pressure LOS.

Epidemiology

Achalasia is a rare disease, historically believed to have an incidence of 0.5 to 1 per 100,000 per year. However, recent reports have suggested that incidence may be increasing, up to 1.6 per 100,000 per year in some populations. It can occur at any age, but most typically occurs in middle age.

Causes

The cause is degeneration of the ganglia in the distal oesophagus and LOS (related to disturbed nitric oxide synthesis). Destruction of the myenteric plexus, causing a similar clinical syndrome, is seen with oesophageal cancer and Chagas' disease (a tropical parasitic disease caused by the protozoan *Trypanosoma cruzi*).

Clinical features

See Table 12.2. A rare complication is squamous carcinoma of the oesophagus.

Table 12.2 Clinical features of achalasia.

Dysphagia:

- Insidious, initially intermittent
- For solids, eased by liquids
- Worse if swallowing while slouched

Heartburn (may occur despite increased LOS pressure)

Chest pain

Regurgitation   } in late stages

Pulmonary aspiration   } of the disease

LOS, lower oesophageal sphincter.

Investigations

- Oesophageal manometry is diagnostic (Figure 12.2):
  - Absent peristalsis (always).
  - Poor LOS relaxation (frequent).
  - High LOS pressure (occasional).
- High-resolution manometry has allowed further subclassification of achalasia:
  - Type 1 classic achalasia, type 2 achalasia with compression and pressurisation effects, and type 3 spastic achalasia.
- Barium swallow (tapered, narrowing, 'bird's beak' appearance of distal oesophagus with proximal dilatation and aperistalsis).
- Upper GI endoscopy is mandatory (to exclude carcinoma '*pseudo-achalasia*').

Management

Medical

- Drugs that reduce LOS pressure (calcium channel antagonists, nitrates) are not usually clinically helpful.

Endoscopic

- Forced pneumatic dilatation: this benefits 80% of patients, but may need to be repeated. The perforation rate for each procedure is 1–2%.
- LOS botulinum toxin injection: benefits as many, but short-lived efficacy. Both procedures are complicated by the development of GORD, and so co-prescription of a PPI is needed.

Surgical

- Heller's myotomy (performed 'open' or laparoscopically) is indicated in young patients or those requiring multiple dilatations. As with endoscopic procedures, reflux is common, so fundoplication is also often undertaken.

Prognosis

Despite an increased risk of developing aspiration pneumonia, megaoesophagus and oesophageal squamous cell carcinoma and adenocarcinoma, achalasia patients have a similar overall life expectancy to the general population. Most longitudinal studies of surgical and endoscopic therapy for achalasia show good success (up to 90% at 2 years), but many patients require repeated treatments and follow-up studies tend to be of relatively short duration.

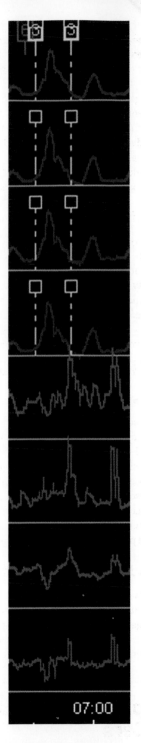

Figure 12.2 Stationary oesophageal manometry study showing simultaneous contractions in upper four traces and non-relaxing high-pressure **lower oesophageal sphincter** (LOS) in lower four traces.

Diffuse oesophageal spasm

This typically presents with angina-like chest pain (with or without dysphagia) in middle age. The pain is thought to be triggered by smooth muscle spasm in response to reflux. Oesophageal manometry (see Chapter 6) and 24-hour pH are required for diagnosis. Treatment therefore depends on the use of a PPI. Nitrates and calcium channel antagonists may also relieve pain. Endoscopic dilatation and surgical myotomy are not often effective.

'Nutcracker' oesophagus

Extremely high-amplitude contractions can cause chest pain and dysphagia. Diagnosis is by manometry. Treatment is with nitrates and calcium channel antagonists.

Non-specific motility disorders

A variety of manometric abnormalities are observed in one-third of patients (especially the elderly) with chest pain and dysphagia. These abnormalities (e.g. ineffective peristalsis, high-pressure LOS, low-pressure LOS) do not necessarily relate to symptoms, and no specific treatment is indicated.

Systemic sclerosis (and to a lesser extent other connective tissue disorders) can involve the oesophagus, resulting in failure of peristalsis, and hence dysphagia and heartburn. Long-term treatment is with PPIs to prevent peptic strictures.

Oesophageal tumours

Gastrointestinal stromal tumours (GISTs)

These are rare benign lesions that are usually asymptomatic and observed at endoscopy performed for another reason. No treatment is required as long as they do not cause symptoms.

Oesophageal carcinoma

Epidemiology and causes

- **Adenocarcinoma**: typically lower third of the oesophagus (see Barrett's oesophagus earlier). Its incidence is increasing (5 in 100,000 in the UK).
- **Squamous carcinoma**: can occur anywhere along the oesophagus. Less common than adenocarcinoma in the Western world; very common in Iran and the Far East. *Risk factors*: smoking, alcohol, betel nut and tobacco chewing, achalasia, post-cricoid web, coeliac and post-corrosive ingestion.
- **Small cell cancer**: very rare.

Clinical features

- Painless, rapidly progressive dysphagia is classic.
- Weight loss.
- Chest pain (usually late, suggests local invasion).
- Hoarse voice (usually late, suggests local invasion).
- Coughing after swallowing, pneumonia or pleural effusion suggests oesophagobronchial fistula.
- *Acutely*: bolus obstruction.
- Examination may be normal until late – look for cervical nodes.

Investigations

- Upper GI endoscopy: demonstrates site and allows histological sampling.
- Barium swallow: demonstrates length of stricture if the tumour could not be intubated at endoscopy.
- CT of the thorax and abdomen: for staging.
- Endoscopic ultrasound: best staging modality.

Management

- 30% have 'operable' disease (not spread beyond the oesophagus):
  ○ Oesophagectomy.
  ○ Preoperative chemotherapy.
- 70% have inoperable disease at presentation:
  ○ Palliation of dysphagia by endoscopic stenting or laser.
  ○ Palliation of pain with potent analgesia.
  ○ Squamous cancers (and to a lesser extent adenocarcinomas) may be palliated by radiotherapy.
  ○ Provision of nutritional supplementation.

Prognosis

Overall 5-year survival is <10%. If the tumour is operable, 5-year survival is 30%.

Oesophageal endoscopic abnormalities

Pharyngeal pouch

See Box 12.2. Also known as Zenker's diverticulum. The major importance of this condition is that it is a potential cause of perforation at endoscopy; if suspected, the first-line investigation is a barium swallow.

- Proton pump inhibitor therapy has a role in some patients with oesophageal eosinophilia, either by treating acid reflux in those with concomitant reflux disease, or perhaps by immune effects independent of their acid-suppressing action.
- Steroid therapy is indicated in diet-refractory patients, with systemic steroids more effective than topical.
- Rarely, patients presenting with oesophageal strictures may need endoscopic dilatation.

Eosinophilic oesophagitis

Eosinophilic oesophagitis is a condition characterised by eosinophilic infiltration of the mucosal layer of the oesophagus. It can be due to an allergic trigger and usually occurs in isolation, but may form part of a generalised eosinophilic gastroenteritis.

Epidemiology

Initially thought to be rare, the incidence of eosinophilic oesophagitis appears to have increased over the past 15 years, in most part due to an increased awareness among endoscopists and pathologists. It is now recognised as one of the most prevalent causes of oesophageal dysphagia in adults.

Males are affected twice as often as females. There are two age peaks at diagnosis: in children and in the early 30s. Recent estimates of incidence have been as high as 10 per 100,000 per year.

Causes

Eosinophilic oesophagitis is recognised as a largely allergic disease, however the precise pathways by which the disease arises remain unclear.

Clinical features

- Paediatric cases typically present with vomiting, and adults with dysphagia.
- Diagnosis is based on the presence of >20 eosinophils/high power field (hpf), since reflux oesophagitis is associated with up to 10 eosinophils/hpf.

Management

- Treatment with elemental or elimination diets is beneficial in children. It may also be efficacious in adults if they adhere to it.

Prognosis

In children, eosinophilic oesophagitis is associated with a significant reduction in health-related quality of life. The rate at which patients progress to food impaction, oesophageal stricture, narrow-calibre oesophagus, oesophageal tears and perforations is not well defined, however. In adults there is an increasing body of evidence suggesting that eosinophilic oesophagitis might be a progressive fibrosing disease, akin to Crohn's disease. However, the effect that different therapies might have on preventing this progression remains unclear.

Oesophageal rings and webs

These are typically seen at radiology rather than at endoscopy. Schatzki's ring is a circumferential narrowing in the mid or lower third of the oesophagus, while oesophageal webs are not circumferential and proximal. If iron-deficiency anaemia is associated with an oesophageal web, the condition is known as Plummer–Vinson syndrome. Oesophageal rings and webs are usually asymptomatic. They may cause intermittent dysphagia to solids over many years, in which case dilatation is required.

Mallory–Weiss tear

This is a cause of **haematemesis** (see Chapter 7). It is caused by recurrent retching or forceful vomiting (typically after alcohol binges), resulting in a mucosal tear of the oesophagogastric junction. The characteristic history is that the initial vomitus does not contain blood. Most cases settle spontaneously. Acid-suppression medication and endoscopic therapy are only rarely necessary.

KEY POINTS

- Gastro-oesophageal reflux is one of the most prevalent symptoms, with 10–20% of the population in the developed world experiencing at least weekly heartburn.
  - Endoscopy is the first-line investigation (to exclude other conditions causing similar symptoms).
  - 24-hour (or longer) pH measurement is helpful if surgery is being considered or the exact diagnosis is unknown.
- Barrett's oesophagus is the presence of a columnar-lined oesophagus thought to arise as an adaptive response to chronic acid exposure. It is associated with the development of oesophageal adenocarcinoma and surveillance for the development of dysplasia is widely recommended.
- Achalasia is is characterised endoscopically and manometrically by:
  - Failure of propagation of peristalsis in the body of the oesophagus.
  - Progressive dilatation of the body of the oesophagus.
  - Failure of relaxation of the LOS.
  - High-pressure LOS.
- The incidence of oesophageal carcinoma is increasing. Only 30% have 'operable' disease at the time of diagnosis.
- Eosinophilic oesophagitis now recognised as one of the most prevalent causes of oesophageal dysphagia in adults.
  - Characteristic endoscopic abnormalities are frequently seen.
  - Diagnosis is based on the presence of >20 eosinophils/high power field (hpf).

 SELF-ASSESSMENT QUESTION

(The answer to this question is given on p. 267)

A 60-year-old woman presented with a 1-year history of intermittent dysphagia, which was gradually worsening. This was always to both solid and liquid meals, and it was taking her longer to manage her meals. She was often woken from sleep with paroxysms of coughing. She had lost 3 kg in weight.

Regarding the most likely diagnosis in this patient, which of the following statements is most correct?

(a) Liquid dysphagia makes an oesophageal stricture more likely than achalasia.

(b) Typically a 'bird's beak' appearance of the oesophagus is seen on barium swallow.

(c) Endoscopy is very likely to be the only test required for diagnosis.

(d) The problem is likely to be confined to the lower oesophageal sphincter and oesophageal peristalsis will be unaffected.

(e) Dilatation of the oesophagus on barium swallow indicates a fixed lower oesophageal stricture.

13

Stomach and duodenum

Gastritis

Strictly speaking, gastritis is a histological diagnosis, and there is poor correlation with endoscopic appearances.

Classification is according to:

- Type (acute, chronic, special form).
- Site (antrum, body, whole stomach).
- Morphology (inflammation, atrophy, metaplasia, *Helicobacter pylori*).
- Aetiology (*H. pylori*, autoimmune, alcohol, NSAID, post gastrectomy).

Its features are summarised in Table 13.1.

Ménétrier's disease

This is a rare condition presenting classically with weight loss and diarrhoea (due to protein-losing enteropathy). It is aetiologically linked to *H. pylori*, leading to achlorhydria. Endoscopically there is hypertrophy of mucosal folds of the body and fundus. Histologically, mucus-secreting cells replace parietal cells. Treatment is to eradicate *H. pylori*, reduce secretion (PPIs) and monitor endoscopically due to risk of gastric cancer.

Peptic ulcer disease

Peptic ulcers are caused by an imbalance between luminal acid and mucosal defences. Hydrochloric acid (pH 1) and pepsin are secreted from the gastric pits, but do not damage the mucosa in health because of a layer of overlying unstirred mucus. This mucus layer has bicarbonate secreted into it, maintaining a pH of 7.

Prostaglandin and a good capillary blood flow are essential for this mucus and bicarbonate secretion, explaining how NSAIDs and smoking may predispose to ulcers. Peptic ulcers are becoming less frequent in the developed world due to widespread *H. pylori* eradication.

Peptic ulcers may occur in the distal oesophagus, stomach, duodenum, near a Meckel's diverticulum or any small bowel anastomosis. Pathologically, they are distinct from erosions in that they penetrate the muscularis mucosae. They may be acute or chronic (the latter bearing the pathological hallmark of submucosal fibrosis).

Gastric and duodenal ulcer

The differences between duodenal and gastric ulcers are summarised in Table 13.2.

Gastroenterology and Hepatology: Lecture Notes, Second Edition. Stephen Inns and Anton Emmanuel.
© 2017 John Wiley & Sons, Ltd. Published 2017 by John Wiley & Sons, Ltd.
Companion website: www.lecturenoteseries.com/gastroenterology

Table 13.1 Features of gastritides.

	Acute gastritis	Chronic gastritis		Special forms
Aetiology	NSAIDs Alcohol Other drugs Stress (burns, ITU patients) Bile reflux (post-gastrectomy) *H. pylori* Infections (CMV or HSV)	• *H. pylori* (commonest by far) • Autoimmune		Infections (CMV, TB) Crohn's disease Systemic disease (sarcoid, GVHD) Granulomatous gastritis
Presentation		***H. pylori***	***Autoimmune***	
	Asymptomatic usually Rarely dyspepsia, anorexia, retching, haematemesis	Asymptomatic usually	Asymptomatic usually	Asymptomatic usually
Site	Anywhere in stomach	Antral usually	Body usually	Anywhere – can be focal or whole stomach
Histology	Neutrophil infiltrate	Lymphocyte and plasma cell infiltrate	Diffuse inflammation, atrophy, intestinal metaplasia	Depends on cause
Other features	–	Antral predisposes to duodenal ulcer, body predisposes to gastric ulcer (*H. pylori*) May cause mucosal erosions ('erosive gastritis')	Circulating antibodies to parietal cells With severe atrophy there is achlorhydria and loss of intrinsic factor leading to pernicious anaemia	–
Cancer risk	–	Increased risk	Increased risk	–
Treatment	Treat cause Antacids Acid suppression Antiemetics	*H. pylori* eradication	Correct anaemia Look for other autoimmune disease	Treat cause

CMV, cytomegalovirus; GVHD, graft-versus-host disease; HSV, herpes simplex virus; ITU, intensive therapy unit; NSAIDs, non-steroidal anti-inflammatory drugs; TB, tuberculosis.

Epidemiology

The annual incidence of peptic ulcer diagnosis in developed countries is in the range of 2 per 1000 patient years. The incidence rates for duodenal and gastric ulcers are similar. Incidence increases with age and is strongly affected by environmental factors, including *Helicobacter pylori*, non-steroidal anti-inflammatory use, smoking and alcohol.

Gastric ulcer

These are usually benign, but gastric adenocarcinoma may present as an ulcer.

Causes

- *H. pylori*.
- NSAID use (especially if also *H. pylori* positive).
- Steroid use.
- Stress (which more often causes gastric erosions than ulcers).

Clinical features

- Simple ulcers present as described in Table 13.2.
- Complications such as haematemesis or perforation are commoner in the elderly.

Table 13.2 Features differentiating gastric and duodenal peptic ulcers.

	Gastric	Duodenal
Pathophysiology		
Acid secretion	Normal	Increased
Epidemiology		
Age	Elderly especially	Under 40-year-olds especially
Male:female	2:1	4:1
Clinical		
Epigastric pain	Soon after eating, relieved by antacids	Nocturnal and hunger pain
Vomiting	Not uncommon	Rare, only with proximal cap ulcers
Other symptoms	Loss of appetite and weight common	No loss of appetite or weight
Endoscopy		
Necessity	Diagnosis *and* repeat to check healing at 8–12 weeks	Diagnosis only
Biopsy	Edge of ulcer to exclude malignancy	Antral biopsy for *H. pylori*
Treatment		
Simple ulcer	*H. pylori* eradication if infection present. Add 4 weeks PPI	*H. pylori* eradication only Add 4 weeks PPI
Ulcer presenting with GI bleed	Get surgical opinion	

Management

- Eradication of *H. pylori* (or 50% will recur) and 4 weeks of PPI (preferred to H_2 receptor antagonists).
- Smoking cessation and alcohol moderation advice.
- Stop NSAIDs if possible.
- Maintenance PPI is indicated if there is major comorbidity or presentation with bleeding.
- Consider surgery (Billroth partial gastrectomy) if there is:
  - Haemorrhage (seen in 25%).
  - Perforation (in 10%).
  - Failure to heal.
  - Gastric outlet obstruction (with prepyloric ulcers).

Duodenal ulcer

Causes

- *H. pylori* (infection of the antrum depletes somatostatin production, which results in hypergastrinaemia and hence increased acid secretion, which in turn results in gastric metaplasia of the duodenum and ulceration).
- NSAID use (especially if also *H. pylori* positive).
- Smoking.
- Stress (especially with chronic illness – renal failure, cirrhosis).

Clinical features

- Simple ulcers present as described in Table 13.2.
- Perforation as a complication is commoner than with gastric ulcer.

Management

- Eradication of *H. pylori* – routine use of PPI is only indicated if there is haemorrhage or recurrence of ulcer symptoms after eradication.
- Smoking cessation and alcohol moderation advice. Stop ulcerogenic drugs (NSAIDs, bisphosphonates) if possible.

Complications

Perforation

- Especially with acute ulcers and NSAID-associated ulcers.
- Acute presentation (see Chapter 1) with severe upper abdominal pain, rapidly becoming generalised.
- Rigid, silent abdomen.
- Free air under diaphragm on upright chest X-ray; if not seen, water-soluble contrast examination will show abnormality.
- Resuscitation and surgery (over-sew of defect or resection).
- 25% mortality.

Gastric outlet obstruction

- May occur with pyloric gastric ulcers, or proximal cap duodenal ulcers.
- May also be caused by gastric antral carcinoma, adult hypertrophic pyloric stenosis.
- Vomiting of 'old' food, abdominal distension.
- Sucussion splash, visible gastric peristalsis and dehydration.
- Hypokalaemic alkalosis (due to luminal loss of K^+ and acid).
- Endoscopic diagnosis after stomach content has been aspirated by a nasogastric tube.
- Initial management is '*drip and suck*' – intravenous rehydration and nasogastric aspiration.
- Later management is with balloon dilatation (if possible) or surgical resection/gastroenterostomy.

Prognosis of peptic ulcer disease

The prognosis of peptic ulcer disease is very good as long as complications do not ensue. Treatment of *H. pylori* and use of PPI almost invariably result in ulcer healing.

Zollinger–Ellison syndrome

Epidemiology and cause

This is a rare disorder, but may affect over 1% of peptic ulcer patients.

It is characterised by the triad of:

- Severe (i.e. multiple or complicated) or recurrent peptic ulceration (may be throughout upper gut).
- Increased gastric acid secretion.
- Hypergastrinaemia due to secretion from a non-beta cell islet pancreatic tumour.

Clinical features

Diarrhoea and steatorrhoea often occur (due to acid destruction of lipase). 60% of tumours are malignant (albeit slow growing), 50% are multiple and 25% have other endocrine tumours (part of a multiple endocrine neoplasia type I).

Investigations

- **Condition**:
  - Gastric acid secretion: grossly elevated at baseline with little increment following intravenous pentagastrin.
  - Serum gastrin: grossly elevated.
- **Cause**: locate tumour by endoscopic ultrasound or Octreoscan (radiolabelled somatostatin receptor scan).

Management

- 30% resectable (small, single, localisable).
- Lifelong PPI in high doses.
- Octreotide (a somatostatin analogue) may help.

Prognosis

The presence of hepatic metastasis is the most important determinant of survival. In all patients with gastrinoma the 5-year survival is between 62% and 75%, whereas the 5-year survival for patients with hepatic metastases is about 20%, with a 10-year survival of about 10%.

Gastroparesis

This refers to delayed gastric emptying without mechanical obstruction. It may occur as a primary (idiopathic) condition, but may be secondary to autonomic neuropathy (especially secondary to diabetes) or gastroduodenal myopathy (systemic sclerosis, amyloidosis). Early satiety, recurrent vomiting, abdominal bloating and distension are characteristic. Peripherally acting antiemetics (metoclopramide, domperidone) may help, as may erythromycin (as a motilin analogue). If malnutrition develops, jejunostomy feeding or parenteral nutrition is indicated. Rarely, surgical enterostomy may be needed. Prognosis depends on the cause. Where there is a reversible or treatable condition, such as diabetes or pancreatitis, underlying the motility disturbance the outcome is often good. In other situations the disorder can be progressive and disabling.

Gastric carcinoma

Epidemiology

Gastric carcinoma is the commonest cause of cancer death worldwide (especially in China and Japan), but is falling in incidence in the UK. It occurs more often in men and those over 50 years old. In the UK in 2011 there were 15 new stomach cancer cases for every 100,000 males, and 8 for every 100,000 females.

Causes

- Chronic *H. pylori* infection (especially the cagA strain) is probably responsible for two-thirds of cases.

- Familial: blood group A is associated, and there are rare gastric cancer families.
- Genetic (rare polyposis syndromes – familial adenomatous polyposis, Peutz–Jegher's syndrome; familial form associated with e-cadherin mutation [New Zealand Maori]).
- Diet containing *N*-nitrosamines (pickled or smoked foods), diets low in fruit and vegetables.
- Environmental factors such as smoking and alcohol.
- Rarely, organic disorders: Menetrier's disease, previous partial gastrectomy.

Pathology

Adenocarcinoma develops from regions of intestinal metaplasia in the stomach, which themselves develop secondary to chronic atrophic gastritis. The spectrum of pathology ranges from polypoid lesions to diffuse infiltration (*linitis plastica*). The term *early gastric cancer* refers to adenocarcinoma confined to the mucosa or submucosa. It is diagnosed, and can often be cured, endoscopically.

Clinical features

- Epigastric pain (non-specific, unrelated to meals and relieved by acid suppressants), loss of appetite and weight are common.
- Haematemesis is rare and physical signs are rare except in late disease.
- A supraclavicular lymph node (*Troisier's sign*) and migratory thrombophlebitis (*Trousseau's sign*) are rare but classic signs.

Investigations

- **Condition**: endoscopy – rolled irregular-edged ulcers (biopsy the edges).
- **Complications** = staging: FBC and LFTs, chest X-ray, abdominal CT and endoscopic ultrasound; laparoscopy is often required.

Management

- **Surgery**: resection is only possible in a minority of cases, and most surgery is palliative.
- **Chemotherapy**: postoperatively this may improve survival, and can also be used palliatively.

Prognosis

While the prognosis for early gastric cancer is good (90% 5-year survival), overall the outlook is dismal (10% 5-year survival). Prognosis would be improved by improved public awareness and early diagnosis.

Gastric lymphoma

The stomach is the commonest site for non-nodal non-Hodgkin's lymphoma.

Primary gastric lymphoma

This affects mostly males over 50 and relative risk is increased in patients with AIDS. The annual incidence is less than 1 per 100,000 population per year. These are B-cell tumours, most of which are aggressive large-cell lymphomas, with a minority being low-grade mucosal associated lymphoid tissue tumours ('MALT lymphomas'). Clinical and endoscopic features are similar to gastric adenocarcinoma. Diagnosis rests on histology, from deep mucosal biopsies or laparoscopy. Endoscopic ultrasound and abdominal CT help with staging. Early disease is managed surgically, later disease by chemoradiotherapy. The prognosis is better with younger age and lower grade and stage of disease. The overall 5-year survival approaches 50%.

MALT lymphoma

The annual incidence of gastric mucosally associated lymphoid tissue lymphomas in Western countries is less than 0.5 per 100,000 per year and seems to be decreasing with time, perhaps due to reducing prevalence of *H. pylori* infection. This is a B-cell tumour caused by an immune response to chronic *H. pylori* infection with cagA strains. It is a histologically distinct disease, with lympho-epithelial lesions and reactive lymphoid follicles. *H. pylori* eradication leads to remission in 75%. Endoscopic mucosal resection, chemoradiotherapy and resectional surgery are only rarely needed. Long-term follow-up with endoscopy is required because of an ongoing risk of recurrence even after many years free of disease. The outcome from low-grade MALT lymphoma is excellent, with overall 10-year survival of 95%.

Other gastric tumours

Gastrointestinal stromal tumours (GISTs)

GISTs are rare tumours with an annual incidence of less than 1 per 100,000. They can occur anywhere along the GI tract, but most commonly occur in the stomach (60%) or small intestine (30%). They arise from the interstitial cells of Cajal, and their origin can be identified immunohistochemically by expression of the *c-kit* oncogene, which encodes the tyrosine kinase receptor. GISTs originate from the muscularis propria and submucosa. They are often found coincidentally at endoscopy, but may ulcerate and bleed. Tumour size, mitotic rate and presence of the *c-kit* oncogene predict malignant potential. Resection and chemoradiotherapy are traditional treatments.

The development of treatments that act as specific inhibitors of tyrosine kinase (imatinib and more recently sunitinib for imatinib-resistant disease) has revolutionised the treatment of malignant GISTs. Median survival rates have gone from less than 2 years to more than 5 years since the advent of imatinib therapy.

Gastric polyps

Hyperplastic or cystic fundal polyps are lesions of no clinical significance, whose only significance is to be differentiated from early gastric cancer. Rarely, adenomatous polyps are found. They are premalignant and associated with colonic polyps; they need resection and colonoscopic examination.

 KEY POINTS

- Gastritis is a histological diagnosis and is classified according to chronicity, site, morphology and aetiology.
- Peptic ulcer disease is common in developed countries, in the range of 2 per 1000 patient years.
- Zollinger–Ellison syndrome is rare in the general population but may affect over 1% of peptic ulcer patients and should be considered with severe or recurrent disease.
- Gastroparesis refers to delayed gastric emptying without mechanical obstruction.
  - Where there is an underlying, treatable condition the outcome is often good.
  - In other situations the disorder can be progressive and disabling.
- Gastric carcinoma is the commonest cause of cancer death worldwide, but is falling in incidence in the UK.
  - While the prognosis for early gastric cancer is good (90% 5-year survival), overall the outlook is dismal (10% 5-year survival).
- The stomach is the commonest site for non-nodal non-Hodgkin's lymphoma.
- Treatments that act as specific inhibitors of tyrosine kinase have revolutionised the treatment of malignant gastrointestinal stromal tumours.

 SELF-ASSESSMENT QUESTION

(The answer to this question is given on p. 267)

A 39-year-old New Zealander of Māori descent presents with nausea and vomiting for the last 2 months. He has lost 5 kg in weight in that period. Gastroscopy reveals retained food and fluid in the stomach and ulceration of the pre-pyloric region with pyloric stenosis. The endoscope cannot be passed through the pylorus. There is antral redness and erosions, but no ulceration proximal to the pylorus.

Regarding this situation, which of the following statements is most correct?

(a) The family history is unlikely to be useful in this situation.

(b) The predominantly antral location of the gastritis suggests that the cause is more likely to be autoimmune.

(c) If gastric adenocarcinoma is proven, testing for germ-line e-cadherin mutation might be worthwhile.

(d) If gastric adenocarcinoma is proven, testing for mutation of the c-kit oncogene might be worthwhile.

(e) Gastric ulcers can be treated empirically with a proton pump inhibitor and do not require routine follow-up.

Small intestine

Malabsorption

Causes

- Structural disorder (pancreas, small bowel, biliary tree).
- Mucosal disorder (pancreas, small bowel, biliary tree).
- Abnormal luminal digestion (metabolic defect).

Metabolic defects are unusual in causing isolated defects, whereas most other defects cause combined deficiencies (macronutrients – *carbohydrate, fat, protein*; or micronutrients – *vitamins, minerals*).

Clinical features

- **General**:
  - Malaise.
  - Anorexia, abdominal bloating.
  - Diarrhoea (especially stool bulk rather than frequency compared with colonic disease).
  - Weight loss (document body mass index, BMI).
- **Specific**:
  - Steatorrhoea = *fat malabsorption* (more severe in pancreatic disease than small bowel disease).
  - Oedema, ascites = *protein* malabsorption.
  - Paraesthesiae, tetany = Ca^{2+} or Mg^{2+} malabsorption.
  - Skin rash = Zn^{2+} or *vitamin B* malabsorption.
  - Cheilitis, glossitis = *vitamin B* malabsorption.
  - Neuropathy, psychological effects = *vitamin B_{12}* malabsorption.
  - Night blindness = *vitamin A* malabsorption.
  - Bruising = *vitamin K* or *vitamin C* malabsorption.
  - Bone pain, myopathy, osteoporosis = *vitamin D* malabsorption.

Investigations

Investigation can take the form of blood tests to assess the consequences of malabsorption and its underlying cause, tests to investigate the structure of the gastrointestinal organs, and tests of gastrointestinal physiological function. Table 14.1 is an aide mémoire to investigating the patient with suspected malabsorption. The intention is to:

- Establish the condition.
- Identify the site of abnormality.
- Identify the severity.

Intestinal failure

Sometimes called **short bowel syndrome**, this situation occurs when there is insufficient functioning small intestine to allow normal digestion and absorption. Typically, when there is <100 cm of small bowel, malabsorption will occur (resulting in malnutrition and weight loss, as mentioned earlier); when the colon is also missing, severe dehydration and malabsorption occur. The stomach and intestine produce about 6 l of secretions, so reabsorption of this fluid is critical in intestinal failure.

Gastroenterology and Hepatology: Lecture Notes, Second Edition. Stephen Inns and Anton Emmanuel.
© 2017 John Wiley & Sons, Ltd. Published 2017 by John Wiley & Sons, Ltd.
Companion website: www.lecturenoteseries.com/gastroenterology

Table 14.1 Potential investigations in patients with malabsorption (malabsorption factor being assessed, if not obvious, given in parentheses).

	Condition	Cause
Serology	Full blood count Folate, B_{12}, iron studies INR (vitamin K) Albumin Ca^{2+}, Mg^{2+}	Coeliac antibodies Amylase is *not* a useful test of chronic pancreatitis* HIV antibody
Structural		Duodenal biopsy (see Box 14.1) Jejunal aspirate for *Giardia** CT or MRI enterography (to identify Crohn's disease, diverticula, stricture, tumours) Capsule endoscopy (to identify Crohn's disease, lymphangiectasia*) CT, MRCP (to identify chronic pancreatitis)
Functional	Faecal elastase (pancreatic exocrine insufficiency and fat malabsorption) Xylose absorption (carbohydrate malabsorption in the small bowel*) Faecal radioactivity after ^{131}I-albumin (protein malabsorption in the small bowel*)	Lactose hydrogen breath test – small bowel lactase deficiency Glucose hydrogen breath test – small bowel bacterial overgrowth Schilling test – to detect small bowel disease* Basal acid output to identify Zollinger–Ellison*

*Rarely performed test.
CT, computer tomography; INR, international normalised ratio; MRCP, magnetic resonance cholangiopancreatography; MRI, magnetic resonance imaging.

Causes

- Extensive surgery.
- Crohn's disease.
- Mesenteric ischaemia.
- Radiation damage.
- Volvulus.
- *In children*, congenital abnormalities.

Management

- **Short term**:
  - Correct malnutrition (total parenteral nutrition).
  - Reduce gut secretions (loperamide, codeine and PPI).
- **Medium term**:
  - Gradual reintroduction of enteral feeding.
- **Long term**:
  - Monitor nutrition and ensure adequate calorie intake.
  - Monitor hydration status – especially if stoma output >1.5 l – and replace with oral rehydration solution.
  - Replace vitamins (B_{12}, D) and minerals (Ca^{2+}, Mg^{2+}).
  - Reduce gut secretions (loperamide, codeine and PPI; rarely octreotide).
  - Treat small intestinal bacterial overgrowth (see Chapter 6).

- Cholecystectomy if gallstones develop (greater risk due to bile acid depletion, see Chapter 19).
- Small bowel transplantation (in very rare situations).

Coeliac disease

Cause and epidemiology

This is an immune-mediated disorder resulting in *small intestinal villous atrophy*, which *resolves on gluten withdrawal from the diet*.

Gluten is a family of proteins found in cereals (but not rice or oats) and its main toxic antigenic component is α-gliadin.

This protein causes a T-cell-mediated inflammatory response of the small bowel. Prevalence in the UK is about 1:200 (least common in black and Oriental people), with a slight female preponderance. Estimates suggest that about 50% of cases are 'silent' (diagnosed on routine testing).

Clinical features

- **Infants**:
  - Diarrhoea.
  - Malabsorption.
  - Failure to thrive at weaning time.

- **Older children**:
  - Abdominal pain.
  - Anaemia.
  - Short stature.
  - Delayed puberty.
- **Adults**:
  - Abdominal bloating.
  - Lethargy.
  - Diarrhoea or constipation.
  - Iron-deficiency anaemia.
  - Occasionally malabsorption.
  - Rarely oral ulcers and psychiatric disturbance.

 Coeliac disease is linked to HLA-DQ2, so is often associated with other autoimmune diseases, most commonly dermatitis herpetiformis (itchy blistering rash on extensor surfaces), insulin-dependent diabetes, thyroid disease, primary biliary cirrhosis (see Chapter 19), Sjögren's syndrome.

Investigations

- **Confirm diagnosis** (*condition*):
  - Duodenal biopsy – *gold standard for diagnosis* – villous atrophy (Box 14.1) *and* crypt hyperplasia *and* intraepithelial lymphocytosis (IEL; although seen in as many as 2% of routine small bowel biopsies, is present in 40% of coeliac patients).
  - IgA antibodies to tissue transglutaminase (TTG), endomysial and gliadin antigen. (NB: False negative if patient has selective IgA deficiency.) These are valuable *screening tests* and help *monitor treatment response*.
  - Because coeliac disease is associated with HLA-DQ2 and -DQ8, the disease can effectively be excluded if these are negative (useful when wanting to avoid biopsy). It must be noted, however, that these haplotypes are very common in the unaffected population.
  - IgG antibodies can be used in IgA deficiency.
- **Look for consequences** (*complications*):
  - FBC (micro- or macro-cytic anaemia) and blood film (features of hyposplenism = target cells, Howell–Jolly bodies).
  - Haematinics (low folate, B_{12}, iron status).
  - Clotting screen (vitamin K malabsorption).
  - Bone investigation (potentially low Ca^{2+}, vitamin D and albumin; osteopaenia on DEXA bone scan).
- **Supportive factors**: rarely needed (*coincidences*):
  - Liver enzymes (elevated transaminases).
  - Small bowel radiology (altered mucosal appearances, clumping of contrast).
  - Intestinal permeability (increased).
  - Faecal fat (increased due to fat malabsorption); see Figure 14.1.

Management

- Lifelong gluten-free diet (supported by dietician): this prevents the ongoing antigen provocation of the inflammatory response.
- Correct deficiencies (haematinics, vitamins and minerals).
- Aggressive management of any bone disease.
- If patient remains refractory:
  - Check compliance with diet; if compliant, consider immunosuppression.
  - Consider co-morbidity: giardiasis, lactase deficiency, microscopic colitis (see Chapter 15), IBS (see Chapter 15).
  - Consider complications: small intestinal bacterial overgrowth (common), small intestine T-cell lymphoma (rare), ulcerative jejunitis (very rare).

Prognosis

The prognosis for patients with coeliac disease is good. Most, up to 90% in some studies, will have complete and lasting resolution of symptoms on a gluten-free diet alone. For the 10% with persistent symptoms, most of these will be attributed to ongoing gluten exposure, lactose intolerance and irritable bowel syndrome. Less than 1% can be expected to develop refractory coeliac disease.

Tropical sprue

This extremely rare condition is associated with small intestine villous atrophy and is thought to be post-infectious. It affects primarily residents of (rather than

> **Box 14.1 Causes of villous atrophy**
>
> *Common*
> - Coeliac disease
> - Dermatitis herpetiformis
> - Giardiasis
> - Acute infectious enteritis
> - Bacterial overgrowth
>
> *Rare*
> - Lymphoma
> - AIDS enteropathy
> - Tropical sprue
> - Hypogammaglobulinaemia
> - Radiation enteropathy
> - Whipple's disease
> - NSAID enteropathy
> - Lactose intolerance
> - Zollinger–Ellison syndrome

(a)

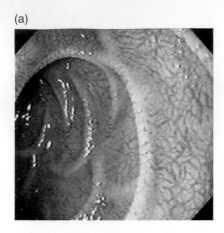

(b)

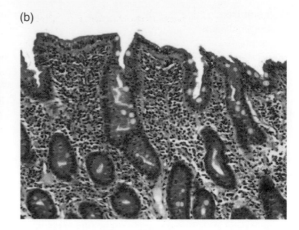

Figure 14.1 Endoscopic (a) and histopathologic view (b) of coeliac disease. Source: Shepherd NA, Warren BF, Williams GT et al. 2013. Morson and Dawson's gastrointestinal pathology, 5th edn, Chichester: John Wiley & Sons, Figures 21.5 and 21.7. Reproduced with permission of John Wiley & Sons.

travellers to) tropical countries. Diarrhoea and abdominal distension are common, and malabsorption may occur, especially if there is concomitant bacterial overgrowth. The main differential is giardiasis. Treatment is with long-term tetracycline and folic acid.

Small intestinal bacterial overgrowth

Epidemiology

Small intestinal bacterial overgrowth (SIBO) occurs rarely in the healthy population. Its prevalence depends on that of the underlying causes.

Causes and clinical features

Colonisation of the small intestine by colonic flora results in their:

- Deconjugating bile salts (resulting in diarrhoea).
- Metabolising vitamin B_{12} (resulting in anaemia).
- Metabolising carbohydrate (resulting in calorie malnutrition and halitosis).

Small intestinal bacterial overgrowth almost always occurs secondary to another cause (Table 14.2).

Investigations

- **Condition**:
  ∘ Jejunal aspirate – gold standard, but rarely required.
  ∘ Hydrogen breath test after ingesting glucose or lactulose.

- **Cause**: small bowel radiology (to identify structural or communication abnormalities).
- **Complications**: – low B_{12} and normal folate.

Management

- Antibiotics directed towards colonic flora – may need repeated courses.
- Replace vitamin B_{12}.
- Definitive treatment if possible – surgery for structural abnormalities, prokinetics for motility disorders.

Prognosis

The response of the symptoms of SIBO to antibiotics is generally good, but many of the conditions that predispose to SIBO are intractable and the burden of ongoing symptoms and complications of treatment are high in this population.

Bile acid malabsorption

This is a condition characterised by postprandial diarrhoea due to:

- Osmotic effect of bile salts in the colon.
- Steatorrhoea.

Bile acid malabsorption may be a primary abnormality or, if secondary, is most commonly due to Crohn's disease, ileal resection or intestinal failure.

A positive diagnosis depends on identifying reduced retention after administration of Se-HCAT

Table 14.2 Causes of small bowel bacterial overgrowth.

Site	Mechanism	Clinical condition
Stomach	Reduced gastric acidity	Gastric atrophy Partial gastrectomy Long-term PPI usage Old age
Small intestine	Structural abnormality	Small intestine diverticulosis Post Billroth II surgery ('blind loop syndrome') Strictures (Crohn's disease)
	Abnormal communication between proximal and distal gut	Enterocolic fistula Ileocolonic resection
	Impaired motility	Systemic sclerosis Diabetic autonomic neuropathy Chronic intestinal pseudo-obstruction
	Altered immune function	Immunodeficiency syndromes
Miscellaneous		Liver cirrhosis Chronic pancreatitis

PPI, proton pump inhibitor.

(a synthetic radiolabelled bile acid analogue). Treatment is with cholestyramine, a bile acid sequestrant.

Whipple's disease

This is a rare disease characterised by malabsorption, seronegative large-joint arthropathy, skin pigmentation, finger clubbing and fevers. It especially affects men.

Diagnosis is established by identifying 'foamy' macrophages that stain positive with periodic acid-Schiff (PAS) on jejunal biopsy. Electron microscopy may show the pathogenic actinomycete *Tropheryma whippelii*. Treatment is with co-trimoxazole or tetracycline for 1 year. One-third of patients relapse.

Protein-losing enteropathy

This is defined as gut loss of protein sufficient to reduce serum albumin. Patients therefore present with oedema in the absence of proteinuria or signs of heart failure, and in the presence of normal LFTs. Investigation is towards identifying the condition (faecal α-antitrypsin) and the potential cause (Table 14.3).

Intestinal infections

See Chapter 5.

Small intestine tumours

These are rare, accounting for <5% of all GI tumours. Carcinoid and lymphoma are the two most important.

Carcinoid tumours (neuro-endocrine tumours)

Gastro-intestinal carcinoid tumours or neuro-endocrine tumours (NETs) are slow growing and arise most commonly from the appendix (45%), small intestine (30%) or rectum (20%). **Carcinoid syndrome** occurs only if the tumour metastasises, occurring in 2% of cases with tumours >2 cm in size. The carcinoid syndrome (Box 14.2) is caused by systemic release of serotonin, prostaglandins and bradykinins.

Diagnosis is made by measuring urinary 5-HIAA (a serotonin metabolite), although many tumours are detected incidentally at appendicectomy. Carcinoid tumours need surgical resection; carcinoid syndrome implies that hepatic metastases have occurred. Hepatic resection or arterial embolisation reduces the metastatic mass of tumour and improves symptoms. Octreotide (a synthetic somatostatin analogue)

Table 14.3 Conditions causing protein-losing enteropathy.

Mechanism	Site	Clinical condition	Comments
Mucosa intact	Stomach	Ménétrier's disease	See p. 101
	Small intestine	Bacterial overgrowth	See p. 111
		Coeliac disease	See p. 108
		Eosinophilic gastroenteritis	Peripheral blood and mucosal/serosal eosinophilia in absence of parasite infection Treat with prednisolone or mast cell stabiliser (Na cromoglycate)
Mucosal ulcerated	Stomach	Cancer	See p. 104
	Small intestine	Cancer or lymphoma	See p. 112
		Crohn's disease	See p. 115
		Radiation enteritis	
	Colon	Ulcerative colitis	See p. 115
Lymphatic obstruction	Small intestine	Intestinal lymphangiectasia	Primary (congenital) or secondary (lymphatic obstruction)
		Lymphoma	Treat with low-fat diet and medium-chain triglycerides
		Whipple's disease	See p. 111
		Constrictive pericarditis	Causes back pressure on lymph vessels

may help palliate symptoms if debulking is not possible. Octreotide can be used in other ways also: radiolabelled octreotide scans can help delineate lesions, and radioactive octreotide has been used to treat disseminated lesions.

Lymphoma

These are rare tumours, but may complicate:

- Poorly managed coeliac disease (T-cell > B-cell tumours).
- AIDS and immunodeficiency states (B-cell > T-cell tumours).

Presentation is most commonly with obstructive symptoms, though haemorrhage or perforation may occur. Weight loss is common, but malabsorption syndromes are unusual. Abdominal CT scanning is usually diagnostic (luminal imaging is rarely required) and staging laparotomies are often required to decide treatment. Surgical resection is the treatment of choice, occasionally complemented with chemoradiotherapy.

Immunoproliferative small intestinal disease

A rare condition, also known as alpha heavy chain disease, this affects especially Mediterranean and Arab races. There is proliferation, ranging in severity from benign proliferation to malignant transformation, of IgA-producing small bowel immunocytes (in response to chronic bacterial antigen stimulation). There is a dense, diffuse proximal small bowel infiltration. Patients present typically as young adults with diarrhoea, malabsorption, clubbing and weight loss (differential diagnosis includes Crohn's and Whipple's disease). Serum electrophoresis shows α-heavy chains (the F_c portion of IgA) and hypo-γ-globulinaemia. Treatment is with long-term antibiotics, with only a minority of patients needing chemotherapy.

Polyps

- **Single polyps**: extremely rare, often malignant. May be secondaries from melanoma or lung.
- **Multiple polyps**: commoner. They are either:
  - Nodular lymphoid hyperplasia (in children, with hypo-γ-globulinaemia).

- Hamartomas (Peutz–Jegher syndrome, with labial pigmentation and intussusception).
- Adenomatous (Cronkhite–Canada syndrome, with alopecia and nail dystrophy).

Adenocarcinoma

This is exceptionally rare, but may be associated with coeliac disease, Crohn's disease, Lynch syndrome or familial adenomatous polyposis. It usually presents with obstruction or chronic blood loss, and surgical resection is the definitive treatment.

Miscellaneous intestinal disorders

Chronic intestinal pseudo-obstruction

This term refers to a spectrum of rare disorders characterised by the signs and symptoms of intestinal obstruction in the absence of true obstruction. It is caused by pathology of either gut smooth muscle ('visceral myopathy') or nerves ('visceral neuropathy'); see Table 14.4.

In the early stages vomiting, abdominal distension and constipation occur episodically, with no symptoms between acute episodes. With disease progression, symptoms become more chronic and weight loss and malnutrition develop. Myopathic forms are commonly associated with urinary tract symptoms. The diagnosis

Table 14.4 Classification of chronic intestinal pseudo-obstruction. Those in bold have myopathic causation; others have neuropathic causation.

Primary	Secondary
Familial visceral myopathy	Infiltrative – sarcoid, amyloid
Familial visceral neuropathy	**Myopathic – mitochondrial disorders**
	Myenteric plexitis – inflammatory
	Myenteric plexitis – paraneoplastic (small cell lung cancer)
	CNS disorders (Parkinson's, autonomic failure)
	Endocrine – hypothyroidism, porphyria

CNS, central nervous system.

requires radiological demonstration of a dilated proximal small bowel. Laparoscopic full-thickness biopsies of the small bowel confirm both the diagnosis and whether it is myopathic or neuropathic in origin.

Management comprises symptom relief during acute episodes, care being taken to avoid inducing opiate dependence. In the long term parenteral nutrition is often required and surgery should be avoided.

Meckel's diverticulum

This affects approximately 2% of the population, but is symptomatic in only 2% of those individuals. It is the commonest congenital gut abnormality, resulting from failure to close the vitelline duct. It is typically 60 cm (2 feet) proximal to the ileo-caecal valve and 5 cm (2 inches) long. If symptomatic, patients present before age 2, and males are twice as likely to be affected. Histologically, the mucosa is either gastric or pancreatic.

The classic symptoms are of painless melaena, with intestinal obstruction or intussusception being rare. Diagnosis is by a Meckel's scan (injecting a radioisotope, which is taken up ectopic parietal cells). Surgical removal is rarely necessary.

Lactase deficiency

Brush border lactase digests lactose in milk to create glucose and galactose. Whereas Caucasians are very rarely deficient of the enzyme, 90% of Africans and Asians have hypolactasia. Secondary lactase deficiency may occur following gastroenteritides and if undigested lactose enters the colon, it becomes a substrate for colonic bacterial fermentation, causing an osmotic diarrhoea, flatulence, abdominal pain and borborygmi after eating milk products. Diagnosis is with a lactose substrate hydrogen breath test (see Chapter 6), and treatment is by minimising (not necessarily absolutely avoiding) milk products. Commercially available lactase may be added to the diet.

Food allergy

Immune-mediated reactions to particular foods are experienced by 5% of children (cow's milk and soya especially) and 1% of adults (peanuts and shellfish especially). Typically this is a type I hypersensitivity reaction and there is an instantaneous reaction on ingestion, which may be unpleasant but self-resolving. Rarely, there is a life-threatening anaphylaxis. Skin-prick tests and assay of serum IgE levels are not helpful in diagnosis, which rests on double-blind placebo-controlled food challenge. Treatment is by appropriate dietary avoidance and anaphylaxis may require constant availability of an epinephrine syringe.

NSAID-associated enteropathy

NSAID-induced erosions, ulcers, webs and strictures of the small bowel occur more often than NSAID gastropathy. These mucosal changes may result in bleeding and protein loss. While many of these are mild, the serious events (major haemorrhage, perforation, obstruction and sudden death) occur as often as that reported for NSAID gastropathy. The diagnosis of NSAID enteropathy has been greatly aided by the introduction of capsule enteroscopy.

 KEY POINTS

- Malabsorption can be caused by structural disease, mucosal disorders or abnormal luminal digestion.

- Intestinal failure typically occurs when there is <100 cm of small bowel. Treatment involves ensuring adequate calorie intake, managing hydration status and replacing vitamins and minerals.

- Coeliac disease is screened for using IgA antibodies to tissue transglutaminase, endomysial and gliadin antigen. Duodenal biopsy is the gold standard for diagnosis. HLA-DQ2 and -DQ8 and IgG antibodies can also be used. Treatment involves a lifelong gluten-free diet.

- Small intestinal bacterial overgrowth is almost always secondary to structural disease. Antibiotics are used, and often repeated courses are needed. Definitive treatment of the underlying cause should be undertaken if possible.

- Carcinoid tumours (gastrointestinal neuroendocrine tumours) are generally benign. They result in carcinoid syndrome only if metastatic.

- Small bowel adenocarcinoma, while rare, is associated with coeliac disease, Crohn's disease, Lynch syndrome and familial adenomatous polyposis.

- Chronic intestinal pseudo-obstruction is a chronic disabling disorder characterised by the signs and symptoms of intestinal obstruction in the absence of true obstruction.

- Meckel's diverticulum occurs in 2% of the population, but is symptomatic in only 2% of those individuals. Surgical removal is rarely necessary.

 SELF-ASSESSMENT QUESTION

(The answer to this question is given on p. 267)

A 69-year-old woman presents because of difficulties with ileostomy function. She had a panproctocolectomy 10 years ago because of a Dukes B colonic carcinoma in the setting of ulcerative colitis and a family history of Lynch syndrome. For many years she has had excellent ileostomy function, but did have repeated admissions to hospital with mechanical small bowel obstructions, the cause for which was never determined. Over the last year she has suffered with bloating, flatulence and high stomal outputs as well as intermittent, colicky, central abdominal pain. She has noticed that a course of antibiotics used to treat a skin infection did seem to markedly improve her ileostomy function.

With regard to her clinical situation, which of the following statements is most correct?

(a) She is at no increased risk of small bowel adenocarcinoma compared with the general population.

(b) The improvement that she experienced with antibiotics is likely to be coincidental.

(c) HLA-DQ2 and –DQ8 testing should be performed to exclude coeliac disease.

(d) It is likely that her serum folate will be normal but her B_{12} reduced.

(e) Her previous surgery to remove the entire colon puts her at risk of intestinal failure.

15

Small and large bowel disorders

Inflammatory bowel diseases (IBDs)

These are a family of related diseases, which follow a relapsing and remitting course. They share the pathological hallmark of chronic inflammation, with environmental, genetic and immunological factors interacting to cause these diseases. The two major members of the family are Crohn's disease and ulcerative colitis (UC). The term indeterminate colitis is often used where an apparently idiopathic colitis demonstrates features consistent with both Crohn's disease and ulcerative colitis. Often with time the underlying diagnosis becomes clearer. Microscopic colitis is sometimes considered under the umbrella of IBD.

Causes

Genetic factors

Twin studies have pointed to a *genetic predisposition* in a subset of IBD patients, specifically Crohn's disease (concordance ~50%, compared to ~10% for ulcerative colitis). The disease is more common in Ashkenazi Jews and second-generation Asians in developed countries. Early in the history of IBD genetic studies, the *CARD15/NOD2 gene* on chromosome 16 was linked to the development of Crohn's disease, probably by altering the way bacterial antigens are presented to the ileal mucosa. Since then genome-wide association scanning studies have demonstrated in excess of 160 different IBD associated genes, more than for any other disease.

IBD is a polygenic disorder and generally more than one genetic association is needed to produce disease in an individual.

Environmental factors

The greatest prevalence of IBD is in developed countries, specifically where there is improved *sanitation*. It has been hypothesised that exposure to unhygienic conditions in early years can result in the development of intestinal immune defence mechanisms. *Dietary* influences on the epidemiology of IBD are evident, in particular the move from a diet based on oily fish to animal fat in some societies and an associated increase in IBD incidence. *Smoking* is another important factor, and curiously has contrasting effects in Crohn's disease and ulcerative colitis: increasing the risk of relapse in Crohn's and reducing the risk in ulcerative colitis.

Immunological factors

Recent evidence points to the role of the host bacterial environment in exerting a protective or stimulatory effect on the mucosal inflammation in IBD. This bacterial profile depends on early-life factors (breast feeding, sanitation). Debate continues as to whether a single pathological agent might be responsible for causation in some individuals or whether it is interactions between the organisms that make up the intestinal microbiota that are important.

Gastroenterology and Hepatology: Lecture Notes, Second Edition. Stephen Inns and Anton Emmanuel.
© 2017 John Wiley & Sons, Ltd. Published 2017 by John Wiley & Sons, Ltd.
Companion website: www.lecturenoteseries.com/gastroenterology

Pathogenesis

The gut tissue damage results from the interplay of circulating and gut immune cells (lymphocytes and neutrophils) and non-immune cells (mast cells and fibroblasts). It is clear that dietary antigens and host bacteria play a key initiating role in this inflammatory process. The antigens are taken up through breaches in the mucosa and specialised antigen-presenting cells (APCs) liberate a variety of pro-inflammatory cytokines, such as tumour necrosis factor-α (TNF-α) and interleukin-12 (IL-12). These APCs pass on the antigen to CD4+ T-lymphocytes, which themselves then differentiate down specific pathways.

Classically **Crohn's disease** was thought to be predominantly a *Th1-driven* immune response, characterised initially by further release of pro-inflammatory cytokines, including TNF-α and interferon-γ. In contrast, **ulcerative colitis** was thought to be a *Th2-driven* immune response, with increased release of pro-inflammatory cytokines, including IL-5. However, crossover between the cytokine profiles of both pathways and the contribution of the Th17/IL-23 pathway and T regulatory cells has been increasingly recognised.

Whichever immune process is followed, the net result is recruitment of further inflammatory cells (through increased adhesion of neutrophils to vascular endothelium) and activation of non-immune cells (mast cells, fibroblasts). This in turn results in tissue damage, and hence further ingress of antigen from the lumen into the gut mucosa.

Finally, in predisposed individuals, this inflammatory process can extend beyond the gut, resulting in the extraintestinal features of Crohn's disease and ulcerative colitis.

Epidemiology

The incidence of Crohn's disease, which is increasing, is ~7 in 100,000 in the developed world, with a prevalence of ~70 in 100,000. There is marked geographical variation, with New Zealand having one of the highest reported incidences in the world.

Unlike Crohn's, the incidence of ulcerative colitis is stable in the developed world, at ~12 in 100,000 with a prevalence of ~120 in 100,000. Both diseases show two age peaks, one in the third and fourth decades and the other in the sixth and seventh.

Clinical features

Distribution of disease

Although it can be difficult to differentiate Crohn's disease from ulcerative colitis, there are important differences in the distribution of the diseases. As well

as the severity and nature of the disease (i.e. inflammatory vs structuring), the distribution of disease has a large influence on what symptoms are exhibited.

Crohn's disease

Crohn's disease affects the gut in a *non-continuous* way, causing characteristic 'skip' lesions with normal mucosa in between. Involvement is ileal or ileocolonic (40%), small intestinal (30%), purely colonic (20%) and purely perianal (10%). In children, proximal gut inflammation is more common. Inflammation involves the *full thickness* of the gut wall with deep ulcers, causing a 'cobblestone' appearance. Ulcers may be so deep as to penetrate the bowel wall, causing fistulae and abscesses. The fistulae may be from the gut to adjacent viscera (bladder, vagina, other regions of the gut) or through the skin. The histological hallmark is of **giant cell granuloma**.

Ulcerative colitis

Ulcerative colitis always involves the rectum, and may extend in a *confluent* manner to involve the sigmoid colon and rectum (proctosigmoiditis) in 40%. About 20% have involvement of the entire colon (pan-colitis) and the remaining approximately 40% have an 'extensive colitis', which does not involve the whole colon but extends proximal to the sigmoid. Only the colonic mucosa is involved, and the inflammation is confined to the mucosa.

It should be noted that ulcerative colitis, particularly pancolitis, is associated with mild inflammation in the terminal ileum (backwash ileitis) in 17% of cases, and left-sided colitis can demonstrate limited inflammation around the appendiceal orifice (caecal patch) in between 3% and 8% of patients.

Histologically, there is inflammation with **acute and chronic inflammatory cells, crypt distortion** and **crypt abscesses**. Increased dysplasia with chronic inflammation predisposes to colorectal carcinoma.

Extraintestinal disease

About 35% of patients develop extraintestinal manifestations of IBD, and some (but not all) of these relate to the activity of disease in the gut (Table 15.1). HLA-B27 positivity predisposes to joint manifestations.

Crohn's disease clinical features

Crohn's disease is characterised by **abdominal pain** and **diarrhoea**, but specific symptoms depend on the *region* of gut involved.

Table 15.1 Extraintestinal manifestations of IBD.

System	Disorder	Relationship to disease activity?	Relationship with colonic involvement?	Relationship with Crohn's disease?
Ophthalmology	Conjunctivitis	+	+	
	Iritis/uveitis	+	+	
	Episcleritis/scleritis	+	+	
Oral	Aphthous mouth ulcers	+		+
	Angular stomatitis		+	
Dermatology	Erythema nodosum	+	+	
	Pyoderma gangrenosum	+	+	
	Erythema multiforme	+	+	
	Metastatic Crohn's disease	+		+
Musculoskeletal	Ankylosing spondylitis		+	
	Sacroiliitis		+	
	Peripheral arthropathy		+	
	Osteoporosis/osteomalacia		+	+
Genitourinary	Kidney stones (oxalate)			+
	Amyloidosis			+
	Glomerulonephritis			
Hepatobiliary	Gallstones			
	Autoimmune hepatitis			
	Primary sclerosing cholangitis (PSC)		+	
	Cholangiocarcinoma		+	
	Fatty liver	+		
	Liver abscess	+	+	
Cardiovascular	Venous thrombosis	+		
	Pleuropericarditis			
Respiratory	Fibrosing alveolitis			
	Pulmonary vasculitis			
Neurology	Neuropathy			
	Myopathy			

- **Ileal Crohn's** may cause small bowel obstruction and an inflammatory mass or abscess, resulting in abdominal pain (commonly post-prandial). This results in anorexia coupled with non-bloody diarrhoea. Weight loss is common. Inflammation of the small intestine may cause malabsorption, resulting in anaemia (classically B_{12} or folate deficiency) or malnutrition.
- **Proximal intestinal Crohn's disease** is more often associated with vomiting.
- **Crohn's colitis** presents with bloody diarrhoea, loss of mucus and constitutional symptoms (malaise and fever). In contrast to ulcerative colitis, which has similar symptoms, there is typically 'rectal sparing' on sigmoidoscopy.

- **Perianal Crohn's** may cause perianal soiling of mucus or faeces, and examination reveals skin tags, anal fissures or fistulous openings (see Figure 17.1 for classification of fistulae).

Ulcerative colitis clinical features

Ulcerative colitis is characterised by *bloody diarrhoea*. Specific symptoms depend on the *extent* and *severity* of colonic involvement.

- **Proctitis** and **proctosigmoiditis** cause fresh rectal bleeding, loss of mucus per rectum and tenesmus. Constitutional symptoms are absent unless *severe* inflammation occurs.

Table 15.2 Truelove and Witts' criteria for assessing acute colitis severity. Source: Truelove SC, Witts LJ. Cortisone in ulcerative colitis. BMJ 1955;2, Table III. Reproduced with the permission of BMJ Publishing Group Ltd.

	mild	severe
stools	<5/d, trace blood	>5/d, bloody
temperature	No fever	>37.8
pulse	<90	>90
Hb	Normal	<10.5
ESR	<30	>30

ESR, erythrocyte sedimentation rate; Hb, haemoglobin.

- **Extensive** or **pancolitis** present with more prominent constitutional symptoms, abdominal pain and bloody diarrhoea. *Severity* is indicated by bowel frequency (>6 per 24 h), degree of blood loss in stools, pulse >90 bpm and temperature (Truelove and Witts' criteria, see Table 15.2).

In rare cases, the colon may dilate (**toxic megacolon**) with symptoms of a severe colitis, marked constitutional symptoms and abdominal distension. Because of the high risk of perforation, joint management between medical and surgical teams is essential. This complication can occur with Crohn's colitis, but is most frequent in first presentations of ulcerative colitis.

Malignancy complicating IBD

Cancer complicating colitis may occur with both ulcerative colitis and Crohn's disease. Risk is related to:

- Extent of disease (especially extensive UC).
- Duration of disease (>8 years).
- Comorbidity of primary sclerosing cholangitis (PSC).
- Coexistent family history of colorectal cancer.

Colonoscopic surveillance is reserved for left-sided and extensive colitis. Surveillance begins 10 years after the onset of disease and the interval depends on the activity of the disease, the family history of colon cancer, the presence of primary sclerosing cholangitis and any finding of dysplasia.

Small bowel adenocarcinoma is a very rare complication of extensive small bowel Crohn's disease.

Investigations

Investigations are directed towards confirming the condition (i.e. diagnosis, defining extent of disease and activity of disease), identifying cause (infection) and assessing for complications (toxic megacolon).

Condition

The differential diagnosis of small bowel Crohn's includes:

- Caecal carcinoma.
- Appendix abscess.
- Intestinal TB or lymphoma.
- Pelvic inflammatory disease.
- Radiation enteritis.

For colitis symptoms, the differential includes:

- Bacterial infections.
- Microscopic colitis.
- Colorectal carcinoma.
- Pseudo-membranous colitis diverticulitis.
- Ischaemic colitis.
- NSAID colitis.
- Radiation enteritis.
- **Lab tests**: anaemia, iron deficiency, leucocytosis, thrombocytosis, hypokalaemia, hypoalbuminaemia, ESR and CRP reflect disease activity. LFTs may be abnormal if PSC is present. *Clostridium difficile* toxin assay will exclude pseudo-membranous colitis.
- **Endoscopy**: sigmoidoscopy will identify an inflamed rectum in active ulcerative colitis (but may be normal in Crohn's colitis). In active disease the mucosa is friable and oedematous, and with more severe inflammation ulceration and mucopus are present. With chronic disease there is a loss of vascular pattern and a granular appearance of the mucosa. The key thing is to establish whether there is active mucosal disease, as if it is normal, the differential diagnosis needs to be considered. Thus, full colonoscopy is rarely needed in the acute setting; performed in the chronic setting, it informs about the extent of colonic ulceration, and indicates whether there is terminal ileal Crohn's disease.
- **Abdominal X-ray**: essential if toxic megacolon is suspected (see later discussion). In Crohn's ileitis it may show small bowel obstruction.
- **Small bowel studies**: fluoroscopic studies using intestinal contrast have largely been supplanted by cross-sectional studies. CT has the advantage of being quick and is often more accessible than MRI. MRI has the advantage of not using ionising radiation, and thus being more appropriate in young patients who may require repeated scans over time. The small bowel is distended by fluid, usually administered orally. These are *not* often required in the acute situation, but do have a role in defining the extent of disease. Capsule endoscopy is rarely required, except in cases where small bowel changes may be too subtle for identification by CT or MRI enterography.

Cause

- Stool culture: as infective exacerbations are common. *Clostridium difficile* is a commonly involved organism and stool testing should include analysis for this.

Complications

- **Abdominal X-ray**: in toxic megacolon, in addition to the colonic dilatation, there may also be mucosal oedema ('thumb-printing'), areas of necrosis ('mucosal islands') or evidence of perforation.
- **Abdominal ultrasound**: of value if an abdominal mass is suspected, and may also give information about bowel wall thickness (and hence activity).
- **Colonoscopy**: will identify colorectal cancer complicating chronic IBD as well as terminal ileal or colonic stricturing.
- **Abdominopelvic CT or MRI**: invaluable acutely to identify colonic wall thickness, suspected perforation, extraluminal features of Crohn's disease. Pelvic MRI is particularly helpful for imaging perianal Crohn's disease.
- **Examination under anaesthetic** (EUA) of the perianal region is a very useful diagnostic and therapeutic tool for fistulating perianal Crohn's disease.

Management

Different approaches are needed when attempting to induce remission of disease compared to maintaining remission once induced (see Table 15.3). Because of their speed of onset, corticosteroids may be appropriate to help induce remission and act as a *bridge* to a longer-term immunosuppressive strategy, but their side-effect profile and lack of long-term efficacy make them inappropriate as a maintenance therapy.

Introduction to IBD medicines

The therapeutic approach to different forms and severities of IBD are outlined later in this chapter. This section briefly considers the medicines commonly used in IBD, their mechanism and risks. The order used here is the same as the order in which they would often (but not always) be used in clinical practice.

5-aminosalicylic acid preparations (5ASA)

These agents can be considered 'ointment for the bowel'. They act as topical anti-inflammatories and can be administered either orally or rectally. Combining oral and rectal therapy is the most effective strategy for inducing remission.

Because of their topical action when taken orally, they need to be released in the inflamed area. Multiple mechanisms exist for achieving this (Table 15.4). The main limiting adverse effects include nausea, diarrhoea (rarely 5ASA induced colonic inflammation), skin rashes and headaches. A dose-dependant nephritis occurs in up to 1 in 1000 patients and most experts recommend monitoring for renal dysfunction by monitoring creatinine. Adherence to 5ASA treatment is poor, at least in part because the tablet burden is high. Using the medicine once per day improves this.

Corticosteroids

The oral preparation used is generally prednisolone in the UK and prednisone in Australasia. Hydrocortisone is the most frequent intravenous preparation used in hospitalised patients with severe disease. Corticosteroid use should be limited to active IBD; there is no role for maintenance use of corticosteroids.

Table 15.3 Therapies used to induce remission vs maintain remission.

Remission induction	Remission maintenance
Corticosteroids	5-aminosalicylates (5ASA)
Cyclosporin	Azathioprine/ 6-mercaptopurine
Anti-TNF-alpha antibodies	Methotrexate
Surgery	Anti-TNF-alpha antibodies
	Lifestyle (smoking)

Table 15.4 Characteristics of 5-ASA compounds. As 5-ASA is easily absorbed from the small bowel, the molecule needs modification to be released at the site of inflammation.

Sulphasalazine	5-ASA linked to sulphapyridine (hence adverse effects) – well absorbed, so good for co-existent joint disease
Mesalazine	Coated and slow-release forms available, released according to luminal pH; used as oral and rectal preparations for colonic action
Olsalazine	Two 5-ASA molecules released in presence of colonic bacteria
Balsalzide	5-ASA molecule especially well released in distal colon

While they are effective for the treatment of inflammation, they do slow mucosal healing and for this reason recurrence is common if they are reduced too quickly. The optimal dose is not known, but a commonly used regimen in IBD is 40 to 60 mg of prednisolone, reduced by 5 mg every 1 to 2 weeks as tolerated. Budesonide is a steroid that exhibits limited absorption in the gut and is used orally as a topical alternative to prednisolone in Crohn's disease.

Corticosteroids are poorly tolerated by many patients and have extensive side-effects, including weight gain, skin changes, dysphoria, glaucoma/cataracts, hypertension, and predisposition to infection, diabetes and osteoporosis. The latter is one of the more feared consequences of long-term corticosteroid use and should be monitored for carefully and treated appropriately.

Thiopurines

Azathioprine and 6-mercaptopurine (6MP) act by multiple mechanisms, including the inhibition of purine synthesis, to reduce the number and activity of lymphocytes, particularly T cells. Azathioprine itself is a prodrug of 6MP and is converted to 6MP in the liver. Further metabolism to active and inactive substrates occurs in the liver and, while it is incompletely understood, does in large part rely on the enzyme thiopurine methyltransferase (TPMT). This enzyme exhibits genetic polymorphism, which can affect its activity. This activity can be measured in the blood, as can the presence of polymorphisms in the gene encoding TPMT. This measurement is used in clinical practice to guide dosing and determine safety.

In addition, the active metabolites of 6MP can be measured. 6-thioguanine nucleotides (6TGN) are largely responsible for the immunosuppressive effects of azathioprine/6MP and 6-methylmercaptopurine (6MMP) for toxic effects in the liver. The overproduction of 6MMP compared to 6TGN is commonly termed 'shunting' and is associated with poor response to therapy. The addition of allopurinol, via its inhibition of xanthine oxidase – another important enzyme in the metabolism of azathioprine/6MP – can restore this balance and improve the outcome of disease.

The immunosuppressive effect of azathioprine/6MP is slow, taking up to 17 weeks for full effect. This limits their use for induction of remission. While, as with any immunosuppressive medicine, the side-effect profile of azathioprine/6MP is daunting, all of the side-effects are reversible if discovered early. The main limiting side-effect is nausea. This prevents up to 10% of people from using the medicine. Swapping from azathioprine to 6MP (or vice versa) can benefit some patients

with this side-effect. Otherwise the concerning side-effects are idiosyncratic (unpredictable) allergic reactions, rashes, pancreatitis and hepatitis. Marrow suppression is rare, particularly if dosing is tailored to the TPMT, but should be monitored for. Generally it is recommended that patients have weekly bloods, including full blood count, liver biochemistry, creatinine and amylase. In the long term there are concerns regarding increasing the predisposition to cancer. This is likely to be true for non-melanomatous skin cancers, but debated for other lesions. It may well be that there is a small increase in the relative risk of non-Hodgkin's lymphoma. However, it must be noted that with such an uncommon disease an increase in incidence from approximately 2:10,000 people to 10:10,000, while it represents a fivefold increase in relative risk, is still a very low absolute risk for an individual.

Methotrexate

Methotrexate is a folate antimetabolite and in cancer treatment acts largely by inhibiting dihydrofolate reductase. In IBD, however, its action is thought to be via multiple mechanisms, the main one being inhibition of purine metabolism. Thus, as with azathioprine, its main action is via inhibition of T cell function. While methotrexate is highly bioavailable, there is evidence of unreliable absorption in the presence of Crohn's disease, so it is often given parenterally, generally subcutaneously, in this situation.

Methotrexate is teratogenic and in women must be discontinued at least 6 weeks prior to conception. Although it is debated whether conception where the man is taking methotrexate poses a risk to the foetus, many experts continue to recommend that contraception be used. Other side-effects include allergic reaction and bone marrow suppression. Methotrexate can cause oral ulceration and gastrointestinal upset, but giving oral folic acid the day after taking it reduces these effects. Pulmonary fibrosis and hepatic fibrosis have been reported with methotrexate, but are rare in IBD and are not generally specifically monitored for. Similar blood test monitoring to that performed with azathioprine is used with methotrexate.

Anti-tumour necrosis factor (TNF) alpha antibodies

Several treatments exist using antibodies, or antibody fragments, directed against TNF-alpha. The main two used in IBD treatment are infliximab, a chimeric murine–human monoclonal antibody, and adalimumab, which is fully humanised. These treatments are not orally bioavailable and must be given parenterally, generally by 8-weekly infusion in the case of infliximab and fortnightly subcutaneous injection for adalimumab. They are prone to the effect of neutralising antibodies produced by the recipient over time and are often used with another immunosuppressant, typically azathioprine, to counter this effect.

Infusion reactions are common, but are lessened by continuous therapy and concomitant immunosuppression. Rare side-effects include exacerbation of heart failure, neurological complications and aplastic anaemia. Paradoxical inflammation, where a previously mild or unrecognised inflammatory condition (e.g. psoriasis) is exacerbated by an anti-TNF agent, is not infrequent, but does not often result in discontinuation. Although the association with lymphoma is not well understood, it is thought to be similar to that seen with azathioprine.

Novel approaches to IBD therapy

As our understanding of the pathogenesis of IBD improves, so new targets for therapy become available. Many new therapies for IBD are in the development pipeline, so some may have become widely available by the time you read this book. This section briefly outlines just a few of them.

IL-12 and IL-23 are important cytokines in the production of IBD. Their shared ligand subunit is named p40. **Ustekinumab** is a monoclonal antibody to the p40 subunit, which blocks the effect of IL-12/23 and has effect against IBD.

In order to cause IBD, T-lymphocytes must access the gut and cross the vascular endothelium by way of adhesion molecules called integrins on the vessel wall. Monoclonal antibodies to these molecules can block this interaction and prevent activated T-lymphocytes gaining access to the gut, thus treating disease. Examples of this class of agent include **natalizumab**, an antibody to alpha-4 integrin, **vedolizumab,** which acts on alpha-4 beta-7 integrin, and **etrolizumab**, which targets the beta-7 integrin subunit.

A similar approach uses small molecules, rather than monoclonal antibodies, to block this 'trafficking' of lymphocytes to the gut. Examples of this are the **chemokine receptor 9 (CCR9) antagonists**. For T-lymphocytes to access the small intestine from blood, interaction between CCR9 on the cell surface and its ligand, chemokine ligand 25 (CCL25), is required. This 'gut-homing' behaviour can be blocked using small molecules designed to interfere with this interaction.

Janus Kinase (JAK) tyrosine kinases are responsible for the signalling in immune cells that eventually produces such cytokines as IL-2, IL-4, IL-7, IL-9, IL-15 and IL-21. Blockage of this effect using small molecules might have an effect against IBD. The first of these agents, **tofacitinib**, an oral inhibitor of JAK 1, 2 and 3, has shown effect in ulcerative colitis. Other agents acting on different parts of the JAK associated signalling mechanism are under development.

Crohn's disease

Treatment is tailored to the *extent* and *severity* of disease. Note that azathioprine/6MP are generally added whenever prednisolone or budesonide is required, as they take up to 17 weeks to have their full effect, may assist with induction of remission and are very likely to be required for maintenance of remission. In addition, it is generally accepted that anti-TNF therapies should be used in combination with an immunomodulator (such as azathioprine), as the combination seems to be more effective than either therapy alone.

Inducing remission

- Localised terminal ileal or ileo-caecal disease:
  - Medical first line: course of oral prednisolone (>40 mg reducing over 4–6 weeks) or budesonide (a less well-absorbed steroid, hence causing fewer side-effects).
  - In mild disease high-dose 5ASA can be considered as a first-line therapy in this group (Table 15.4).
  - Medical second line: infliximab/adalimumab – these are monoclonal antibodies targeting TNF-α that can induce rapid healing (beware adverse effects of severe infection, anaphylaxis and immune reaction).
  - Surgical: limited ileal resection (may be preferred by patients as first-line therapy, and should be considered in all patients if frequent relapses occur; patients will need B_{12} replacement long term).
- Extensive small bowel disease: careful enteral nutrition is often needed:
  - First line: prednisolone or budesonide.
  - Second line: infliximab/adalimumab.
  - Third line: enteral nutrition using polymeric formula.
- Colonic disease:
  - Proctitis or left-sided colitis – determine severity: Mild: 5-ASA or prednisolone suppositories for proctitis, enemas for left-sided disease. Severe: 5-ASA or prednisolone enemas; if refractory, course of oral prednisolone.
  - Extensive colitis – determine severity: Mild: high-dose oral 5-ASA and 5-ASA enemas. Severe: course of oral prednisolone.
- Perianal Crohn's disease:
  - Fissure: topical glyceryl trinitrate and/or 5-ASA or prednisolone suppository.

Box 15.1 Examination under anaesthetic (EUA) in fistulating perianal Crohn's disease

EUA of the perianal region is a very useful diagnostic and therapeutic tool for fistulating perianal Crohn's disease. Generally surgery is aimed at controlling sepsis by allowing drainage of abscesses, rather than attempting to close fistulae. This is often achieved using soft silastic rubber sutures called Seton sutures, which are threaded through the internal and external fistula opening, allowing drainage of any sepsis and promoting healing of the inflamed fistula tract. These are then removed once drainage has stopped with the hope of spontaneous closure of the fistula, usually under the influence of anti-TNF therapies.

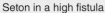

Seton in a high fistula

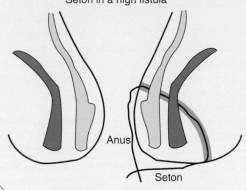

Anus

Seton

○ Fistula: oral metronidazole and perianal MRI; if complex (multiple fistulae or abscess formation) for EUA and non-cutting seton suture (see Box 15.1). Once sepsis controlled, treat with infliximab +/− azathioprine/6MP.
- Abscess: surgical or radiologically guided drainage.

Maintaining remission

- Localised terminal ileal disease:
  ○ With mild disease treatment may be able to be stopped, but if relapses occur despite continuous high-dose oral 5-ASA, treatment is as for moderate-severe disease and more extensive disease.
- Moderate-severe terminal ileal disease and more extensive disease:
  ○ First line: azathioprine/6MP.
  ○ Second line: methotrexate, particularly for steroid-dependent disease.
  ○ Third line: anti-TNF therapy.
- Perianal disease: if frequent relapses or severe inflammation occur, then treat with infliximab +/− azathioprine/6MP.

Box 15.2 Operative options in ulcerative colitis

Indications
- Failure of medical therapy (steroid dependence or drug side-effects)
- Acute severe colitis and toxic megacolon
- Impaired quality of life
- Disease complications (severe haemorrhage, pyoderma gangrenosum)
- Colorectal cancer

Operations
- Proctocolectomy and ileostomy
- Proctocolectomy and ileoanal pouch (but 20% risk of this pouch becoming inflamed)
- Colectomy and ileorectal anastomosis (not favoured)

Ulcerative colitis

Inducing remission

- Proctitis and left-sided colitis – determine severity:
  ○ Mild: 5-ASA suppositories for proctitis, enema for left-sided.
  ○ Moderate: 5-ASA suppositories/enema + oral therapy.
  ○ Severe: 5-ASA suppositories and oral therapy and oral/topical steroids.
    If severe refractory disease: consider intravenous cyclosporin or infliximab or surgery (Box 15.2).
- Extensive colitis – determine severity:
  ○ Mild/moderate: high-dose oral and rectal 5-ASA.
  ○ Severe: add course of oral prednisolone:
    If remains refractory: consider intravenous cyclosporin or infliximab.
    If still refractory: surgery.

Maintaining remission

- Proctitis or proctosigmoiditis:
  ○ Mild cases may not need anything, or oral 5-ASA.
  ○ Severe cases may need azathioprine or 6-MP.
- Extensive colitis:
  ○ Mild: oral 5-ASA.
  ○ Severe: azathioprine or 6-MP.

Osteoporosis

Crohn's disease patients in particular, and the use of steroids in all IBD, means that patients are predisposed to metabolic bone disease. Diagnosis is with a DEXA bone scan. Treatment of mild cases is with calcium and vitamin D, and of severe cases is with bisphosphonates.

IBD in children, pregnancy and lactation

Maintaining nutrition is vital to ensure normal puberty and growth (malnutrition is predisposed towards by chronic illness and treatments). For **Crohn's disease**, polymeric diets are preferred to steroids in children and adolescents to avoid growth retardation induced by the latter. Treatment with steroids, immunosuppression or surgery is otherwise similar to that in adults.

Pregnancy, labour and lactation are not associated with any greater risk of relapse. Equally, with the obvious exception of methotrexate, treatment options generally need not be altered by pregnancy or lactation, but should be closely monitored by a specialist. The guiding principle in pregnancy medicine is 'do what is right for the mother and that will be best for the baby too'. The harm that active IBD can do to the mother and baby must be included in the assessment of any risks that IBD medicines might pose.

Prognosis

Advances in medical and surgical treatment since the 1950s have resulted in the life expectancy of IBD patients now being the same as the general population. About 90% of ileal Crohn's patients will have at least one operation, as opposed to only about 40% of colonic Crohn's patients. With ulcerative colitis, 90% will run a relapsing–remitting course, while 10% have chronic active disease, the latter being especially likely to undergo surgery. Surgery for ulcerative colitis is most common in the first 5 years after diagnosis.

Microscopic colitis

This term microscopic colitis comprises two histologically distinct conditions, **collagenous colitis** and **lymphocytic colitis**.

Epidemiology

The annual incidence is 5 to 10 per 100,000, and it is more common in patients with coeliac disease, autoimmune disorders and those taking drugs (particularly PPIs and NSAIDs). There is a peak incidence in 60- to 70-year-old individuals and a predominance of female patients in collagenous colitis.

Cause

The cause is unknown but is likely to be multifactorial and represents specific mucosal responses to different, thus far unidentified luminal agents in predisposed individuals, resulting in an uncontrolled mucosal immune response. No clear genetic association with microscopic colitis has been identified. Smoking has been shown to be a risk factor for microscopic colitis. It does seem that drugs can induce microscopic colitis and there is a strong association with acarbose, aspirin, Cyclo3 Fort, non-steroidal anti-inflammatory drugs, proton pump inhibitors, ranitidine, sertraline and ticlopidine.

Clinical features and investigation

Clinically, the hallmark is watery diarrhoea variably associated with abdominal pain and weight loss. In both conditions, the endoscopic appearance of the mucosa is normal. Histologically, changes are seen more often on right- than left-colon biopsies: collagenous colitis is characterised by a thickened subepithelial collagen layer, while in lymphocytic colitis there is an increased infiltrate of intraepithelial lymphocytes.

Management

Mild cases respond to loperamide used as required. For more severe cases, the first choice is budesonide. Alternative options include immunosuppressives such as azathioprine, infliximab and adalimumab (Figure 15.1).

Prognosis

There is no evidence that microscopic colitis adversely affects survival, but there is increasing evidence that it is associated with reduced health-related quality of life (HRQoL). This effect is mainly associated with symptom severity, and those with three or more stools/day or one or more watery stools/day had impaired HRQoL compared to those with fewer than three stools/day and no watery stools/day.

Functional gastrointestinal disorders

This is a collective term for the spectrum of disorders labelled functional heartburn, functional dyspepsia and irritable bowel syndrome (IBS). These are interrelated conditions involving the foregut, midgut and hindgut, respectively. All are marked by the complaint of pain associated with dysfunction of that region of the gut.

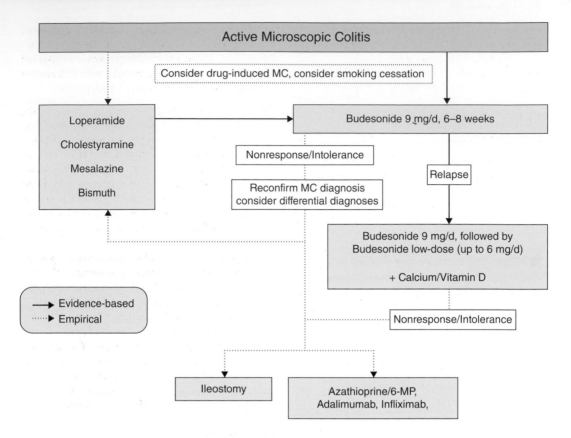

Figure 15.1 Algorithm for the treatment of microscopic colitis proposed by the European Microscopic Colitis Group. Source: Münch A, Aust D, Bohr J, et al. Microscopic colitis: current status, present and future challenges: statements of the European Microscopic Colitis Group. J Crohns Colitis. 2012;6(9):932–945, Figure 4. Reproduced by permission of Elsevier.

Epidemiology

These are common conditions (the most frequent disorders seen by gastroenterologists) with many overlapping symptoms, and up to 20% of the general population fulfil diagnostic criteria for these conditions. However, only about 10% present to medical services, women more often than men. Patients can present at any age, typically during childbearing years. Diagnosis is arrived at having excluded organic diseases presenting with the same symptoms, typically blood tests (including testing for coeliac disease, see Chapter 14), endoscopy or radiology.

Not only do these patients show overlap between gut symptoms, they also frequently report symptoms of functional disorders in other parts of the body (chronic fatigue syndrome, functional backache etc.).

Causes

The aetiopathogenesis of these disorders is multifactorial:

- **Psychological factors** contribute to the perception of gut stimuli and also influence gastric motility. This has been proven in both acute stress and in chronic depression and anxiety.
- **Visceral hypersensitivity and abnormal gut motility** are physiological phenomena that are often interrelated and contribute to causing gut symptoms. These visceral changes are in turn influenced by psychological factors. A variety of neurotransmitters have been implicated in these alterations of gut sensitivity and motility.
- **Alterations of mucosal immunology** function are also thought to contribute. About 25% of IBS cases begin after a gut infection, although again the risk

of subsequently developing IBS is related to certain psychological traits. These patients with so-called postinfectious IBS have altered mast cell and cytokine function.

Clinical syndromes and management

- **Functional heartburn**: defined as the presence of a retrosternal burning sensation in the absence of pathological gastro-oesophageal reflux. Treatment is generally supportive; a subset of patients may respond to intensive antireflux treatment, but antireflux surgery is not generally recommended.
- **Functional dyspepsia** comprises two distinct subgroups: the postprandial distress syndrome (with postprandial fullness and early satiety) and the epigastric pain syndrome (chronic and less meal-related pain syndrome). PPIs are usually ineffective in this setting, treatment again being supportive. Cognitive behavioural therapy, where available, is effective.
- **Irritable bowel syndrome**: categorised as being either constipation-predominant (c-IBS), diarrhoea-predominant (d-IBS) or mixed stool pattern (m-IBS). The prevalence of these forms is approximately 40%, 20% and 40%, respectively. All forms have cramping abdominal pain as the central feature and symptoms do *not* occur at night. Associated symptoms of rectal mucus loss and incomplete evacuation are common. Treatment centres on making a positive diagnosis and offering empathic reassurance. It should be tailored to the patient and their symptoms:
  - Diet is often of little help, perhaps with the exception of a diet low in fermentable carbohydrates (FODMAPs) in d-IBS.
  - Probiotics have not been proven to be beneficial.
  - Antispasmodics may help some patients with postprandial cramp.
  - Tricyclic antidepressants in low dose are of proven efficacy.
  - Occasional patients need hypnotherapy or cognitive behavioural therapy.
- **Functional constipation** (see also Chapter 3). Constipation is a symptom, not a diagnosis. The cause needs to be investigated to exclude the exhaustive list of possible causes (see Table 3.3), but – in contrast to diarrhoea – in most cases a cause is not found, and the final diagnosis is of a functional disorder. The symptom is defined broadly: bowel opening <3 times per week, or need to strain frequently, or passage of hard stools, or excessive time spent on toileting, or a sensation of incomplete voiding. With this loose definition, approximately 15% of the general Western population are said to be affected. Patients can be classified as having slow transit constipation, a defaecation disorder, or a combination of the two.

  - Slow transit constipation mostly affects young women with characteristically infrequent urge, infrequent bowel opening and abdominal bloating. The colon is not dilated, and the diagnosis can be confirmed by a radio-opaque marker transit study. Specific management is to avoid a high-fibre diet and consider use of an osmotic laxative or, as required, stimulant laxative. Biofeedback may help toileting behaviour. Colectomy is almost never indicated.
  - Defaecation disorder affects patients of all ages and is characterised by straining to evacuate the rectum, the need to use digital assistance to expel stool and a sensation of incomplete voiding. Diagnosis is confirmed by defaecography (barium or MR). Management is with suppositories or enemas and biofeedback to improve defaecatory coordination. If proctography shows an anatomical abnormality, such as rectal prolapse or a rectocoele (a protrusion of the rectum into the posterior wall of the vagina), this may need surgical correction.

Prognosis

By definition the functional diseases are not associated with structural disturbance of the gastrointestinal tract and longevity is unaffected. They are, however, often chronic relapsing–remitting diseases associated with significant effects on health-related quality of life and with significant costs to patients and the healthcare system.

Ischaemia of the gut

Causes

The vessels supplying the foregut, midgut and hindgut are, respectively, the coeliac, superior mesenteric and inferior mesenteric. The former is the least vulnerable to ischaemia, and the 'watershed' area between the supply of the latter two (namely the splenic flexure of the colon) is the most vulnerable. Causes of gut ischaemia in order of frequency of occurrence are:

- Arterial thromboembolism – by far the commonest.
- Venous insufficiency (as part of a thrombophilic tendency).

- Profound hypotension.
- Vasculitis.

Acute small bowel ischaemia

This is a (rare) medical emergency, characterised by severe abdominal pain with minimal physical signs. In fact in the early stages, when the bowel is most salvageable, the only physical signs are abdominal distension and reduced bowel sounds. The features of the causative condition may be present (generalised atherosclerosis, atrial fibrillation, vasculitis). Epigastric bruits are diagnostic but rare. Rectal bleeding and peritonism are late, and often preterminal, features. Lab features are of a leucocytosis, raised amylase and metabolic acidosis.

Management is with aggressive resuscitation, analgesia and correction of acidosis. CT or mesenteric angiography may show the causative occlusion, but should not delay *early* laparotomy to resect infarcted gut. Mortality is over 80%, and long-term parenteral nutrition is often required in survivors due to the quantity of gut resected.

Chronic intestinal ischaemia

This is a rare condition, characterised by abdominal pain postprandially in an arteriopathic patient. The pain typically starts 30 min after eating and continues for up to 4 hours. Anorexia and weight loss are the sequelae to this meal-related pain. Epigastric bruits are rarely heard.

A variety of radiological techniques are available to image the intestinal arteries. The gold standard is angiography, but less invasive options include duplex ultrasound, CT and MR angiography. Angioplasty or arterial reconstruction is rarely appropriate in these patients, who often have major atherosclerotic comorbidity. Small, frequent meals are advised.

Ischaemic colitis

This is a condition that affects arteriopathic individuals. The typical symptoms are abdominal pain (unrelated to meals), rectal bleeding and occasionally diarrhoea. A more severe, and rarer, fulminant form of the condition may occur, with toxic dilatation and a gangrenous colon.

Abdominal X-ray may show mucosal oedema ('thumb-printing') at the splenic flexure, and a gentle limited colonoscopy may show erythematous and ulcerated mucosa. Biopsy findings of haemosiderin-laden macrophages are diagnostic. Management is by resuscitation and early enteral nutritional support. The prognosis is usually excellent, although colonic strictures may develop later in some patients.

Radiation enterocolitis

Acute radiation enteritis

This affects about 70% of patients in the early weeks after first radiotherapy. Symptoms of vomiting, pain and diarrhoea are usually self-limiting.

Chronic enteritis

Approximately 15% of patients undergoing abdominal or pelvic radiotherapy sustain damage to the gut, the risk depending on cumulative dose and site of exposure. Typically symptoms begin within 12 months of exposure, but may first present 20 years later. The pathology is of an obliterative endarteritis with secondary fibrosis. The latter results in ischaemia, and hence ulceration, perforation, fistulisation or stricturing.

A variety of symptom patterns may occur:

- **Recto-sigmoid**: rectal bleeding, tenesmus, rectal pain and loose stools. Sigmoidoscopy reveals friable, inflamed mucosa, with telangiectatic bleeding. Management of rectal bleeding is with argon plasma coagulation of involved mucosa. Topical 5-ASA compounds, prednisolone, sucralfate and even formaldehyde have all been used. Hyperbaric oxygen may be considered in refractory cases. Surgery is avoided.
- **Faecal incontinence**: the internal anal sphincter is especially vulnerable to ionising radiation, and passive faecal soiling should be managed with loperamide and if needed anal plugs.
- **Diarrhoea** may result from bacterial overgrowth in blind segments formed by strictures or bile salt malabsorption, treated respectively by antibiotics or cholestyramine. A rarer cause of diarrhoea is small bowel fistulae managed by nutritional support and loperamide; surgery is again best avoided.

Prevention of damage is the best treatment. Optimising dose and radiation dosing regimens is critical. Surgical lifting of bowel loops out of the field of radiation, with or without use of bioprotective mesh, is used when heavy localised exposure cannot be avoided.

KEY POINTS

- The two major inflammatory bowel diseases are Crohn's disease and ulcerative colitis.
  - Crohn's disease affects the gut in a non-continuous way. Inflammation involves the full thickness and may cause penetration of the bowel wall.
  - Ulcerative colitis involves the rectum and may extend in a confluent manner to involve up to the whole large bowel.
- Different approaches are needed to induce remission of disease compared to maintaining remission.
  - Corticosteroids may be appropriate to help induce remission and act as a bridge to a longer-term immunosuppression, but are inappropriate as maintenance therapy.
  - 5-aminosalicylic acid preparations are topical anti-inflammatories best used with combination oral and rectal therapy.
  - The thiopurines and methotrexate act by multiple mechanisms, including the inhibition

of purine synthesis, to reduce the number and activity of lymphocytes.
  - Tissue necrosis factor alpha antibodies are often used if thiopurines and methotrexate are unsuccessful.
- Microscopic colitis consist of two histologically distinct conditions: collagenous colitis and lymphocytic colitis.
- The functional gastrointestinal disorders are a spectrum of disorders affecting up to 20% of the general population.
- Ischaemia of the gut can be acute or chronic.
  - Acute small bowel ischaemia is a rare medical emergency treated with aggressive resuscitation, analgesia and correction of acidosis.
  - Chronic intestinal ischaemia is characterised by abdominal pain postprandially in an arteriopathic patient.

 SELF-ASSESSMENT QUESTION

(The answer to this question is given on p. 267)

A 42-year-old man presents with 3 weeks of bloody diarrhoea and abdominal pain. Stool culture is negative, but white cells and red cells are present in the stool. Colonoscopy shows inflammation of the whole colon with granularity, erythema and small ulcers, but no involvement of the terminal ileum. Biopsies from the colon show a mixed inflammatory infiltrate with crypt distortion and crypt abscesses, but no granuloma formation.

Regarding this patient's illness, which of the following statements is most correct?

(a) Testing for the *CARD15/NOD2* gene mutation is likely to be positive in this patient.

(b) Measuring thiopurine methyl transferase levels may guide the dose of thiopurine to be used in this case.

(c) Inflammation of the terminal ileum only occurs in Crohn's disease, not ulcerative colitis.

(d) Corticosteroid therapy can be considered first-line therapy for induction and maintenance of remission in this situation.

(e) Rectally administered 5-aminosalicylic acid is the treatment of choice for this patient.

16

Colon

Colorectal tumours

Colonic polyps

Colonic polyps may be classified histologically as neoplastic or non-neoplastic. They cannot yet be distinguished endoscopically with certainty, although advanced endoscopic techniques are being developed and tested that allow much more accurate endoscopic differentiation of polyp type.

- Neoplastic polyps:
  - Adenoma.
  - Sessile serrated polyp/adenoma (SSP/A).
- Non-neoplastic polyps:
  - Hamartoma.
  - Metaplastic ('hyperplastic').
  - Inflammatory.

Colonic adenomas

Causes and epidemiology

All colonic adenocarcinomas originate from colonic adenomas, but only a small minority of adenomas are premalignant. At least 30% of people in the UK develop an adenoma by age 60 and 3% have a lifetime risk of colorectal cancer. The progression from adenoma to carcinoma takes on average 10 years. Adenomas are classified by endoscopic and histological (Box 16.1) appearance:

- Endoscopic:
  - Pedunculated.
  - Sessile.
  - Flat.

- Histological:
  - Tubular.
  - Villous.
  - Tubulo-villous.
  - Serrated ('saw-tooth' histology).

Investigation and management

Adenomas are usually asymptomatic, detected on surveillance or endoscopy. Occasionally they may bleed, and very rarely villous adenomas cause a mucus diarrhoea.

Colonoscopy and removal of polyps are the gold standard (though it is estimated that 25% of polyps are missed by an average colonoscopist). Histology should determine the histological classification and completeness of removal. The need for and timing interval of future colonoscopy are dependent on the malignant potential of the polyp(s).

Prognosis

Complications of polypectomy are:

- 2% early haemorrhage.
- 2% delayed (up to 2 weeks) haemorrhage.
- 0.5% perforation.
- 30% recurrence of polyp at same site (incomplete removal).

Inherited cancer syndromes

Familial adenomatous polyposis (FAP)

FAP is an uncommon disorder characterised by multiple (>100) colonic adenomas that invariably progress to colorectal cancer unless colectomy is performed in

Gastroenterology and Hepatology: Lecture Notes, Second Edition. Stephen Inns and Anton Emmanuel.
© 2017 John Wiley & Sons, Ltd. Published 2017 by John Wiley & Sons, Ltd.
Companion website: www.lectnoteseries.com/gastroenterology

> **Box 16.1 Histological features defining malignant potential of an adenoma**
>
> - Size (especially >2 cm)
> - Multiplicity of polyps (>5)
> - Histological type (villous > tubulo-villous > tubular > serrated)
> - Histological degree of dysplasia

> **Box 16.2 Amsterdam criteria for diagnosing HNPCC**
>
> - ≥ One HNPCC-related cancer diagnosed < age 50
> - ≥ Two generations with colorectal cancer
> - ≥ Three family members with HNPCC-related cancers, at least one being a first-degree relative

the second or third decade of life. It accounts for 1% of colorectal cancers. The cause is a chromosomal (autosomal dominant) disorder arising from a mutation in the *APC* gene (chromosome 5); about 25% of cases are spontaneous new mutations with no family history. Gastric and duodenal adenomas and carcinomas also occur with greater frequency. **Gardner's syndrome** is a variant associated with osteomas.

The cornerstone of management is early diagnosis and family screening by colonoscopy from teenage years until the age of 40. When polyps are detected pan-proctocolectomy is the treatment of choice, with formation of an ileoanal pouch or end ileostomy. Carcinoma of the ampulla should be screened for, and abdominal pain after colectomy should raise the concern of intra-abdominal desmoid tumours.

Hereditary non-polyposis colorectal cancer (HNPCC)

This autosomal dominant disorder, otherwise known as Lynch syndrome, accounts for 10% of colorectal cancers, and is caused by germline mutations of mismatch repair genes. Primarily right-sided colon cancer develops at a mean age of 45, without the generalised polyposis of FAP, although almost half of patients have metachronous lesions. There is an increased risk of other adenocarcinomas (uterus, ovary, stomach and small bowel).

Management centres on family screening based on the Amsterdam criteria (Box 16.2), undertaken by gene testing. Microsatellite instability is a histological feature of HNPCC tumours, and finding it should trigger consideration of HNPCC. Surveillance upper and lower gastrointestinal endoscopy is required.

Hamartomas

There are specific syndromes in which hamartomatous polyps occur. These syndromes are often associated with greater risk of non-gut cancers (breast, thyroid):

- **Peutz–Jegher syndrome**:
  - Multiple small hamartomas in small bowel *and* colon.
  - Buccal and labial melanin pigmentation.
  - Autosomal dominant inheritance.
  - Hamartomas are usually asymptomatic, but may rarely bleed or form the focus of intussusception.
- **Juvenile polyposis**:
  - Large pedunculated vascular polyps in small bowel *and* colon.
  - Specific gene mutations with autosomal dominant inheritance.
  - Colorectal cancer risk of ~40%, gastric cancer risk of ~20%.
  - Treatment is with endoscopic polypectomy if there are a few polyps, but with heavy polyp density colectomy is recommended. Family screening for the gene mutation should be performed.
- **Cowden's disease**:
  - Gastric, small bowel and cutaneous hamartomas.
  - Autosomal dominant inheritance.
  - Multiple congenital abnormalities.
- **Cronkhite–Canada syndrome**:
  - A non-inherited disorder.
  - Diffuse gastrointestinal hamartomas (including gastric).
  - Malabsorption.
  - Alopecia and nail dystrophy.

Metaplastic polyps

These are extremely common, usually small (<5 mm) polyps found in the rectum.

Inflammatory polyps

These are known as 'pseudo-polyps' since they represent exuberant mucosal regrowth after a severe episode of colitis.

Colorectal adenocarcinoma
Epidemiology

This is the second commonest cancer in the UK, with 30,000 cases per year, two-thirds of which result in death. The majority (75%) are sporadic, 10–12% occur in relation to the inherited polyposis syndromes, 10%

have some other family history and 2% are related to inflammatory bowel disease (IBD).

Causes

The adenoma–carcinoma sequence (Figure 16.1) is widely accepted as the mechanism resulting in most colorectal cancers. The main exceptions are IBD-related colorectal cancers, and SSA/P related cancers in which BRAF mutation may play a role.

- **Risk factors**:
  - Genetic (as per sequence described).
  - Dietary:
    - Exacerbating – red meat, saturated animal fats.
    - Protective – dietary fibre (cereal and fruit/vegetable), folic acid.
  - Chronic inflammation (IBD [see Chapter 15], prior ureterosigmoidostomy).
  - Medical conditions (primary sclerosing cholangitis, acromegaly, obesity).
  - Smoking.

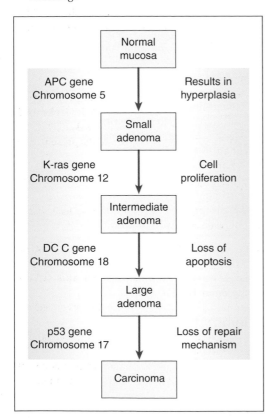

Figure 16.1 Adenoma–carcinoma sequence *APC*, adenomatous polyposis coli; *DCC*, deleted in colon cancer (this *DCC* gene has the least strong evidence of involvement in this sequence).

- **Location**:
  - 65% rectosigmoid.
  - 10% left and transverse colon.
  - 25% right colon.
  - (NB: 5% are synchronous.)
  - Spread occurs early through bowel wall, then into lymphatics, and later by portal and systemic circulations.

Clinical features

Depend on location of the tumour:

- Rectal bleeding, rectal and left colon tumours (remember that presence of haemorrhoids does not preclude the possibility of comorbid cancer).
- Altered bowel habit – especially in distal tumours.
- Anorexia, weight loss, abdominal mass and anaemia – especially caecal cancers.
- Intestinal obstruction or perforation is rare – especially in distal tumours.
- Tenesmus – in rectal cancers.
- Abdominal pain – a non-specific symptom.

Investigations

- **Condition**:
  - Rigid sigmoidoscopy (will detect 30% of tumours).
  - Flexible sigmoidoscopy – for any patients with fresh rectal bleeding.
  - Colonoscopy if:
    - Altered bowel habit.
    - Polyps seen at flexible sigmoidoscopy.
    - Family history of colorectal cancer.
    - Surveillance of IBD or polyps; endoscopic examination allows histological specimens to be collected.
  - Barium enema: apple-core strictures or ulcerated defects may be seen, but sensitivity is less than with colonoscopy.
  - CT colonography ('virtual colonoscopy'): more comfortable than colonoscopy; but does involve radiation exposure, bowel preparation is still needed, histology is not possible and resolution is less than with colonoscopy.
  - FBC and iron studies: supportive of diagnosis.
  - Serum carcinoma embryonic antigen (CEA): of supportive value, but note false positives and negatives are not infrequent.
- **Complications** staging:
  - LFTs.
  - CT abdomen: for local spread and liver metastases.
  - Pelvic MRI: needed for staging of rectal cancers.
- **Staging**: use of Dukes' staging and TNM staging systems (Tables 16.1 and 16.2).

Table 16.1 Dukes' staging for colorectal cancer.

Dukes' stage	Description	Prevalence at diagnosis (%)	5-year survival (%)
Dukes' A (T_{1-2}, N_0, M_0)	Tumour confined to bowel wall	10	95
Dukes' B (T_{3-4}, N_0, M_0)	Tumour extends through bowel wall	35	75
Dukes' C (T_{any}, N_1, M_0)	Tumour through bowel wall and involves lymph nodes	35	35
Dukes' D (T_{any}, N_{either}, M_1)	Distant metastases	20	1

Table 16.2 TNM staging for colorectal cancer.

Stage	Description
T – primary tumour	T_0 – no evidence of tumour
	T_{1-4} – varying depths of invasion
N – lymph nodes	N_0 – no nodes
	N_1 – positive nodes
M – metastases	M_0 – no metastases
	M_1 – metastases

Management

Decided at multidisciplinary team (MDT) meetings.

Surgery

Suitable for Dukes' A and B tumours.

- **Basic principles**:
  - Tumour resection.
  - Direct anastomosis if possible.
  - Clear resection margins.
  - Sampling of lymph nodes.
- **Rectal cancers**: total mesorectal excision reduces recurrence; cancers within 2 cm of the anus require abdominoperineal (AP) resection and colostomy.

Adjuvant therapy

This may be pre- or postoperative, by radiotherapy or chemotherapy.

- **Colon cancer**:
  - Chemotherapy (5-fluoro-uracil or irinotecan) for Dukes' C or B with T_4.
  - Radiotherapy is only used for palliation.
- **Rectal cancer**:
  - Preoperative radiotherapy or chemoradiotherapy is used for Dukes' B and C cancers to downsize the tumour and improve postoperative survival.
  - Postoperative chemotherapy is also widely employed.

Palliation

- **Surgery**:
  - To treat obstruction, intractable bleeding or pain.
  - Liver resection of metastases.
- **Chemotherapy or radiotherapy**:
  - Sometimes used for tenesmus, pain.
- **Endoscopy**:
  - Laser therapy for bleeding (not widely available).
  - Expandable metal stent insertion for obstruction in a non-resectable patient.

Prognosis

This depends on the cancer stage at presentation: 5-year survival for Dukes' A is > 90%, for Dukes' B is 77%, for Dukes' C is 48% and for Dukes' D is 6%. Survival rates are halved if patients present with obstruction.

Prevention

The intention is to detect and destroy lesions at a premalignant stage:

- Faecal occult blood test (FOBT): performed every 1–2 years after age 60 in the UK, increases the proportion of early cancers detected and reduces mortality by 16%.
- Flexible sigmoidoscopy: more invasive, reduces mortality by 35%.
- Colonoscopy: gold standard, but impractical as a screening test.
- Faecal and blood gene mutation testing is not yet sensitive enough to be considered at this time.

Surveillance

- Colonoscopy 6–12 months after colon cancer resection to detect metachronous lesions.
- CT scan of the abdomen to identify resectable liver metastases.

Chemoprevention

- Aspirin reduces risk of recurrent adenomas after colorectal cancer surgery by 35%; COX-2 inhibitors are not indicated.
- Optimising calcium and folic acid intake is generally recommended.

Miscellaneous colonic disorders

Colonic diverticular disease

Epidemiology

Colonic diverticula increase in prevalence with age, and are most common in the developed world. 50% of over 50-year-olds have 'diverticulosis', which are asymptomatic diverticula. In the Western world, diverticula are most prevalent in the sigmoid and left colon, while in Oriental populations and the rare under 40-year-old who develops them, right-sided disease is commoner. Diverticula never occur in the rectum. The term 'diverticular disease' refers to patients having symptomatic diverticula, and 'diverticulitis' refers to diverticula causing complications (bleeding, inflammation, stricturing, perforation). The relationship between these terms is shown in Figure 16.2.

Cause

A diet, especially in early life, which is low in unrefined fibre is the traditional explanation of diverticulosis and explains the geographical variability of the problem, and the changes seen with epidemiological studies of migrant populations. With a low-fibre diet, the resulting stools are small volume and require greater colonic pressure for propulsion, explaining the circular muscle hypertrophy seen in diverticula. The elevated pressures result in mucosal herniation between taenia coli muscles of the colon. Faeces may impact in the neck of these diverticula, resulting in inflammation, which may either spontaneously resolve or more rarely lead to haemorrhage, perforation and so on.

Clinical syndromes and treatment

- **Uncomplicated diverticulosis**: symptoms of colicky left iliac fossa pain eased by defaecation, passage of pellet stools and abdominal bloating are typical. The possibility of colorectal cancer always requires exclusion in view of the prevalence of diverticula. Colonoscopy is diagnostic and helps exclude other lesions, but carries the small risk of perforation. Rigid sigmoidoscopy with histology and a CT colonography is an alternative strategy. Treatment is by increasing dietary fluid and fibre intake, hence improving stool output and preventing further diverticula formation.

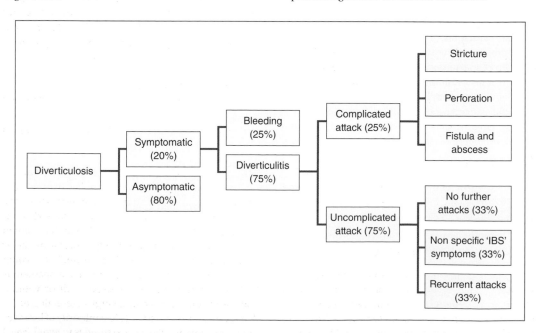

Figure 16.2 Possible presentations with colonic diverticula. IBS, irritable bowel syndrome.

- **Diverticular bleeding**: there is often right-sided bleeding, so visible blood loss may not occur. Greatest risks are in elderly men and those taking NSAIDs or warfarin. Most settle with simple observation. Major haemorrhage occurs in about one-third of cases, and rebleeding rates increase with time and number of prior bleeds. Nevertheless, anaemia and altered bowel habit should *not* be assumed to be due to diverticula until cancer and IBD have been ruled out.
- **Diverticulitis**: characterised by pain, fever, raised white count and inflammatory markers ('left-sided appendicitis'). Colonoscopy is contraindicated acutely, but a CT will demonstrate any abscess:
  - *Mild cases* are managed with oral antibiotics (metronidazole and a cephalosporin or ciprofloxacin) and analgesia.
  - *Severe cases* may need hospitalisation for intravenous antibiotics.
  - *Complicated attacks* (stricture, perforation, fistula, abscess) require surgery. Fistulation (to bladder or vagina) occurs in 20%; mortality following perforation is high.
  - *Uncomplicated attacks* only need consideration of elective surgical therapy if there is:
    - Localised diverticula.
    - Frequent recurrence.
    - Episodes beginning at a young age (known to run a more recurrent course).

Prognosis

Approximately 80–85% of patients remain asymptomatic. The incidence of diverticulitis in patients with diverticulosis is widely debated, but appears to approach 10%. Once diverticulitis develops, the outcome depends on the complications sustained, as outlined earlier.

Megacolon

Congenital (Hirschsprung's disease) and acquired (idiopathic megacolon and megarectum) forms are recognised.

Hirschsprung's disease

Caused by congenital aganglionosis of the colon, resulting from defective migration of neuroblasts into the embryonic hindgut. It is a rare cause of constipation and a family history is present in 35% of cases; some hereditary causes are associated with a specific gene mutation (*RET* tyrosine kinase).

The absence of submucosal ganglia is usually localised to the distal rectum, but may be widespread in the hindgut (sigmoid colon). This results in defective anorectal reflexes, in particular the absence of the internal anal sphincter relaxation in response to rectal filling ('rectoanal inhibitory reflex'). This results in constipation, abdominal distension and vomiting; most cases present in neonatal life, although up to 10% present in adolescents and adults. Diagnosis is established by demonstrating the absence of the rectoanal inhibitory reflex on physiological testing (*condition*). In addition, barium enema will show the narrowed aganglionic segment and dilatation proximal to that. The *cause* may be identified through surgically obtained full-thickness biopsies of the rectum and appropriate immunohistochemistry. Treatment involves resection of the localised segment.

Idiopathic megacolon and megarectum

This condition may be localised to the rectum or may more extensively involve the colon. Constipation with infrequent urge to defaecate is common to both megarectum and megacolon, but the former is more often associated with faecal soiling. Faecal impaction and overflow incontinence are the main complication. In children, the condition is thought to result from disturbed toileting behaviour in toddlers, with voluntary avoidance of toilets and withholding of stools. The differential is with Hirschsprung's disease, from which it is distinct due to:

- Absence of a lifelong history.
- Frequent report of faecal soiling (which does not occur in Hirschsprung's).
- Presence of stool in the rectum on digital examination.

Adult megacolon may be associated with dementia or depression, scleroderma, chronic opiate use and neurological disorders like multiple sclerosis. Diagnosis is confirmed by unprepared contrast study demonstrating continuous colonic dilatation until a point of abrupt transition to proximally normal-diameter colon. (NB: By contrast, in Hirschsprung's, the colon proximal to the narrowing is dilated.) Management is by titrated use of osmotic laxative with or without enemas to empty the rectum. Surgical resection of the dilated colon is required only in a minority of laxative-refractory patients. The cornerstone is to avoid faecal impaction and overflow.

Acute colonic pseudo-obstruction ('Ogilvie's syndrome')

Characterised by sudden, painless distension of the colon in the absence of mechanical obstruction, this is often due to disturbance of the retroperitoneal autonomic nerves (e.g. secondary to abdominal surgery, retroperitoneal tumour invasion, abdominal trauma, diabetic autonomic neuropathy). It may occur secondary to metabolic disturbance (e.g. electrolyte disturbance, uraemia, respiratory failure). Examination reveals abdominal distension and increased bowel sounds. The *condition* is confirmed by plain abdominal X-ray showing the dilated gut, and contrast study will exclude a mechanical cause of obstruction.

Management depends on reversing the cause if possible. The parasympathomimetic neostigmine may help to deflate the colon and ease symptoms. If urgent decompression is required (due to the risk of perforation with gross colonic distension), then a rectally placed flatus tube or careful colonic decompression is preferable to surgical caecostomy.

Pneumatosis cystoides intestinalis

This is a rare condition with multiple gas-filled submucosal cysts in the colon (and rarely small bowel). It is usually asymptomatic, but diarrhoea, rectal bleeding and pain may occur. The cysts may be seen on abdominal X-rays or lower GI endoscopy. If treatment is required for severe symptoms, 70% inspired oxygen for 5 days via a mask and non-rebreather gives long-term benefit. Elemental diets may also help.

 KEY POINTS

- Colonic polyps are either neoplastic or non-neoplastic.
  - Neoplastic polyps are either adenomas or sessile serrated polyp/adenomas.
  - Non-neoplastic polyps include hamartomas, metaplastic ('hyperplastic') and inflammatory polyps.
- All colonic adenocarcinomas originate from colonic adenomas, but only a small minority of adenomas are premalignant.
- Colorectal cancer screening and surveillance are aimed at detecting and destroying lesions at a premalignant stage.
- Hereditary non-polyposis colorectal cancer accounts for 10% of colorectal cancers. It is caused by mutations of the mismatch repair genes. Management centres on genetic screening and endoscopic surveillance in affected families.
- Familial adenomatous polyposis is caused by a mutation of the APC gene (chromosome 5). Endoscopic surveillance is the initial management strategy, but many patients opt for prophylactic colectomy.
- Intestinal hamartomas occur in Peutz–Jegher syndrome, Cowden's disease and Cronkhite–Canada syndrome.
- Colonic diverticular disease is very common and increases in prevalence with age. Approximately 80–85% of patients remain asymptomatic, but diverticulitis occurs in up to 10%.

 SELF-ASSESSMENT QUESTION

(The answer to this question is given on p. 267)

A 43-year-old man is referred by his GP for consideration of colonoscopy. His father died of colorectal cancer aged 51. His uncle is well following a sigmoid colectomy for cancer aged 60. His grandfather also died of colorectal cancer in his 50s. At colonoscopy he is found to have a 4 cm fungating lesion in the sigmoid colon and a 1 cm polyp in the transverse colon. Sigmoid colectomy reveals a Duke's A adenocarcinoma and the excised polyp is a tubular adenoma.

Regarding this man's clinical situation, which of the following statements is most correct?

(a) The most likely familial syndrome in this setting is familial adenomatous polyposis.

(b) You would expect a mutation on chromosome 5 to be the cause of this family's high rate of colon cancer.

(c) This patient should be offered prophylactic colectomy.

(d) This man's tumour should be tested for microsatellite instability.

(e) Lynch syndrome is a variant of familial adenomatous polyposis that is associated with osteomas.

17

Anorectum

Haemorrhoids

These are commonly occurring dilatations of anal veins surrounded by tissue. *Internal* haemorrhoids originate above the dentate line, and comprise a venous branch of the internal haemorrhoidal plexus surrounded by rectal mucosa. *External* haemorrhoids arise below the dentate line and comprise a branch of the inferior venous plexus overlain by anal skin. Over half the population has haemorrhoids, being especially common in situations where there is raised intra abdominal pressure (chronic constipation, pregnancy, chronic cough).

Haemorrhoids most commonly present with the sensation of a lump at the anus. They are classified as:

- First-degree: internal haemorrhoids move into the anal canal.
- Second-degree: haemorrhoids prolapsed out of the anus on straining, but spontaneously reduce.
- Third-degree: as second-degree, but need manual reduction.
- Fourth-degree: as second-degree, but cannot be reduced.

The other classic presentation is with rectal bleeding, typically in small quantities of fresh blood on the toilet tissue. Rarely, haemorrhoids may:

- Cause passive faecal or mucus leakage (and hence pruritus ani).
- Thrombose (causing severe pain).

Diagnosis is usually obvious on anal inspection and asking the patient to strain gently. If no lump is visible, anoscopy may be required.

Management

First- and second-degree haemorrhoids will usually respond to non-surgical approaches as an outpatient, whereas third- and fourth-degree piles usually need haemorrhoidectomy (Table 17.1). Most people have an excellent prognosis and require only intermittent treatment.

Anal fissure

Epidemiology and causes

This is a tear of the skin of the anal canal. Incidence is around 1 in 350 adults. It is equally common in men and women, and often affects young adults aged 15 to 40, although it may be seen in older adults. It may also occur in children due to poor toileting.

Typically anal fissures occur in the posterior midline, where anal blood flow is lowest and the anal skin is least supported. Internal anal sphincter spasm also contributes to the development of an anal fissure.

They occur most often in patients with:

- Constipation (by far the commonest cause).
- Crohn's disease.
- Anorectal infection (TB and HIV patients).
- Haematological malignancy.

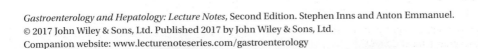

Gastroenterology and Hepatology: Lecture Notes, Second Edition. Stephen Inns and Anton Emmanuel.
© 2017 John Wiley & Sons, Ltd. Published 2017 by John Wiley & Sons, Ltd.
Companion website: www.lecturenoteseries.com/gastroenterology

Table 17.1 Management of haemorrhoids.

General	Non-surgical	Surgical
Correct constipation (especially with diet alteration or bulk laxatives)	Rubber band ligation (complications: pain, bleeding, infection)	Stapled haemorrhoidectomy – with a mini bowel anastomosis device (complications: pain, incomplete excision)
Avoiding straining Local anaesthetic suppositories or creams	Injection sclerotherapy (complications: infection, ulceration)	Open haemorrhoidectomy (complications: pain, anal stenosis, infection)
	Photocoagulation (complications: pain, ulceration)	

Clinical features

Fissures present with pain, which begins with defaecation but then continues afterwards. Blood loss is common, but not invariable. The diagnosis is evident on inspection, but examination can be very uncomfortable for the patient. Typical features are:

- Breach in the anal skin.
- 'Sentinel' pile (actually a skin tag that grows near the fissure).
- Muscle fibres of the internal sphincter (with severe fissuring).

Management

Treatment options are listed in Table 17.2.

Internal anal sphincterotomy surgery is reserved for refractory fissures only, due to the risk of faecal incontinence.

Prognosis

Medical therapy works more than 80% of the time in treating and preventing future anal fissures. If surgery is required, the success rate is often greater than 95% in preventing recurrences.

Anal fistula

Epidemiology and causes

A fistula is a pathological connection between the gut and skin, in this situation the anal canal and perianal skin. They occur more often in men and typically in the third and fourth decades. The true prevalence of anal fistulas is unknown. The incidence of an anal fistula developing from an anal abscess ranges from 26% to 38%.

Table 17.2 Management of anal fissure.

First-line	Second-line	Third-line
Correct constipation (especially with diet alteration or bulk laxatives)	Topical nitroglycerin or diltiazem	Botox injection
Avoiding straining		
Local anaesthetic suppositories or creams		

At-risk groups:

- Crohn's disease.
- Prior anal surgery.
- Prior pelvic radiation.
- Prior pelvic trauma.

Clinical features

Typically there is anal discomfort or itching. Loss of faecal material and pus are more common than bleeding.

Investigations

Inspection reveals the external opening, while endoscopy rarely identifies the internal one. MRI and endoanal ultrasound are essential to help identify the internal sphincter tracks prior to surgery. Classification (see Figure 17.1) is based on whether:

- Track crosses the sphincters (trans-sphincteric), is in between them (inter-sphincteric) or outside them (extrasphincteric), or
- Internal opening is above (high) or below (low) puborectalis muscle.

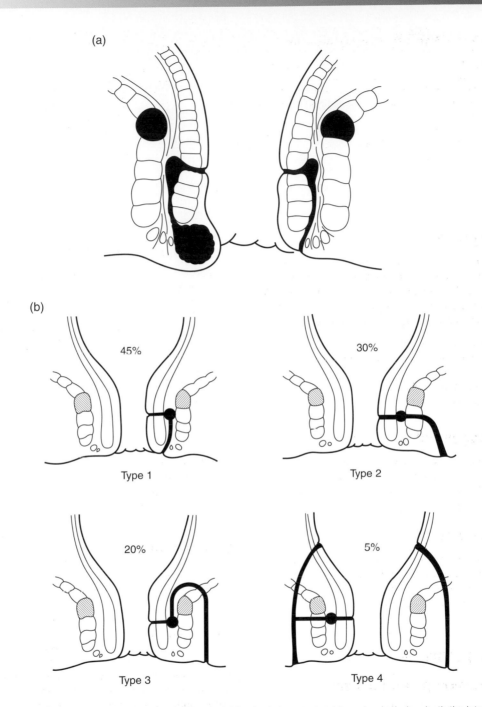

Figure 17.1 Classification of anal fistula. (a) A superficial fistula, the commonest type, tracks below both the internal anal sphincter and external anal sphincter complexes and presents as perianal abscess. (b) Type 1. An intersphincteric fistula tracks between the internal anal sphincter and the external anal sphincter in the intersphincteric space. Type 2. A transsphincteric fistula tracks from the intersphincteric space through the external anal sphincter. Type 3. A suprasphincteric fistula leaves the intersphincteric space over the top of the puborectalis and penetrates the levator muscle before tracking down to the skin. Type 4. An extrasphincteric fistula tracks outside of the external anal sphincter and penetrates the levator muscle into the rectum. Source: Parks AG, Gordon PH, Hardcastle JD. A classification of fistula-in-ano. Br J Surg. 1976 Jan;63(1):1–12. Reproduced with permission of John Wiley & Sons.

Management

The principles of surgery are to obtain drainage of all fistulae and to lay open or cut out the tracks to stop them spreading and causing further fistulae. Rarely, a defunctioning stoma may be needed to cover a complex fistula repair.

Prognosis

Depending on the thickness of sphincter muscle the fistula transgresses, surgery carries a greater or lesser risk of causing incontinence. For this sphincter-preserving techniques have been developed, but in these more complex situations the recurrence rate is 30–50%, often resulting in multiple operations.

Anal pain and itch

Anal pain can be caused by a number of organic conditions:

- Perianal Crohn's disease (see p. XX).
- Anal fissure.
- Thrombosed haemorrhoids (see p. XX).
- Radiation proctitis (see p. XX).
- Anorectal abscess (following blockage of an anal gland).

In addition, there are functional conditions that can cause anal discomfort (Table 17.3).

Anal cancers

Epidemiology and causes

Histologically, a variety of cancers may arise. Each year there is 1 new anal cancer case for every 100,000 males in the UK, and 2 for every 100,000 females. Most patients present in their fifth or sixth decades. Squamous cell carcinoma occurs with the greatest frequency (80%), the rest are rarer:

- Anal squamous cell cancer (of which there are three subtypes: transitional epithelium, squamous epithelium or keratinised perianal skin).
- Anal adenocarcinoma.
- Basal cell carcinoma.
- Bowen's disease.
- Perianal Paget's disease.
- Malignant melanoma.

  Particular at-risk groups for **anal cancer** include:

- HIV infection.
- HPV (human papilloma virus) infection.
- Syphilis.
- People participating in anoreceptive intercourse.
- Prior perianal Crohn's disease or fistulae.
- Prior pelvic irradiation.
- People who have received immunosuppression.
- Smokers.

Table 17.3 Clinical features and management of conditions causing anal pain.

	Proctalgia fugax	Levator ani syndrome	Pruritus ani
Type of pain	Episodic, intense	Episodic, intense	Itch around anus
Duration of pain	Seconds (<20 s)	Minutes (<30 min)	Chronic (worse at night)
Epidemiology	Males especially, under 40s	Females especially, over 40s	Males especially
Associated symptoms	Faecal urgency, syncope	Difficult evacuation	Depend on cause (see below)
Digital examination	Normal tone, painless	Sphincter spasm and puborectalis tenderness	Exclude worms or candida Look for eczema and psoriasis
Treatment	Explanation and reassurance Acute treatment with inhaled salbutamol or topical GTN Chronic treatment with diet or psychotherapy	Explanation and reassurance Pelvic floor physiotherapy and sitz baths	Explanation and reassurance Avoid scratching and over-zealous cleaning Increase diet fibre and use wet-wipes Local anaesthetic cream

GTN, glyceryl trinitrate.

Investigations

Diagnosis often requires examination under anaesthesia and biopsy.

Management

Treatment depends on size of lesion:

- Involving mucosa/submucosa only: wide local excision.
- More advanced lesions: abdominoperineal resection.

Combination chemotherapy and radiotherapy may sometimes be added.

Prognosis

5-year survival rates depend on stage of disease and are better for squamous cancers than non-squamous cancers. They range from 71% for stage I squamous carcinoma down to just 7% for stage IV non-squamous cancer.

Rectal prolapse

Causes and epidemiology

This occurs most frequently in women over the age of 50 who have had children. The prevalence is estimated at 1% in adults over age 65 years. Other *at-risk groups* include:

- Patients who chronically strain.
- Patients with cystic fibrosis (where rectal prolapse can occur in childhood).
- Spina bifida.
- Congenital mesenchymal disorders (e.g. Marfan's syndrome).

Clinical features

In the early stages there is prolapse of the mucosa only, and in more severe forms the whole rectal wall is externalised (and very rarely may be life-threateningly

incarcerated). Patients usually present with the sensation of a mass on wiping. They may passively soil stool, but blood loss and pain are rare.

Examination while straining will reveal the prolapse, and this may need to be done with the patient seated on the toilet.

Management

Mild forms may be managed by biofeedback to retrain defaecatory coordination. More severe prolapse will need surgery, which can be transanal, perineal or transabdominal.

Prognosis

Most children (90%) who develop prolapse will have a spontaneous resolution, but in adults the outcome depends on the severity of prolapse, any underlying causes, age and comorbidities.

Solitary rectal ulcer syndrome

Mucosal ischaemia and ulceration resulting from repeated straining, anal self-digitation and rectal prolapse cause loss of blood and mucus per rectum. This typically occurs in young women, and there will often be a prior history of constipation and psychological distress. The condition is easily identified at sigmoidoscopy with single or multiple ulcers, typically on the anterior rectal wall, in the distal 10 cm.

Management

Treatment is initially through biofeedback, to avoid straining and digitation. Laxatives may be needed, but suppositories and enemas are best not used to avoid the cycle of recurrent digitation. Rarely, surgical therapy may be needed, especially if heavy bleeding occurs or if the problem is recurrent.

KEY POINTS

- Over half the population have haemorrhoids. These are classified according to whether they prolapse through the anal canal and whether they reduce.

- Anal fissure occurs in the posterior midline most often. The commonest predisposition is constipation, but it may be associated with Crohn's disease (less common) and other chronic conditions (rare).

- Anal fistula may be idiopathic but particularly occurs in Crohn's disease, prior anal surgery, prior pelvic radiation and prior pelvic trauma.

- Classification of anal fistulae, and subsequent treatment, is based on whether the track:
  - Crosses the sphincters (trans-sphincteric)
  - Is in between them (inter-sphincteric)
  - Is outside them (extrasphincteric), or
  - The internal opening is above (high) or below (low) puborectalis muscle

- Anal cancers are made up of a variety of cancers, Squamous cell carcinoma being the most common. Treatment is surgical, according to the extent of disease.

- Rectal prolapse occurs in 1% of adults over age 65 years. Examination while straining will reveal the prolapse. Treatment may be conservative or surgical.

- Solitary rectal ulcer syndrome is where mucosal ischaemia and ulceration result from repeated straining and is treated by methods to avoid straining.

SELF-ASSESSMENT QUESTION

(The answer to this question is given on p. 268)

An 80-year-old woman presents complaining of a lump that she feels at her anus after opening her bowels. It is associated with perianal irritation and itch.

Regarding her presenting complaint, which of the following statements is most correct?

(a) Digital rectal examination will quickly rule out anal prolapse.

(b) It is unlikely that she has second-degree haemorrhoids, as these would require manual reduction.

(c) The most likely anal cancer she might have is adenocarcinoma.

(d) Rectal prolapse is a rare condition affecting less than 0.1% of adults over 65 years of age.

(e) Asking her to sit on the toilet and strain may help to differentiate the cause.

18

Pancreatic diseases

The pancreas, through the production of pancreatic secretions, serves vital *exocrine* digestive functions and acts as the site of production of the *endocrine* hormones, insulin and glucagon, controlling glucose homeostasis. Self-digestion by exocrine products is prevented by a carefully balanced suppressor system; disruption of that system by a variety of causes can result in pancreatic inflammation, called pancreatitis. When recurrent, pancreatitis can cause scarring and destruction of pancreatic tissue, with resultant loss of exocrine and/or endocrine functions.

Pancreatic anatomy

The pancreas is made up of distinct lobules, which are connected by loose areolar tissue that also surrounds the entire gland. Each lobule consists of connective tissue surrounding alveoli, or pouches, that are tubular and almost completely filled with secretory cells. These then join with the ducts of the lobules that drain to the pancreatic duct (Figure 18.1). The islands of connective tissue between the alveoli are termed the islets of Langerhan and contain two types of cells, known as A and B cells, depending on the pattern of staining of the secretory granules they contain; they produce the endocrine secretions of the pancreas involved in glucose homeostasis.

The secretory product of the pancreas, the pancreatic juice, is carried by the pancreatic duct to the duodenum and there aids digestion, mainly by lipolysis of fats.

The gland has three parts: the right extremity, being broad, is called the *head*, and is connected to the main portion of the organ, or *body*, by a slight constriction, the neck, while its left extremity gradually tapers to form the *tail*. Its length varies from 12.5–15 cm, and its weight from 60–100 g.

The pancreatic duct commences in the tail, where the small ducts from the pancreatic lobules join. It runs from left to right through the body, receiving further ducts along the way. Finally it comes into relation with the common bile duct and leaves the head of the gland, passing very obliquely through the mucous and muscular coats of the duodenum, and exiting at the orifice of the papilla of Vater in the descending duodenum. There is often also an additional duct, known as the accessory duct, which is given off from the pancreatic duct in the neck of the pancreas and opens into the duodenum about 2.5 cm above the duodenal papilla. (See also Figure 10.1.)

Embryology

The pancreas develops in two parts. The dorsal part arises as a diverticulum from the dorsal side of the duodenum, just proximal to the hepatic diverticulum. This dorsal part forms part of the head, the body and the tail. The ventral part develops from a diverticulum that forms from the bile duct and goes on to form the remainder of the head and uncinate process.

At this stage each part has its own duct. The duct of the dorsal part (later known as the accessory pancreatic duct) opens independently, while the duct of the ventral part opens with the common bile duct. At about 6 weeks the two parts fuse and form a communication between the two ducts. The pancreatic duct continues to increase in diameter with development,

Gastroenterology and Hepatology: Lecture Notes, Second Edition. Stephen Inns and Anton Emmanuel.
© 2017 John Wiley & Sons, Ltd. Published 2017 by John Wiley & Sons, Ltd.
Companion website: www.lecturenoteseries.com/gastroenterology

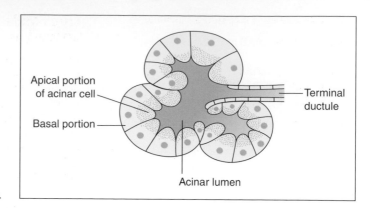

Figure 18.1 Pancreatic acinar structure.

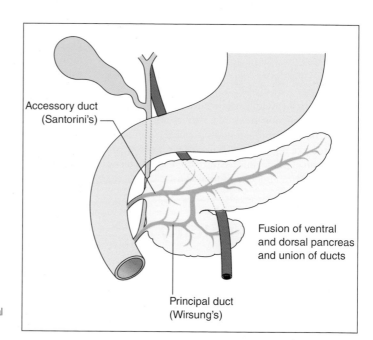

Figure 18.2 Pancreatoduodenal anatomy showing the developing ductal systems.

whereas the accessory duct remains small and its opening may even be obliterated (Figure 18.2).

While initially the pancreas lies intra-peritoneally between the two layers of the dorsal mesogastrium, movement of the stomach draws the dorsal mesogastrium down and to the left. The right surface of the pancreas becomes applied to the posterior abdominal wall, with absorption of the peritoneum covering it, resulting in the posterior aspect of the gland in the adult being devoid of peritoneum and in contact with the aorta, left kidney and its vessels and other retroperitoneal structures.

Physiology

Digestive enzymes

In the acinar cells enzymes are synthesised by the ribosomes of the rough endoplasmic reticulum. These enzymes are then stored, in either active or precursor (pro-enzyme) states, within 'zymogen' granules at the apices of the cell. Cholecystokinin (CCK) release in response to a meal results in release of these enzymes and pro-enzymes into the ductules.

The digestive enzymes produced include:

- Amylase for carbohydrates.
- Lipases for fats.
- Proteases for proteins.
- Nucleases for DNA and RNA.

Luminal digestion of carbohydrate, protein and fat reduces them to smaller molecules, which can be absorbed by the intestinal cells, either directly or following digestion by enzymes on the brush border of these cells.

Amylase

Amylases hydrolyse polysaccharides in starch and glycogen to maltose and other small oligosaccharides, which can then be cleaved to glucose by brush border enzymes in the small intestinal mucosa. Salivary glands also produce amylase.

Lipases

The fatty acids of triglycerides in food are hydrolysed off by lipase, producing free fatty acids. This is aided by the conversion of pro-co-lipase from the acinar cells to co-lipase in the small intestine. Co-lipase prevents bile salts from inhibiting the lipolysis of triglycerides.

Prophospholipase A is converted to phospholipase A by trypsin in the small intestine. This then hydrolyses fatty acids from lecithin and phosphatidyl ethanolamine.

Proteases

Trypsin is secreted from the acinar cells as trypsinogen and activated principally in the upper small intestine brush border by an enterokinase. While the pancreas protects itself from its own proteolytic enzymes by secreting them as inactive proenzymes, trypsin may be 'autoactivated' in the acinar cell. Damage by inappropriately activated trypsin is prevented by a trypsin inhibitor that can inhibit activated trypsin and proteases that can cleave trypsin.

Activated trypsin is important as the common activator of other pancreatic enzymes, including more trypsinogen, chymotrypsinogen, proelastase, procarboxypeptidases and prophospholipase. Trypsin acts to hydrolyse peptide bonds within the polypeptide chain of proteins.

Nucleotidases

Ribonuclease and deoxyribonuclease digest, respectively, RNA and DNA.

Duct cells and bicarbonate secretion

Pancreatic enzymes require a neutral pH to function. This environment is promoted by the secretion of sodium bicarbonate by pancreatic duct cells to neutralise the gastric acid that enters the duodenum. Pancreatic bicarbonate secretion is stimulated by secretin from endocrine cells in the duodenal mucosa. The normal pancreas secretes about 2 l of pancreatic juice per day, containing 9–18 g of bicarbonate, most of which is reabsorbed by the intestine.

There are two main mechanisms for the production of sodium bicarbonate:

- Pancreatic duct cells use carbonic anhydrase to catalyse the conversion of carbon dioxide and water ($H_2O + CO_2 \rightarrow H_2CO_3^- \rightarrow H^+ + HCO_3^-$);
- An Na^+ / HCO_3^- co-transporter located on the basolateral membrane of duct cells can transport sodium into cells followed by transport of HCO_3^- into the duct lumen by a HCO_3^- / Cl^- exchanger.

Chronic pancreatitis

Epidemiology and causes

Chronic pancreatitis has a population incidence of 3.5–10 in 100,000 in industrialised countries. It is more common in men (4:1). In the Western world the major association is with alcohol abuse (80% of cases).

Much rarer factors include:

- Pancreatic duct obstruction (from strictures).
- Metabolic disturbance (hypertriglyceridaemia, hypercalcaemia).
- Genetic mutations:
  - Defects in the cystic fibrosis transmembrane conductance regulator (*CFTR*) gene cause pancreatitis in cystic fibrosis, but may also play a role in predisposing individuals without cystic fibrosis to chronic pancreatitis.
  - In both tropical pancreatitis and pancreatitis in children, mutations in a serine protease inhibitor gene (*SPINK1*) have been demonstrated in a subgroup of cases: the *SPINK 1* gene product normally inhibits up to 20% of trypsin activity and may predispose to pancreatitis by loss of this mechanism.
  - There is a rare genetic form of chronic pancreatitis closely associated with mutations in the cationic trypsinogen gene; inheritance is autosomal dominant with disease penetrance of about 80%.

- Autoimmunity:
  ◦ A steroid-responsive form of chronic pancreatitis has been more clearly characterised and termed autoimmune pancreatitis.

At times no cause can be found and idiopathic chronic pancreatitis is diagnosed, but the incidence of this continues to decrease with improvements in diagnostic techniques.

Clinical features

History taking

In taking a history it is essential that careful attention is paid to alcohol history. Ancillary history from family members may be necessary. Questions should also be asked about any family history of pancreatitis, personal or family history of autoimmune disorders, use of prescription and illicit drugs, and travel history.

Main presenting complaints

The three major clinical features of chronic pancreatitis are:

- **Pain**: often the major and most difficult to manage clinical problem in chronic pancreatitis. The pain is usually epigastric and may radiate to the back. Because severe pain decreases appetite, it can also contribute to anorexia. Pain can be intermittent or continuous. It should be noted that 10–15% of patients never have pain and present with malabsorption.
- **Maldigestion**: recurrent inflammation in chronic pancreatitis may result in so much glandular destruction that the daily endocrine and exocrine requirements of the pancreas cannot be met. In the case of exocrine insufficiency, this usually occurs when lipase and protease secretions decrease below 10% of normal. The resultant malabsorption of carbohydrates, proteins and fats often results in weight loss and steatorrhoea.
- **Diabetes**: pancreatic endocrine insufficiency results in glucose intolerance as insulin production drops below requirements. Polyuria, polydipsia and malaise may occur.

Examination

Examination is often unremarkable. The presence of jaundice should be sought, as it might indicate associated biliary disease. Infrequently pseudocysts may be palpable as an abdominal mass. Nutritional assessment is essential, as advanced chronic pancreatitis is often associated with malnutrition.

Investigation

Investigations are aimed first at establishing the diagnosis of pancreatitis and the underlying cause(s), and second at assessing the degree of pancreatic damage.

In particular, the presence of cholelithiasis as a precipitating cause should be sought and treated, and the diagnosis of autoimmune pancreatitis should be considered because of the responsiveness of this condition to steroid therapy. Finally, patients with chronic pancreatitis are at increased risk of pancreatic cancer, particularly with increasing age and in smokers, and these groups of patients should be considered for surveillance for the development of pancreatic lesions.

Diagnosis can be difficult because amylase and lipase levels are frequently normal. Diagnosis then relies on the detection of structural changes and, late in the disease, exocrine and endocrine abnormalities. Initial blood tests (taken in the convalescent phase, as episodes of acute pancreatitis may falsely alter blood chemistry) should look for hypertriglyceridaemia and hypercalcaemia, as well as evidence of biliary obstruction by measuring bilirubin, ALP and GGT (see biliary physiology, Chapter 19). Late in the disease, endocrine dysfunction should be tested for by fasting glucose and glucose tolerance testing if indicated. Exocrine function is most commonly tested for using faecal elastase, reduced levels indicating reduced exocrine function.

Radiological investigation should include ultrasound of the abdomen wherever biliary disease might be suspected. CT provides the best means of assessing the degree of calcification of the pancreas (see Figure 18.3). MRCP provides information about the pancreatic parenchyma and ductal system as well as the biliary tree. ERCP is reserved for cases in which the investigations outlined cannot convincingly rule out cholelithiasis, or where the pattern of radiological change suggests that there may be isolated main pancreatic duct stones, the endoscopic removal of which might benefit the patient. Finally, obtaining tissue from pancreatic masses is increasingly important in differentiating between benign and malignant lesions and, as well as open surgical and laparoscopic biopsy, endoscopic ultrasound and fine-needle aspiration are increasingly being used.

Management

Treatment is largely symptomatic and aimed at managing pain, and exocrine and endocrine insufficiency, as well as nutritional support. The most important factor overall is the abstinence from alcohol and smoking in alcoholic pancreatitis. Other precipitating factors should be sought and corrected, such as anatomical abnormalities or metabolic disease. Surgery

and other interventional procedures are mostly reserved for the treatment of underlying anatomical causes or complications of chronic pancreatitis (see Figure 18.4).

Pain management

Pain compromises quality of life in chronic pancreatitis and is of primary concern. Use of analgesia should always start with a conventional analgesic, including paracetamol, but often opiates are required. When prescribing opiates the prominent side-effects of CNS depression, alterations of GI motility and induction of dependence must be kept in mind.

Other strategies of pain relief are used but remain unproven, including inhibition of pancreatic enzyme secretion using pancreatic enzyme therapy and the use of antioxidants, coeliac plexus block, endoscopic procedures and surgical drainage and resection.

Exocrine insufficiency

Steatorrhoea is defined as faecal fat >7 g/day. However, in practice, faecal fat measurement is rarely used and the decision to treat with pancreatic enzymes is based on faecal elastase, nutritional status and subjective reports of steatorrhoea. The aim of treatment is to treat the steatorrhoea and correct the nutritional consequences of fat malabsorption, but a significant increase in body weight is rarely achieved. Generally a dose of 25,000–50,000 U lipase/meal is recommended, but a higher dose or combination

Figure 18.3 CT of chronic pancreatitis. CT showing pancreatic calculi in an atrophic pancreas (long arrow) and a pseudocyst at the tail of the pancreas (short arrow). Source: Braganza JM, Lee SH, McCloy RF, McMahon MJ. Chronic pancreatitis. Lancet. 2011;377(9772):1184–1197. Reproduced by permission of Elsevier.

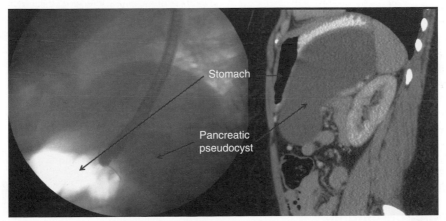

Stomach

Pancreatic pseudocyst

Figure 18.4 CT showing large pancreatic pseudocyst and endoscopic procedure to drain it. This large pancreatic pseudocyst developed after an episode of severe gallstone pancreatitis. The pseudocyst was putting pressure on the stomach and causing early satiety and pain. It was drained by endoscopically puncturing the pseudocyst, using contrast to outline the cyst as in the X-ray shown here, and placing multiple plastic stents through the wall of the stomach and into the cyst. The cyst decompressed very quickly and on repeat CT 3 months later, the stents had fallen out and the pseudocyst resolved.

with a proton pump inhibitor may be required (proton pump inhibitors prevent acid breakdown of the pancreatic enzyme supplement).

Diabetes

Treatment is no different from patients with type 1 diabetes, but it must be recalled that the coexisting deficiency of glucagon puts chronic pancreatitis patients at increased risk of hypoglycaemia. This is particularly true when compliance is poor and/or there is continued alcohol consumption or autonomic neuropathy. Given that the survival of such patients is limited, the aim should be adequate control of glucose and avoidance of hypoglycaemia. Aggressive glucose management should be reserved for patients with good compliance and cessation of alcohol.

Nutrition

There is no specific diet known to be beneficial in chronic pancreatitis, but abstinence from alcohol and the intake of smaller but more frequent meals are recommended. Fat restriction is not recommended and steatorrhoea should instead be treated with pancreatic supplements. Fat-soluble vitamin deficiencies occur particularly with ongoing alcohol use and should be screened for and treated.

Prognosis

Chronic pancreatitis is associated with increased morbidity and mortality. One third of patients die within 10 years of diagnosis. The ongoing destruction can often be stopped or slowed if the inciting cause is removed. However, the end result is often complete loss of exocrine and endocrine pancreatic function. This end-stage consequence may be associated with reduction in pain as the last of the pancreatic tissue is destroyed. The risk of pancreatic cancer is significant and the clinician must remain alert to this.

Pancreatic tumours

Pancreatic carcinoma

The majority of pancreatic cancers are adenocarcinomas that arise from ductal and acinar cells.

They are twice as common in men compared to women and occur at a mean age of 55 years. Risk factors for pancreatic carcinoma include smoking and chronic pancreatitis.

Epidemiology and causes

The age-standardised incidence of pancreatic cancer in Europe and the UK is about 9 per 100,000. This gives a lifetime risk of about 1 in 74 people. This rate has been constant in the UK since 1996, but declined prior to this at least in part due to the decline in smoking prevalence, as smoking accounts for up to 30% of the cancer cases.

Around 95% of pancreatic tumours are adenocarcinomas, nearly all of which are ductal adenocarcinomas. Endocrine tumours of the pancreas can arise from the islets of Langerhans, but are rare. Multiple genetic predispositions to pancreatic cancer have been discovered and pancreatic cancer forms a part of a number of inherited cancer syndromes, including BRCA2, FAMMM, PalB2 and the Peutz–Jegher syndrome. As well as smoking, age, diabetes, obesity and diets high in meat and cholesterol are associated with increased risk.

Clinical features

At initial presentation the majority of patients have advanced disease:

- Most patients have severe abdominal pain, often radiating to the back.
- Weight loss is common.
- Obstructive jaundice is a frequent result of lesions in the head of the pancreas.
- Cancer in the body and tail may cause splenic vein obstruction with resultant splenomegaly, gastric and oesophageal varices, and GI haemorrhage.
- Glandular destruction by the tumour may lead to diabetes and/or pancreatic exocrine insufficiency.

Investigations

- Laboratory tests show elevated ALP and bilirubin in bile duct obstruction. Ca 19-9 is not useful in diagnosis but, if positive, may be used to monitor response to treatment.
- Helical CT or MRCP is the preferred test.
- In the case of obstructive jaundice, it is reasonable to use ERCP as the initial investigation.
- Fine-needle aspiration is usually required for confirmation of the diagnosis, using CT or endoscopic ultrasound guidance.

Management

Unfortunately, the majority of patients have incurable disease, thus symptomatic management is of the utmost importance. Moderate to severe pain should be treated with oral opioid analgesics at sufficient dose. Concerns about addiction should not prevent this. In difficult-to-control pain, percutaneous or operative splanchnic (coeliac) block may be used. Pruritus is best treated by relieving obstruction with palliative surgery or endoscopic biliary stenting. Where this is not possible, cholestyramine or phenobarbitol may be of some benefit. Pancreatic insufficiency is treated with pancreatic supplements.

Prognosis

The overall survival rate for pancreatic cancer is <6%, making it the worst of all the solid organ cancers. The only chance for cure is complete resection of the tumour. However, only 30% of patients with tumours in the head of the pancreas, and only 10% of those with cancer in the body and tail, can be offered curative resection at presentation. Adjuvant chemotherapy and radiation therapy are commonly used.

Cystadenocarcinoma

This rare adenomatous tumour results from malignant degeneration of a mucous cystadenoma. Patients present with upper abdominal pain and a palpable mass. CT or MRI demonstrates a cystic mass that contains debris. The tumour is slow growing and slow to metastasise, and prognosis following surgical excision is good.

Intraductal papillary-mucinous tumour

This rare tumour most commonly occurs in women, in the tail of the pancreas. The tumour over-secretes mucin, causing pain and recurrent bouts of pancreatitis. Disease may range from benign to malignant and cannot be differentiated without surgical removal. Initial diagnosis is made by CT, MRCP or ERCP. ERCP may show the typical 'fish eye' appearance, where the duodenal papilla is seen to be gaping, with 'shiny' mucus bulging through the terminal duct. Following surgical resection, prognosis is excellent for benign disease. Malignant disease has a 5-year survival of 50–75%.

Pancreatic endocrine tumours

These rare tumours arise from the islet and gastrin-producing cells of the pancreas. They may be non-functioning and present with biliary obstruction, bleeding or abdominal masses; or functioning (hormone secreting) and present with an endocrine syndrome, depending on the hormone produced.

KEY POINTS

- The pancreas produces vital exocrine enzymes as well as endocrine hormones responsible for glucose homeostasis.
- Enzymes are synthesised by the ribosomes of the rough endoplasmic reticulum and released in response to cholecystokinin and include:
  ○ Amylase for carbohydrates.
  ○ Lipases for fats.
  ○ Proteases for proteins.
  ○ Nucleases for DNA and RNA.
- Chronic pancreatitis is associated with alcohol abuse in 80% of cases. Much rarer factors include duct obstruction, metabolic disease, genetic predispositions and autoimmune disease.
- Because of its steroid responsiveness, identification of autoimmune pancreatitis has become increasingly important.
- The three major clinical features of chronic pancreatitis are pain, maldigestion and diabetes. Treatment is aimed at managing these.
- At initial presentation the majority of patients with pancreatic carcinoma have advanced disease. The overall survival rate for pancreatic cancer is <6%, making it the worst of all the solid organ cancers.

? **SELF-ASSESSMENT QUESTION**

(The answer to this question is given on p. 268)

A 53-year-old man presents with longstanding intermittent abdominal pain and steatorrhoea. He is known to have a heavy alcohol history. CT shows marked calcification and atrophy of the pancreas and a 2 cm mass in the pancreatic head, which was not seen on a scan done 3 years ago.

Regarding this man's condition, which of the following statements is most true?

(a) Amylase may not be a useful diagnostic test in this situation.

(b) A Ca 19-9 tumour marker is useful to confirm or refute the presence of pancreatic cancer.

(c) A 24-h faecal collection showing a fat level of greater than 7 g/day is required to confirm pancreatic exocrine insufficiency.

(d) Treatment with a proton pump inhibitor should improve any pancreatic exocrine insufficiency contributing to the diarrhoea.

(e) Aggressive control of blood sugars is essential in patients with endocrine pancreatic failure due to chronic pancreatitis.

19

Biliary diseases

The biliary system is concerned with the transport of bile from the liver into the duodenum, including timely release and en route concentration. Disruption of the flow of bile has consequences in the form of pain, inflammation, colonisation by micro-organisms and infection. There may also be loss of essential digestive functions of bile. Disruption of bile flow most commonly occurs because of mechanical blockage caused by biliary stones. However, other acquired and congenital causes also contribute.

Embryology

The liver arises as a hollow outgrowth from the portion of the gut that goes on to become the descending part of the duodenum. This diverticulum gives off two buds of cells that become the right and left lobes of the liver. The original diverticulum from the duodenum forms the common bile duct, and from this the cystic duct and gallbladder arise as a solid outgrowth. This outgrowth later acquires a lumen (Figure 19.1).

Biliary anatomy

Intrahepatic bile ducts

The bile ducts arise as tiny passages in the liver cells that communicate with the **intercellular biliary passages** (bile capillaries or canaliculi). These passages radiate to the circumference of the lobule, and open into the interlobular bile ducts, accompanying

the portal vein and hepatic artery (see Figure 19.2). They then join with other ducts to form two main trunks, which leave the liver at the porta hepatis and join to form the **hepatic duct**.

The large biliary ducts have an external or fibrous and an internal or mucous layer. The mucous coat is continuous with the lining membrane of the hepatic ducts and gallbladder, and also with that of the duodenum. The mucous membrane is a columnar epithelium, with numerous mucous glands.

Gallbladder and cystic duct

About 4 cm after the union of the two main trunks to form the hepatic duct, it is joined at an acute angle by the cystic duct, and so forms the common bile duct. The hepatic duct is accompanied by the hepatic artery and portal vein.

The gallbladder is divided into a fundus, body and neck, and consists of three coats: an external serous coat derived from the peritoneum, a fibromuscular coat that forms the framework of the sac and an internal mucus layer that is elevated into minute rugae (folds). Opposite the neck of the gallbladder, the mucous membrane projects inward in the form of oblique ridges or folds, forming a sort of spiral valve.

The **cystic duct**, which is about 4 cm long, has a mucous lining that is thrown into a series of crescentic folds, from 5 to 12 in number, similar to those found in the neck of the gallbladder. They form a continuous spiral valve, which, when the duct is distended, results in dilatation of the spaces between the fold, so as to give the cystic duct a twisted appearance.

Gastroenterology and Hepatology: Lecture Notes, Second Edition. Stephen Inns and Anton Emmanuel.
© 2017 John Wiley & Sons, Ltd. Published 2017 by John Wiley & Sons, Ltd.
Companion website: www.lecturenoteseries.com/gastroenterology

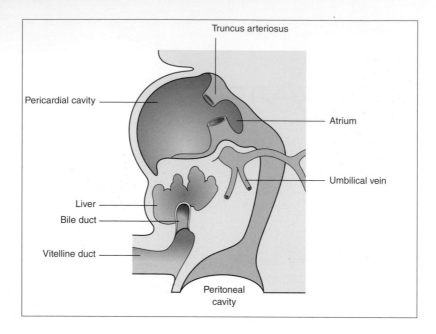

Figure 19.1 Human embryo at 3 mm length stage, showing developmental structures of the biliary tree.

Common bile duct

The **common bile duct**, formed by the junction of the cystic and hepatic ducts, is about 7.5 cm long and <7 mm in diameter (this may increase with age: approximately 1 mm each decade above the age of 50 years). Near its distal end, it lies alongside the terminal part of the pancreatic duct. The two ducts unite and share an opening at the tip of the duodenal papilla. The short tube formed by the union of the two ducts is dilated into the **ampulla of Vater** (Figure 19.2).

Biliary physiology

Over a 24-hour period, a normal adult human produces 400–1100 ml of hepatic bile. Bile is composed of:

- Water (the primary component).
- Electrolytes.
- Bile salts, synonymous with bile acids (they induce influx of water and electrolytes in the canaliculi by active transport and passive diffusion).
- Bilirubin (from degradation of haem compounds from degenerative red blood cells).
- Phospholipids and cholesterol.
- Proteins that regulate GI function.
- Drugs and drug metabolites (including potentially toxic compounds).

From the canaliculi bile passes into the interlobular ducts, then the common hepatic duct. About 50% of the bile secreted while fasting is collected in the gallbladder. The gallbladder then absorbs up to 90% of the water, concentrating and storing bile. Eating results in the release of gut hormones and cholinergic stimulation. These initiate gallbladder contraction and biliary sphincter relaxation, promoting the passage of bile from the gallbladder into the duodenum. The concentrated bile thus released solubilises intestinal fats and fat-soluble vitamins, facilitating their absorption. During fasting an increase in sphincter tone facilitates gallbladder filling.

The proximal small intestine allows limited passive diffusion of bile salts such that 90% of bile salts reach the terminal ileum. Here there is active absorption of bile salts into the portal venous circulation. Bile salts are thus returned to the liver and circulate through this pathway – the enterohepatic circulation – 10–12 times/day.

Biliary microbiology

Biliary infection occurs often in association with cholelithiasis. It can take acute and chronic forms and predominantly involves the gallbladder (cholecystitis) or the bile ducts (cholangitis), discussed separately later.

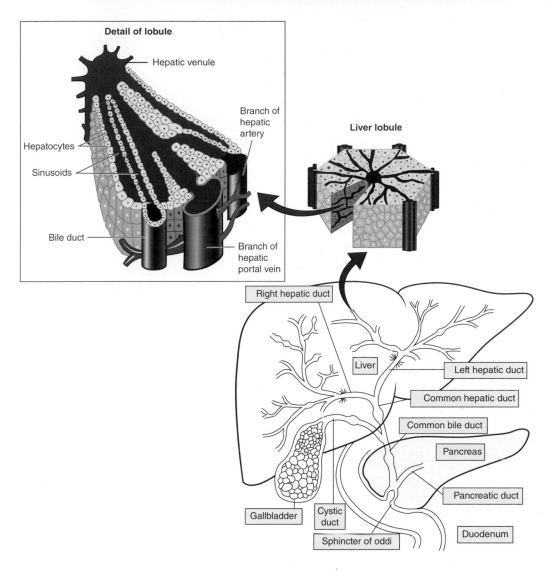

Figure 19.2 Anatomy of biliary system with detail of liver lobule.

The organisms involved are generally intestinal commensals:

- Commonest are Gram negatives (e.g. *Escherichia coli, Klebsiella, Enterobacter*).
- Less common are Gram positives (e.g. *Enterococcus* spp.) and mixed anaerobes (e.g. *Bacteroides, Clostridia*).

Cholelithiasis

Cholelithiasis, or the presence of gallstones, is common. However, the majority of patients (60–80%) do not develop symptoms associated with gallstones.

Management centres on population measures to reduce rates of gallstone formation and, in the individual patient, stratification as to the risk of symptoms and complications in those with asymptomatic, incidentally discovered gallstones. Generally patients with symptomatic gallstones should have cholecystectomy if tolerated.

Pathophysiology of gallstone formation

Gallstones are made up of poorly soluble components of bile precipitated on a three-dimensional matrix of mucins and proteins. The three main types

Table 19.1 Characteristics of different gallstone types.

Characteristic	Cholesterol	Black pigment	Brown pigment
Composition	Cholesterol with calcium bilirubinates	Black pigment polymer with calcium bilirubinates and phosphates	Calcium bilirubinates with cholesterol and calcium palmitate
Colour	Yellow–white	Black to dark brown	Yellow to orange
Shape and texture	Hard and shiny, round or faceted	Shiny or dull, faceted	Soft and greasy, ovoid
Number	Single or multiple	Multiple and numerous	Single or multiple
Location	Usually gallbladder	Usually gallbladder	Usually bile ducts
Associations	Female gender, multiparity Diabetes Oral contraceptives Obesity or rapid weight loss Family history	Haemolysis Cirrhosis Crohn's disease Total parenteral nutrition	Structural biliary disease (strictures, sclerosing cholangitis, surgery)
Cause	Increased cholesterol with or without decreased bile salt excretion	Increased bilirubin and calcium excretion into bile Increased bile pH	Bacterial infection causes hydrolysis of bilirubin conjugates

of gallstones are cholesterol stones, black pigment stones and brown pigment stones (Table 19.1). For gallstone formation to occur there must be:

- Supersaturation.
- Excess of promoters over inhibitors of crystallisation.
- A matrix template on which crystallisation can occur.
- Bile stasis (retention in the gallbladder to allow time to grow).

The major precipitates are cholesterol, calcium bilirubinates and calcium salts of phosphate, carbonate and palmitate.

The vast majority of gallstones in Western countries are cholesterol or mixed type. It is interesting to note that, while pigment gallstones predominate in Asian countries, Asians who take up a Western diet become more prone to cholesterol stones.

Normally, in the gallbladder, bile is concentrated by active absorption of water and electrolytes. Phospholipids and biliary cholesterol are absorbed so that the concentration of cholesterol relative to bile salts is actually lower than in hepatic bile. Supersaturation with cholesterol therefore can occur only if the bile secreted by hepatocytes is already supersaturated and/or the composition or pH of bile is altered in the extrahepatic bile ducts or gallbladder.

When there is supersaturation, if a suitable matrix is present, the minerals crystallise on a matrix template to form a miniature calculus or nidus. The matrix is made up of proteins and glycoproteins. For this nidus then to grow to form a gallstone, there needs to be bile stasis due to impairment of emptying of the gallbladder or bile flow in the ducts.

Epidemiology and causes

Gallstones are an important health problem in the Western world, affecting 10–15% of the adult population.

Risk factors for cholesterol gallstones include:

- Demographic factors:
  - Family history.
  - Older age.
  - Female gender.
  - Pregnancy and multiparity.
- Abnormal eating behaviours:
  - Obesity.
  - Rapid weight loss.
  - Prolonged fasting.
- Systemic diseases:
  - Diabetes mellitus.
  - Crohn's disease.
  - Spinal cord injury.
- Iatrogenic causes:
  - Somatostatin(-analogue) treatment.
  - Sex hormone treatment.
  - Total parenteral nutrition.

Possible *preventative factors* include:

- High-fibre diet.
- Low consumption of saturated fatty acids.

- High relative amounts of cis- *versus* trans-fatty acids.
- Nut consumption.
- Moderate physical activity.

Clinical features

- Pain: typically right hypochondrial or epigastric.
- Radiates to the upper back or right shoulder.
- Steady and intense, occurs more than an hour after meals (especially fried or fatty foods).
- Often associated with an urge to walk (75% of patients).
- Each episode lasts 1–24 h.
- More likely to be gallstone related when there is no associated heartburn and no relief with bowel movements.
- Murphy's sign (deep inspiration exacerbates the pain during palpation of the right upper quadrant [RUQ] and halts inspiration) develops with involuntary guarding of right-sided abdominal muscles.
- Fever (common): usually low grade.
- In the elderly, fever may not develop, and the first or only symptoms may be systemic and non-specific (e.g. anorexia, vomiting, malaise, weakness).

Investigations

- **Routine tests:** because only 10% of gallstones are calcified, plain abdominal X-ray is infrequently helpful. In addition, given the intermittent nature of symptoms, nor are routine blood tests, although repeated liver tests timed to the onset of pain may give extra clues as to the cause of pain.
- **Advanced tests:** magnetic resonance cholangio-pancreatography (MRCP) has high specificity and sensitivity in choledocholithiasis, giving it an accuracy very similar to ERCP. However, it has limitations in the detection of small gallstones (<4 mm) and gallstones that sit close to the ampulla of Vater. Endoscopic ultrasonography (EUS) has proven useful in detecting very small gallstones (<3 mm) and may be needed if other studies are equivocal.

Risk stratification of patients with asymptomatic gallstones

The average risk of someone with gallstones developing symptomatic gallstones is low at approximately 2% per year, the yearly incidence of complications is 0.3% and the risk for gallbladder cancer is 0.02%. Hence most patients need no therapy. However, the subgroup with high risk of symptoms and/or gallbladder cancer will generally benefit from prophylactic cholecystectomy.

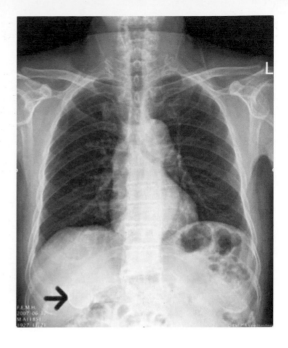

Figure 19.3 Plain abdominal X-ray showing porcelain gallbladder. Source: Liang H-P, Cheung W-K, Su F-H, Chu F-Y. 2008. Porcelain gallbladder. J Am Geriatr Soc, Figure 1. Reproduced with permission of John Wiley & Sons.

Indications for cholecystectomy:

- Gallbladder polyps that are rapidly growing or that are >1 cm.
- 'Porcelain gallbladder,' a radiological sign (Figure 19.3).
- Solitary stone or total stone burden >3 cm.
- Sickle cell anaemia.
- Morbidly obese patients undergoing bariatric surgery.

Primary prevention of gallstones in high-risk groups

High-risk groups can benefit from modulation of therapy to avoid gallstones.

- During weight loss:
  - Limitation of weight loss to a maximum rate of 1.5 kg/week.
  - Addition of 10 g of fat to a low-calorie diet.
  - Evidence for NSAIDs is contradictory.
  - Ursodeoxycholic acid (UDCA) is efficacious and cost beneficial.
- Daily intravenous cholecystokinin or amino acids during total parenteral nutrition.
- UDCA during somatostatin analogue therapy.

Management of symptomatic gallstones

Cholecystectomy

After symptoms develop, the risk of recurrent symptoms decreases with time:

- Within 1 year from the first pain attack, about 50% have a second attack.
- About 30% of patients will have only one pain attack.
- After 5 years symptom free, the risk returns to that of asymptomatic patients.

Symptomatic patients are at higher risk of complications (i.e. acute cholecystitis, acute pancreatitis, cholangitis); the risk is about 1–2%, as compared to 0.1–0.2% in asymptomatic patients. Open cholecystectomy, previously the treatment of choice, is safe and effective, with an overall mortality of 0.1–0.5%. However, laparoscopic cholecystectomy has become the treatment of choice because it is associated with shorter convalescence, decreased postoperative discomfort, improved cosmetic results and no increase in morbidity or mortality. In about 5% of cases the procedure must be converted to an open one.

Non-surgical alternatives

Where surgery is declined or surgical risks are high, UDCA can sometimes dissolve gallbladder stones:

- Treatment given for many months.
- Must be cholesterol stones.
- Stones cannot be too large (<1.5 cm).
- Gallbladder should be free of obstruction.

However, after UDCA stones recur in about half of patients by 5 years, and it is not successful when used in patients with highly symptomatic gallstones.

ERCP and sphincterotomy may be sufficient treatment for patients with gallstones who are not suitable for surgery.

Prognosis

There is an association between gallstones and cancer of the gallbladder, but the risk remains low at less than 1 in 10,000. Most people have no further problems following cholecystectomy. If complications such as cholangitis and pancreatitis develop, the prognosis depends on the severity of the complication.

Cholecystitis

Causes

Cholecystitis is caused by obstruction of the cystic duct, usually by a gallstone, leading to distension and subsequent chemical or bacterial inflammation of the gallbladder. 95% of people with acute cholecystitis have gallstones (**calculous cholecystitis**) and 5% lack gallstones (**acalculous cholecystitis**). Positive cultures of the bile or gallbladder wall are found in 50–75% of cases of acute cholecystitis. The cause of acalculous cholecystitis is uncertain and may be multifactorial.

Epidemiology

Of those admitted to hospital for biliary tract disease, 20% have acute cholecystitis, and the number of cholecystectomies carried out is steadily increasing, especially in elderly people. Acute calculous cholecystitis is three times more common in women up to the age of 50 years and about 1.5 times more common in women thereafter.

Clinical features

Patients present with unremitting RUQ pain, anorexia, nausea, vomiting and fever. Severe acute cholecystitis can lead to necrosis of the gallbladder wall, known as **gangrenous cholecystitis**. The complications of cholecystitis include perforation of the gallbladder, pericholecystic abscess and fistula.

Management

The treatment of choice for cholecystitis is open or laparoscopic cholecystectomy (Box 19.1) undertaken *early* (within 7 days of onset of symptoms) rather than *delayed* (≥6 weeks after onset of symptoms), as it reduces the duration of hospital stay.

Box 19.1 Comparing laparoscopic *versus* open cholecystectomy

- Reduces hospital stay, duration of surgery and intra- and postoperative complications
- Conversion from laparoscopic to open cholecystectomy is necessary in 4–27% of cases
- Laparoscopic cholecystectomy carries a higher incidence of bile duct injury

Observation alone has a failure rate after 8 years of 30%, but there is no difference in the rate of gallstone-related complications (recurrent cholecystitis, pancreatitis, intractable pain) or emergency admissions for pain. For this reason, those with acute cholecystitis who have multiple comorbid conditions and relative contraindications for cholecystectomy may be treated with antibiotics, a low-fat diet and, in some instances, a cholecystostomy tube. If the comorbidity becomes better controlled, delayed cholecystectomy is appropriate.

Prognosis

In the absence of complications, the prognosis is excellent. However, if complications such as perforation or gangrene of the gallbladder develop, the prognosis is significantly worse. Interestingly, calculous cholecystitis has a higher (10–50%) mortality than calculous cholecystitis (4%).

Acalculous biliary pain

Recurrent biliary-type abdominal pain in patients with no evidence of cholelithiasis is a perplexing clinical dilemma, and evaluation and treatment of these patients are controversial. Synonyms for the term acalculous biliary pain include gallbladder dysfunction, functional gallbladder and sphincter of Oddi dysfunction (SOD), gallbladder dyskinesia, biliary dyskinesia, chronic acalculous cholecystitis and chronic acalculous gallbladder disease.

Epidemiology

The frequency of biliary-type pain without gallstones in the population may be as high as 7% in men and 20% in women.

Causes

These remain incompletely understood:

- Altered gallbladder motility is the most commonly accepted abnormality.
- Impairment of gallbladder filling.
- Gallbladder hyperalgesia.

Functional disorders of adjacent structures, classically SOD (Box 19.2), have been implicated in the pathogenesis of recurrent epigastric or RUQ abdominal pain following cholecystectomy. That SOD might exist in patients with an intact gallbladder has been suggested but remains controversial.

> **Box 19.2 Classification of sphincter of Oddi dysfunction**
>
> *Type 1*
> - Biliary pain
> - Abnormal liver enzyme levels
> - Fixed sphincter of Oddi stenosis on radiograph
>
> *Type 2*
> - Biliary pain and transient elevation of enzyme level and/or
> - Dilated bile duct and/or
> - Delay in emptying of bile duct
>
> *Type 3*
> - Biliary pain only

> **Box 19.3 Diagnostic criteria for gallbladder and sphincter of Oddi disorders**
>
> *Must include episodes of pain located in the epigastrium and/or right upper quadrant and all of the following:*
> - Episodes lasting 30 min or longer
> - Recurrent symptoms occurring at different intervals (not daily)
> - Pain building up to a steady level
> - Pain severe enough to interrupt patient's daily activities or lead to an emergency department visit
> - Pain not relieved by bowel movements
> - Pain not relieved by postural change
> - Pain not relieved by antacids
> - Exclusion of other structural disease that would explain the symptoms
>
> *Supportive criteria: the pain may present with one or more of the following:*
> - Pain associated with nausea and vomiting
> - Pain radiating to back and/or right infrascapular region
> - Pain that awakens patient from sleep in the middle of the night

Clinical features

The clinical features of this pain are summarised in Box 19.3.

Investigations

Gallstone disease and structural abnormalities must be excluded before the diagnosis of a functional disorder can be considered.

- Cholecystokinin cholescintigraphy to measure the gallbladder ejection fraction (GEF) has been advocated as a way to select patients with acalculous biliary pain who would benefit from cholecystectomy.

- ERCP with sphincter of Oddi manometry (SOM) has been used to identify patients who might respond to biliary endoscopic sphincterotomy (ES). It must be noted that SOD increases the risk for post-ES pancreatitis, occurring in as many as 22% of patients.
- More recently botulinum toxin (administered directly by endoscopic injection) has been used to paralyse the sphincter of Oddi in order to treat SOD and to select those patients most likely to benefit from ES.

Management

Given the risks of cholecystectomy and ES, and the lack of clear evidence of benefit in the majority of patients, a conservative approach is advocated except where the symptoms are intractable and affecting quality of life, and the level of certainty as to the underlying cause is high. Careful evaluation of psychological issues is essential, and treatments targeting chronic visceral pain (such as tricyclic antidepressants) should be considered.

Prognosis

The condition itself confers no risk of progression to more serious conditions, such as acute cholecystitis. The morbidity and mortality of this condition instead relate to the investigations and surgical interventions used. While cholecystectomy has a good rate of immediate relief, the long-term response is lower than that in calculous disease, and the postoperative mortality rate is higher.

Structural bile duct abnormalities

The three major adult manifestations of cholestasis due to biliary pathology are primary biliary cirrhosis (PBC), primary sclerosing cholangitis (PSC) and cholangiocarcinoma. Drug-related and congenital biliary abnormalities are discussed in Chapters 25 and 30, respectively.

Primary sclerosing cholangitis
Epidemiology and causes

PSC has a male predominance, typically affecting young men around age 40 years. There is a strong association with inflammatory bowel disease (IBD), especially ulcerative colitis. The estimated prevalence is 6 in 100,000. PSC is an idiopathic, chronic, progressive liver disease that causes inflammation, fibrosis and strictures in the intrahepatic and extrahepatic bile ducts.

Clinical features

These include jaundice, steatorrhoea, pruritus, weight loss and failure of proper absorption of calcium and fat-soluble vitamins. However, many patients have no symptoms or vague symptoms of fatigue and upper abdominal pain. Examination may reveal xanthomas of the eyes, neck, chest, back and extensor surfaces.

Investigations

Laboratory tests show elevated conjugated bilirubin, alkaline phosphatase (ALP) that is often more than three times the upper limit of normal and elevated gamma-glutamyl transferase (GGT). MRCP is the most useful diagnostic tool. ERCP is usually reserved for therapeutic intervention where a dominant biliary stricture has developed that might benefit from stent placement or where choledocholithiasis has developed (Figure 19.4).

Management

This primarily involves symptom management. Liver transplantation is the only life-extending therapy. Surveillance for cholangiocarcinoma is warranted; however, there is no consensus as to how this should

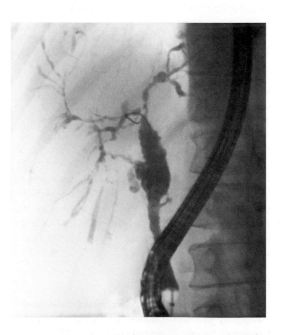

Figure 19.4 ERCP picture showing primary sclerosing cholangitis.

be conducted. Patients with PSC complicating IBD require more frequent colonic surveillance than those with IBD alone because of an increased risk of colon cancer.

Prognosis

Because of the lack of an effective medical therapy for PSC, the prognosis is guarded. The median survival time from diagnosis to death or liver transplantation has been estimated to be as low as 10 years. Cholangiocarcinoma complicates PSC in approximately 10% of cases. If PSC occurs in the setting of ulcerative colitis, the rate of colonic malignancy is very high and increased colonoscopic surveillance is advocated in those patients.

Primary biliary cirrhosis

Epidemiology and causes

PBC is an autoimmune cholestatic liver disease in which the epithelial cells lining the intrahepatic bile ducts are damaged by the immune system. Estimates of annual incidence and prevalence range from 2 to 24 cases per million and 19 to 240 cases per million people, respectively. It predominantly affects women aged 30–65 years, but can occur in those as young as their late teens. The male-to-female ratio is 1:10. There is a wide geographical variation, suggesting that environmental factors may contribute to the development of the disease.

Investigation

Serology is the mainstay of diagnosis; liver biopsy is reserved for situations where there is diagnostic uncertainty, or information regarding liver damage is needed. The antimitochondrial antibody (AMA) is the hallmark serological marker. AMA is not specific for the disease, but is sensitive (98%). Antinuclear antibody (ANA) and smooth muscle antibody (SMA), typically markers of autoimmune hepatitis, do occur in 35% and 66% of patients with PBC, respectively. Ultrasound is useful for defining strictures in the extrahepatic biliary tree and MRCP is able to demonstrate extra- and intrahepatic lesions. ERCP is not usually necessary.

Clinical features

These typically include fatigue, intense pruritus, cutaneous hyperpigmentation, xanthelasmas and hepatosplenomegaly. The rate of progression is slow. PBC is often associated with various autoimmune diseases, such as scleroderma, thyroiditis and Sjögren's syndrome.

Management

UDCA is the first-line treatment early in disease and can slow its progression, but is less effective later in disease. Liver transplant is the only treatment that prolongs life in PBC.

Prognosis

The prognosis in PBC relates to the amount of hepatocellular damage incurred. Bilirubin can be used as an indicator of this, with levels of 34–102 µmol/L (2–6 mg/dL) being associated with a mean survival of 4 years, 102–171 µmol/L (6–10 mg/dL) 2 years, and above 171 µmol/L (10 mg/dL) a mean survival of 1.4 years. PBC is also associated with an increased risk of hepatocellular carcinoma.

Cholangiocarcinoma

Epidemiology and causes

Cholangiocarcinoma is a slow-growing malignancy of the bile duct. It is the second most common primary hepatic tumour (after hepatoma). Worldwide incidence varies widely, the highest rates being in northeast Thailand (96 per 100,000 men), about 100 times greater than in the West. Groups at high risk include:

- Gallstones (20–50% of cases, probably coincidental).
- PSC (10% of cases).
- IBD (10-fold increased risk).
- History of other malignancy (10% of cases).
- Autosomal dominant polycystic kidney disease.
- Previous surgery for choledochal cyst or biliary atresia.
- Alpha-1-antitrypsin deficiency.
- Congenital choledochal cysts.
- Papillomatosis of the bile ducts.
- Chronic typhoid carrier status.
- Parasitic diseases of the biliary tract (*Clonorchis sinensis* or *Opisthorchis viverrini*).
- Thorotrast exposure.

Clinical features

Intrahepatic tumours may cause abdominal pain, palpable masses and weight loss, with progressive obstructive jaundice in 90%. Painless jaundice occurs in 12%. Advanced disease may be complicated by cholangitis or acute cholecystitis, or anaemia (due to chronic blood loss secondary to papillary tumours). Physical examination may demonstrate hepatomegaly and a palpable mass in 18% of patients (the gallbladder may be palpable with distal tumours).

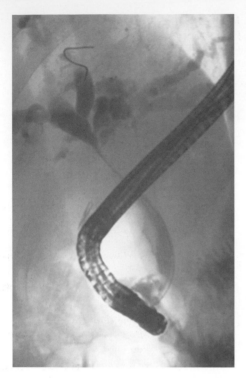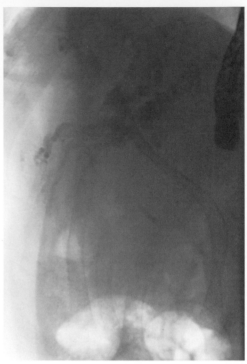

Figure 19.5 ERCP picture showing Klatskin cholangiocarcinoma causing biliary stricturing at the level of the porta-hepatis and following insertion of an expanding metal stent for palliation.

Investigations

Tumours, which may be nodular or diffuse, are classified as:

- Intrahepatic (10% of cases).
- Extrahepatic (25% of cases).
- Perihilar bile duct tumours (65% of cases). If they involve the bifurcation of the hepatic duct, they are known as Klatskin tumours.

The modality most likely to show tumour depends on the type of tumour:

- Ultrasonography is the first-line investigation.
- Abdominal CT may demonstrate the tumour if the malignancy is nodular and mass-like.
- MRCP demonstrates stricture-causing tumours, but does not allow distension of the duct and may not detect long segments and minimal narrowing in diffuse sclerosing tumours.
- ERCP is a more definitive investigation that can depict the periampullary tumour.

Management

- **Complete surgical resection** is the only therapy to afford a chance of cure:
  - <20% of intrahepatic tumours are resectable, and 5-year survival rate in those undergoing resection is 5–15%.
  - Resection is more often possible in patients with mid-ductal (33%) or distal tumours (56%), with a 5-year survival rate of 39%.
- **Palliation**:
  - ERCP drainage with or without endoluminal stenting is preferred (Figure 19.5).
  - Percutaneous radiological drainage may be needed for proximal lesions.
  - Chemotherapy (often as a radiosensitising agent, before palliative radiotherapy).
  - Surgical bypass can also be used for palliation (but most patients die within a year of diagnosis).
- **Orthotopic liver transplantation** is rarely used, primarily because cholangiocarcinoma almost invariably recurs in the transplanted liver.

Prognosis

The treatment options for cholangiocarcinoma are generally limited. The mortality rate is similar to the incidence rate. The majority of patients present with unresectable disease and have a survival of less than 12 months following diagnosis. Careful selection of patients for treatment options, including resection, with routine use of more aggressive resections, has improved survival in those patients.

 KEY POINTS

- The biliary system is concerned with the transport of bile from the liver into the duodenum and disruption of the flow of bile has consequences in the form of pain, inflammation, colonisation by microorganisms and infection
  - over a 24-h period, a normal adult human produces 400–1100 ml of hepatic bile
  - the concentrated bile released into the duodenum solubilises intestinal fats and fat-soluble vitamins, facilitating their absorption
  - 90% of bile salts reach the terminal ileum and are actively absorbed into the portal venous circulation
- The majority of patients with gallstones (60–80%) do not develop symptoms
  - the risk of developing symptomatic gallstones is approximately 2.0% per year,
  - the yearly incidence of complications is 0.3% and
  - the risk for gallbladder cancer is 0.02%.
- Cholecystitis is caused by obstruction of the cystic duct, usually by a gallstone

  - the treatment of choice for cholecystitis is open or laparoscopic cholecystectomy
- The three major adult manifestations of cholestasis due to biliary pathology are primary biliary cirrhosis (PBC), primary sclerosing cholangitis (PSC) and cholangiocarcinoma
  - PSC is complicated by cholangiocarcinoma in approximately 10% of cases.
  - If PSC occurs in the setting of ulcerative colitis the rate of colonic malignancy is very high
  - PBC is diagnosed by serology, anti-mitochondrial antibody (AMA) is the hallmark serological marker.
  - In PBC the first line treatment is UDCA , which can slow its progression, however liver transplant is the only treatment that prolongs life in PBC
  - Cholangiocarcinomas are resectable in <20% of intrahepatic tumours. Resection is more often possible in patients with mid-ductal (33%) or distal tumours (56%).

 SELF-ASSESSMENT QUESTION

(The answer to this question is given on p. 268)

A 55-year-old woman presents with right upper quadrant pain. Initial bloods show bilirubin 45, ALP 190, ALT 93, albumin 35, INR 1.2. She had similar pain in her 30s and had a cholecystectomy for this, with some resolution of pain. She is, however, troubled by variability of bowel habit and abdominal pain. This has been extensively investigated and diagnosed as irritable bowel syndrome and treated as such.

Regarding the investigation of this episode of abdominal pain, which of the following statements is most true?

(a) She exhibits Charcot's triad (RUQ pain, cholestatic liver tests and jaundice) and is likely to have cholangitis.

(b) The most sensitive test to look for cholelithiasis would be a transabdominal ultrasound.

(c) Given the previous cholecystectomy, it is very unlikely that biliary stones are the cause of this episode.

(d) MRCP would be indicated if ultrasound failed to show cholelithiasis.

(e) Given the marked liver test abnormalities and hyperbilirubinaemia, cholelithiasis or type 1 sphincter of Oddi dysfunction are very likely, thus she should proceed directly to ERCP and endoscopic sphincterotomy.

20

Consequences of chronic liver disease

Chronic liver disease results from hepatocellular injury and necrosis, often with a degree of underlying fibrosis of the liver. While the underlying causes of liver damage are diverse, the consequences of damage are held in common. Symptoms may be a result of loss of the:

- Detoxifying function of the liver (jaundice, hepatic encephalopathy).
- Synthetic function of the liver (hypoalbuminaemia, clotting factor deficiencies).
- Portal hypertension (oesophageal and other varices, hypersplenism, ascites).
- Complications of the above (GI bleeding, spontaneous bacterial peritonitis).

This chapter considers each of these, as well as describing the normal anatomy and physiology of the liver, to give a background to liver dysfunction prior to the following chapters on specific liver diseases.

Anatomy of the liver

A description of the embryology of the liver and biliary system can be found in Chapter 19.

Surface anatomy

The liver is a roughly wedge-shaped organ lying in the right upper quadrant of the abdomen that connects with the diaphragm superiorly at the 'bare area', the only part of the liver not covered by visceral peritoneum. This enveloping peritoneum invaginates through the liver, dividing it into right and left lobes and creating the falciform ligament as well as the triangular and coronary ligaments. These ligaments serve no functional purpose, but are easily recognisable anatomical features. The gallbladder sits in a fossa on the infero-anterior surface of the liver and connects, via the cystic duct, to the bile duct, which can be seen to appear at the level of the porta-hepatis, passing inferiorly with the portal vein and hepatic artery. (The vascular anatomy and vascular diseases of the liver are discussed in Chapter 28.)

Functional anatomy

The development of surgical techniques to resect parts of the liver required the development of a functional classification of the parts of the liver independently supplied by a vascular inflow, outflow and biliary drainage. This classification system is called the Couinaud classification (see Figure 20.1). Using this system the middle hepatic vein divides the liver into right and left lobes. The right hepatic vein then divides the right lobe into anterior and posterior segments and the left hepatic vein divides the left lobe into medial and lateral parts. Finally the portal vein divides the liver into upper and lower segments, giving a total of eight independently functioning units, each of which can be resected without damaging those remaining.

Physiology of the liver

The liver can be thought of as containing a single layer of cells that separates blood, which is admixed from the portal vein and hepatic artery, and bile. Neither

Gastroenterology and Hepatology: Lecture Notes, Second Edition. Stephen Inns and Anton Emmanuel.
© 2017 John Wiley & Sons, Ltd. Published 2017 by John Wiley & Sons, Ltd.
Companion website: www.lecturenoteseries.com/gastroenterology

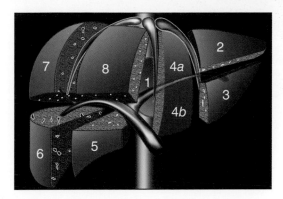

Figure 20.1 Functional anatomy of the liver.

the blood nor the bile is contained within an epithelialised structure; instead, it is essentially in contact with the cells themselves. Anatomically this structure is housed within a symmetrical unit called a lobule, with the venous outflow tract (the hepatic venule) at its centre and the hepatic arteriole, portal venule and bile duct arranged around the outside in portal triads (see Figure 19.2).

This single sheet of cells is responsible for the main functions of the liver: removing and excreting certain (often harmful) substances (detoxification), processing and storing nutrients, synthesising proteins and production of bile to aid digestion. Specialised phagocytic cells, called Kupffer cells, perform the additional role of producing immune factors and removing bacteria and damaged red blood cells.

The physiology of bile formation and excretion is discussed in detail in Chapter 19.

Detoxification

Substances that have entered the blood, either from the outside (by ingestion, injection or absorption) or by production during metabolism, are processed in the liver cells and excreted in bile, or altered so that they can more easily be excreted in urine. One of the main mechanisms by which this occurs is conjugation. One of the main substances detoxified by conjugation is bilirubin (see physiology of bilirubin metabolism in Chapter 30). In addition the liver deaminates amino acids and inactivates some hormones.

Processing and storage of nutrients

The hepatocytes store many types of vitamins and minerals from the blood. These include vitamins A, B12, D, E and K, and minerals like iron and copper.

Carbohydrates, when found in e[...] postprandially), can be stored as gl[...] version by the process of glycogenesis. In tur[...] bohydrate in glycogen is released by glycogenolysis once blood glucose levels fall. In addition, when liver glycogen reserves fall, the liver is responsible for the provision of glucose by gluconeogenesis, converting non-sugars such as amino acids to glucose.

When fat is in excess in the blood the liver prepares it for storage in the subcutaneous tissue and other storage sites. This process is called lipogenesis. Amino acids can also be prepared for storage by conversion to fat. In order for this to occur, the amino acids must first be deaminated (have the nitrogen-containing NH_2 group removed). NH_2 quickly changes to highly toxic NH_3 (ammonia), which must be converted to urea by the liver so that it can be excreted in the urine.

Protein synthesis

The liver is responsible for the synthesis of numerous plasma proteins, which are important for processes around the body. Albumin binds many water-insoluble substances and contributes to osmotic pressure, fibrinogen is key to the clotting process, and globulins are used to transport substances such as cholesterol and iron. Notably, most of the 12 clotting factors are produced in the liver, thus a decline in the synthetic function of the liver is closely paralleled by deterioration in coagulation (often measured using the INR).

Jaundice

Jaundice results when the liver's capacity to convert and excrete bilirubin as bile is exceeded. This can result from:

- Over-production of bilirubin.
- Reduction in the eliminatory capacity of the liver.

Bilirubin is the breakdown product of haem (from haemoglobin and other haemoproteins). It is bound to albumin in the plasma, but at the hepatocyte membrane it dissociates and enters the hepatocyte. It is then conjugated, primarily with glucuronic acid, and excreted as bile.

Thus jaundice can be divided into three main mechanisms (Table 20.1):

- **Prehepatic**: increased degradation of haem (due to haemolysis) leading to haem concentrations

Table 20.1 Classification of jaundice by cause, symptoms and investigation features.

Type of jaundice	Laboratory features	Clinical features	Common causes
Pre-hepatic (haemolytic)	Blood: unconjugated hyperbilirubinaemia Urine: no bilirubin present, urobilinogen increased	Jaundice Normal urine Normal stool	Haemolysis Kidney diseases (e.g. haemolytic uraemic syndrome) Diseases with increased rate of haemolysis (e.g. sickle cell anaemia, glucose-6-phosphate dehydrogenase deficiency, malaria)
Hepatic	Blood: hyperbilirubinaemia unconjugated or mixed conjugated and unconjugated Urine: bilirubin present, urobilinogen may be increased but variable	Jaundice Urine dark Normal stool	Commonest: acute hepatitis, alcoholic liver disease, drug hepatotoxicity Less common causes: primary biliary cirrhosis, Gilbert's syndrome (a genetic disorder of bilirubin metabolism present in 5% of the population, which can result in mild jaundice), metastatic carcinoma
Posthepatic (obstructive/ cholestatic)	Blood: conjugated hyperbilirubinaemia Urine: increased conjugated bilirubin, no urinary urobilinogen	Jaundice Severe itching Urine dark Stools pale	Extrahepatic biliary disease (most commonly, gallstones in the common bile duct and cancer in the head of the pancreas; rarer, strictures of the common bile duct, biliary atresia, ductal carcinoma, pancreatitis and pancreatic pseudocysts, liver flukes in the common bile duct) Intrahepatic cholestasis

that cannot be cleared by the normal conjugative mechanisms, resulting in a predominantly unconjugated hyperbilirubinaemia.
- **Hepatic**: liver damage and/or inflammation affecting the conjugative and excretory ability of the liver so that the normal bilirubin load cannot be excreted, resulting in a predominantly unconjugated, or mixed conjugated and unconjugated, hyperbilirubinaemia.
- **Posthepatic**: obstruction of the biliary outflow tract at any level, leading to an inability to excrete conjugated bilirubin in bile, resulting in a conjugated hyperbilirubinaemia.

Unconjugated bilirubin is water insoluble and thus is not excreted in urine. Conjugated bilirubin excreted in bile is metabolised by bacteria and converted to urobilinogen in the terminal ileum, and then reabsorbed as part of the enterohepatic circulation before being excreted in urine. Urobilinogen is colourless, but that which is not reabsorbed is further converted to urobilin, then stercobilin, which is brown, giving faeces its normal colour. Testing for the different by-products of haem excretion in the blood and urine and observation of the stool give clues as to the cause of jaundice. Obstruction of the biliary system results in pale stools (decreased stercobilin) and dark urine (increased conjugated bilirubin, which is unable to be excreted into bile), but no urobilinogen (because no bilirubin is available for conversion by bacteria in the intestine).

Portal hypertension

Raised pressure in the portal venous system is generally a result of increased resistance classified as occurring within the sinusoids (sinusoidal), proximal to the hepatic sinusoids or distal to the sinusoids (pre- or post-sinusoidal respectively). Another classification system divides the cause into hepatic, pre-hepatic and post-hepatic.

The portal system is formed by the confluence of the splenic and superior mesenteric veins. The critical physiological measure is the 'portal pressure gradient' (the difference in pressure between the portal vein and hepatic veins), and portal hypertension is defined as this gradient reaching 12 mmHg or greater. Increased pressure in the portal system results in (Figure 20.2):

- Collateral vessel formation (in particular varices).
- Ascites.
- Increased risk of hepatorenal syndrome.

- Hepatic encephalophathy.
- Congestion of the gastric mucosa, called portal hypertensive gastropathy (Figure 20.3).
- Splenomegaly (enlargement of the spleen) with consequent sequestration therein of red blood cells, white blood cells and platelets, resulting in pancytopenia (hypersplenism).

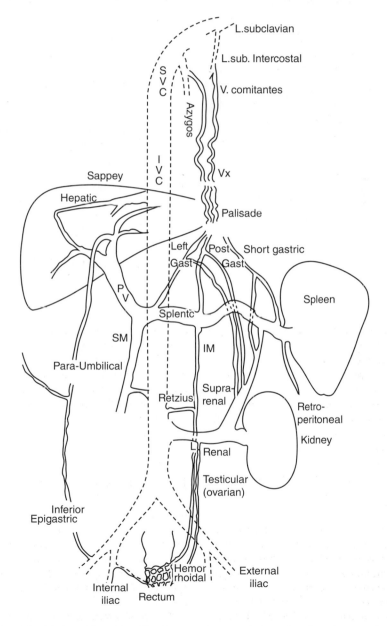

Figure 20.2 Schematic drawing of the major veins that may form portal systemic collateral routes. Source: Okuda K. 1991. Portal-systemic collaterals: anatomy and clinical implications. New York: Springer-Verlag. Reproduced with permission of Springer Science + Business Media.

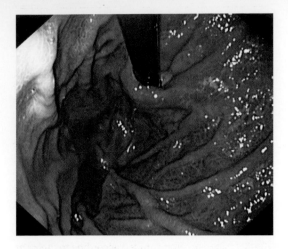

Figure 20.3 Portal hypertensive gastropathy.

Management

First-line treatment is with a non-selective beta-blocker (nadolol or propranolol) to reduce the pressure within the portal system. It is often used as primary prophylaxis once portal hypertension is diagnosed, and should always be considered for secondary prophylaxis after an episode of variceal bleeding.

Ascites

Ascites, the presence of fluid in the peritoneum, has two main pathogenic mechanisms, transudation and exudation.

- **Transudates** result from sequestration of fluid into the peritoneal space due to changes in hydrostatic and oncotic pressures across the peritoneum, or due to fluid retention:
  - Hydrostatic: these are the result of portal hypertension and resultant increases in the pressure in splanchnic vessels.
  - Oncotic: these are the result of lowered serum albumin as the synthetic function of the liver decreases.
  - Fluid retention: renal hypoperfusion resulting from portal hypertension causes release of renin, and hence a secondary hyperaldosteronism; this results in salt and water retention and contributes to ascites.
- **Exudates** result from an inflammatory or neoplastic process at the peritoneal surface, causing increased production of peritoneal secretions. It is the former that is important in hepatic disease, although occasionally

malignant processes that involve the liver may involve the peritoneal surface also.

Investigations

Ascites, when significant, is usually obvious on clinical assessment. The most useful technique to ascertain the presence of ascites is shifting dullness (see Part IV). Ultrasound will clearly delineate the presence and amount of ascites. In addition, ultrasound can be used to detect changes consistent with chronic portal hypertension (portal venous cavernous transformation, splenomegaly). Paracentesis is helpful in determining whether ascitic fluid represents a transudate or exudate and to investigate for the presence of infection or malignant cells.

In order to determine whether ascites is related to transudation or exudation, the serum-to-ascites albumin gradient (SAAG) is calculated:

$$SAAG = \text{Serum albumin concentration} (g/l)$$
$$-\text{Ascites albumin concentration} (g/l)$$

A high gradient (>11 g/l) indicates that the ascites is due to portal hypertension. A low gradient (<11 g/l) indicates ascites of non-portal hypertensive aetiology.

Management

- **General**:
  - Treatment of the underlying liver condition.
  - Improvement of nutritional status in order to maximise serum albumin.
- **Specific**:
  - Reduction of hydrostatic pressure in the splanchnic vasculature with diuretics, particularly spironolactone (an aldosterone antagonist).
  - Abdominal paracentesis (removal of ascitic fluid through a drain placed temporarily in the peritoneal space) when ascites volumes are large. There is an argument for the use of intravenous albumin replacement during paracentesis in order to reduce the haemodynamic consequences of fluid shifts: 10 g of albumin is given for each litre of ascites removed.

Intractable ascites is defined as ascites not responding to aggressive diuretic use. In this setting the options are:

- Repeated paracentesis.
- Radiological placement of intrahepatic portal-venous shunts to reduce splanchnic pressure (transjugular intrahepatic portosystemic shunt [TIPS]).
- Surgical shunt placement (now rarely needed).

Spontaneous bacterial peritonitis

Spontaneous bacterial peritonitis (SBP) is, as the name suggests, the spontaneous onset of bacterial infection of ascitic fluid in the setting of liver disease. Patients with the transudative ascites of liver disease with portal hypertension are particularly at risk of bacterial infection in the peritoneum because of the comorbid loss of the defensive mechanisms present in normal peritoneal secretions, in particular opsonising proteins. Thus, the risk of SBP increases as the protein content of the fluid decreases, the greatest risk being in those with an ascitic albumin concentration <1 g/l.

The bacteria implicated in SBP are enteric organisms. Traditionally, three-quarters of SBP infections are caused by aerobic Gram-negative organisms (mostly *Escherichia coli*), and one-quarter is due to aerobic Gram-positive organisms (especially Streptococcal species). However, the percentage of Gram-positive infections may be increasing, related to quinolone resistance among Gram-positive bacteria.

Investigations

The *diagnosis* of SBP is by paracentesis and identification of ascitic neutrophils >250/mm³. Gram stain and culture of ascitic fluid should also be performed. Culture is aided by direct inoculation of aerobic and anaerobic blood culture bottles, each with 10 ml of ascitic fluid, at the time of collection.

Management

Empiric *therapy* is with:

- Intravenous third-generation cephalosporins, but may be guided by past culture and sensitivity results in the setting of recurrent SBP.
- Concomitant administration of intravenous albumin.

There may be a role for *prophylactic antibiotics* in patients at high risk:

- Ascitic albumin concentration <10 g/l if hospitalised for other reasons.
- Past SBP.
- Patients with fluid protein <15 g/l and either Child–Turcotte–Pugh score of at least 9 or impaired renal function.
- Cirrhotic patients presenting with bleeding oesophageal varices.

Oesophageal and gastric varices

Chronic elevation of the portal pressure results in the formation of collateral venous tract formation between the portal circulation and the systemic venous system. The most troublesome site of collateral formation is around the proximal stomach and distal oesophagus (gastro-oesophageal varices). These varices largely result from collateral flow from the portal system, through the left gastric, posterior gastric and short gastric veins into the azygous vein (Figure 20.2). They lie submucosally and, with minimal trauma and resultant ulceration, can bleed into the GI tract. Varices are graded according to their size and the presence of overlying mucosal lesion (Box 20.1). The grade is a predictor of the likelihood of future variceal bleeding.

Investigation

Oesophageal varices are readily visible at endoscopy (see Figure 20.4). Patients known to have cirrhosis are generally gastroscoped at intervals to monitor for the presence and severity of oesophageal varices. Gastric varices also occur and are visible gastroscopically. Ultrasound and CT can be useful to define the presence of portal venous cavernous transformation, which exists in tandem with varices.

Management

Treatment of varices can take two forms:

- Primary prophylaxis, following diagnosis of varices but prior to the development of a bleeding complication.
- Secondary prophylaxis, instituted after an episode of bleeding.

Currently the favoured initial treatment for primary prophylaxis is with beta-blockers. The risk of variceal bleeding relates to the grade of varices and the severity of liver disease (Figure 20.5).

Box 20.1 Grading for oesophageal varices

Grade 1: Varices that collapse on inflation of the oesophagus with air

Grade 2: Varices between grades 1 and 3

Grade 3: Varices that are large enough to occlude the lumen

(a)   (b)

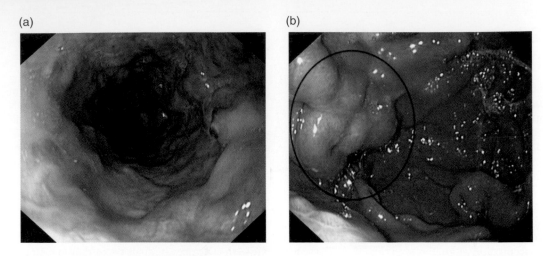

Figure 20.4   (a) Oesophageal varices. (b) Gastric varices at endoscopy.

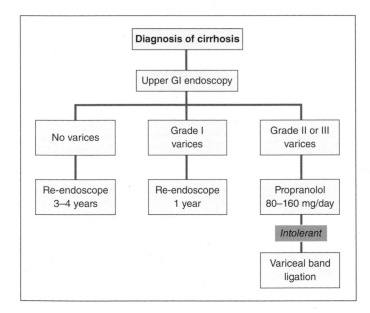

Figure 20.5   Primary management of oesophageal varices.

During an episode of variceal bleeding, endoscopic treatment is required immediately following haemodynamic stabilisation and airway protection:

- The modality of first choice is band ligation.
- Second-line modalities are:
  - Sclerotherapy.
  - Splanchnic vasoconstrictors (vasopressin).
  - Sengstaken tube (an apparatus consisting of a tube with a balloon on the end that is inserted into the oesophagus to tamponade the bleeding vessel; Figure 20.6).

Secondary prophylaxis (Figure 20.7) following an episode of confirmed variceal bleeding is:

- Variceal band ligation in the first instance.
- Beta-blockers in combination with banding or alone.
- Endoscopic variceal injection of tissue glue or thrombin.
- Transluminal intrahepatic portosystemic shunts (TIPPS) and surgical shunts are reserved for patients who do not respond to banding.

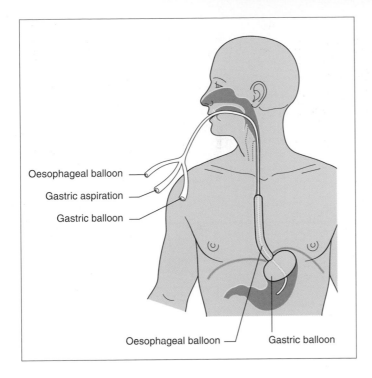

Oesophageal balloon

Gastric aspiration

Gastric balloon

Oesophageal balloon — — Gastric balloon

Figure 20.6 Sengstaken tube for tamponade of bleeding varices.

Hepatic encephalopathy

Hepatic encephalopathy results when toxic metabolites cannot be excreted by the diseased liver; they bypass the liver due to portosystemic shunts and produce direct effects on the brain. The mechanisms underlying this are thought to be multifactorial. Initially it was believed that direct toxic effects of ammonia on the brain were the main factor. However, more recently attention has focused on alterations in plasma amino acid composition leading to accumulation of 'false' neurotransmitters in the brain and increases in neuroinhibitory substances such as manganese, monoamines or endogenous opiates.

Investigations

The differential diagnosis of hepatic encephalopathy is wide (Box 20.2) and its diagnosis at presentation usually requires, in addition to the confirmation and grading of liver failure, exclusion of metabolic disease and toxins (or withdrawal effects) and head CT to exclude intracranial events. Subtle disturbances of cognition can be detected and followed using bedside and more specialised psychometric evaluation (Table 20.2).

Management

Frequently there are factors that precipitate the onset of encephalopathy and correction of these may reverse or at least reduce symptoms. These factors can be classified as direct neurotoxic precipitants, promoters of ammonia formation and factors altering blood–brain barrier function (Table 20.3).

- The mainstay of therapy is the use of non-digestible disaccharides such as lactulose (given orally through a nasogastric tube or through retention enemas). The dose should be adjusted to accomplish three or four soft bowel movements each day.
- Reduction of protein in the diet may be reasonable in the short term but is not a long-term consideration.
- Traditionally, non-absorbable antibiotics were used to detoxify the colon and reduce the production of nitrogenous metabolites. The toxic effects of this meant that it went out of favour for a time, but recent evidence suggests that rifaximin, a semisynthetic antibiotic based on rifamycin that has very poor oral bioavailability, may be useful in preventing recurrence in refractory hepatic encephalopathy.
- L-ornithine L-aspartate (LOLA) is a stable salt of the two constituent amino acids. L-ornithine stimulates the urea cycle, with resulting loss of ammonia. LOLA

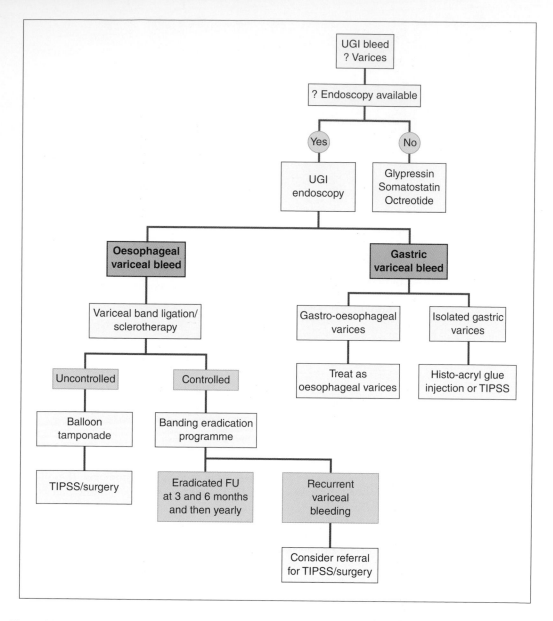

Figure 20.7 Secondary management of oesophageal varices. FU: follow-up.

Box 20.2 Differential diagnosis in hepatic encephalopathy

Metabolic encephalopathies
- Diabetes (hypoglycaemia, ketoacidosis)
- Hypoxia
- Carbon dioxide narcosis

Toxic encephalopathies
- Alcohol (acute alcohol intoxication, delirium tremens, Wernicke–Korsakoff syndrome)
- Drugs

Intracranial events
- Intracerebral bleeding or infarction
- Tumour
- Infections (abscess, meningitis)

Encephalitis

Table 20.2 Grading of hepatic encephalopathy.

Grade	Level of consciousness	Personality and intellect	Neurological signs	Electroencephalogram abnormalities
0	Normal	Normal	None	None
Subclinical	Normal	Normal	Abnormalities only on psychometric testing	None
1	Day/night sleep reversal Restlessness	Forgetfulness Mild confusion Agitation Irritability	Tremor Apraxia Incoordination Impaired handwriting	Triphasic waves (5 Hz)
2	Lethargy Slowed responses	Disorientation to time Loss of inhibition Inappropriate behaviour	Asterixis Dysarthria Ataxia Hypoactive reflexes	Triphasic waves (5 Hz)
3	Somnolence Confusion	Disorientation to place Aggressive behaviour	Asterixis Muscular rigidity Babinski signs Hyperactive reflexes	Triphasic waves (5 Hz)
4	Coma	None	Decerebration	Delta/slow wave activity

Table 20.3 Precipitants of encephalopathy in chronic liver disease.

	Example	Mechanism	Treatment
Neurotoxins	Sedatives, tranquillisers, analgesics	Direct depressant action on brain	Avoid sedatives Lactulose
Increase in serum ammonia	Azotaemia (excess of urea and other nitrogenous compounds in the blood)	Urea production in colon Excessive diuresis Prerenal azotaemia	Lactulose Discontinue diuretics Volume expansion with albumin
	GI bleeding	Colonic protein load leads to ammonia Production Hypovolaemia	Lactulose Blood or plasma transfusion Volume expansion
	Excess dietary protein	Excess nitrogenous substances	Lactulose Reduce protein in diet
	Infection	Peripheral ammonia production Tissue catabolism leading to ammonia production	Treat infection Lactulose
	Constipation	Retention of ammonium in colon More efficient formation of ammonia by colonic bacteria	Laxatives (e.g. lactulose)
Disturbance of blood–brain barrier	Metabolic alkalosis	Diffusion of ammonia across blood–brain barrier	Treat underlying cause

was found to be effective in treating acute refractory hepatic encephalopathy in a number of European trials.

- Occasionally refractory encephalopathy is the main indicator for liver transplantation.

Hepatorenal syndrome

Renal dysfunction in chronic liver disease is often multifactorial: involving hypovolaemia, changes in renal perfusion, infection and use of nephrotoxic drugs. Hepatorenal syndrome (HRS) refers to acute, potentially reversible, oliguric renal failure resulting from intense intrarenal vasoconstriction in otherwise normal kidneys. It occurs in patients with either chronic or acute liver disease. The former group comprises patients with cirrhosis, ascites and liver failure, the latter acute liver failure and alcoholic hepatitis. There are associated gross alterations in cardiovascular function and overactivity of the sympathetic nervous and renin–angiotensin systems, with resultant retention of sodium and water and renal vasoconstriction. It can be classified into early (Type 1) and late (Type 2) hepatorenal syndrome (Table 20.4).

The diagnosis of HRS is one of exclusion (Box 20.3), and it should not be diagnosed until all potentially reversible causes of renal failure have been excluded or treated.

Management

In the first instance treatment is aimed at correcting reversible factors:

- Hypovolaemia.
- Infection.
- Presence of nephrotoxins.

Alternative initial treatment is obviously required in Type 1 HRS:

- Vasoconstrictors, usually terlipressin, in combination with albumin administration.
- TIPSS improve renal function and may improve survival in Type 1 HRS. This has not been shown in Type 2 HRS, but TIPSS may be used to improve the refractory ascites often associated with Type 2 HRS.

Liver transplantation is the only definitive treatment for HRS and remains the treatment of choice. It must be noted, however, that morbidity after liver

Table 20.4 Classification of hepatorenal syndrome (HRS).

Early (Type 1) HRS	Late (Type 2) HRS
Rapidly progressive:	Steady or slowly progressive course
• Usually associated with acute deterioration of circulatory function	
• Characterised by arterial hypotension and activation of endogenous vasoconstrictor	
Severe renal failure: doubling of the initial serum creatinine concentrations to a level >226 µmol/l in <2 weeks	Moderate renal failure: serum creatinine 133–226 µmol/l
May be associated with impaired cardiac and liver functions as well as encephalopathy	Typically associated with refractory ascites
May appear spontaneously, but often develops after a precipitating event, particularly SBP	Appears spontaneously, but can also follow a precipitating event
80% mortality at 2 weeks, only 10% survival at 3 months	70% survival at 3 months, 40% at 1 year

SBP, spontaneous bacterial peritonitis.

Box 20.3 Diagnostic hepatorenal syndrome criteria in cirrhosis

- Cirrhosis with ascites
- Serum creatinine >133 µmol/l
- No improvement of serum creatinine (decrease to a level of 133 µmol/l) after at least 2 days with diuretic withdrawal and volume expansion with albumin
- Absence of shock
- No current or recent treatment with nephrotoxic drugs
- Absence of parenchymal kidney disease as indicated by proteinuria >500 mg/day, microhaematuria (>50 red blood cells per high-power field) and/or abnormal renal ultrasonography

---

Box 20.4 Aa gradient equation

$$Aa\ Gradient = \left(F_iO_2 \left(P_{atm} - P_{H_2O} \right) - \frac{P_aCO_2}{0.8} \right) - P_aO_2$$

F_iO_2: inspired fraction of oxygen; P_{atm}: atmospheric pressure [760 mmHg at sea level]; P_{H_2O}: water vapour pressure [47 mmHg = 100% humidity in the alveoli]; P_aCO_2 and P_aO_2 measured in blood.

---

transplantation is higher in patients with HRS than in those without HRS.

Hepatopulmonary syndrome

Pulmonary dysfunction in association with chronic liver disease is common, with up to 70% of patients complaining of shortness of breath. The differential diagnosis of dyspnoea is extensive in this setting and includes all the common causes of pulmonary dysfunction in those without liver disease. The classic pulmonary condition occurring in chronic liver disease is termed hepatopulmonary syndrome (HPS). This occurs when intrapulmonary vasodilatation impairs arterial oxygenation. It has serious consequences in terms of increasing mortality in the setting of cirrhosis and may influence the frequency and severity of complications of portal hypertension. HPS may co-exist with other cardiopulmonary abnormalities.

Investigations

The diagnosis of HPS relies on the demonstration of:

- Liver disease or portal hypertension,
- Elevated age-adjusted alveolar–arterial oxygen gradient (AaPO$_2$, Box 20.4), *and*
- Evidence of intrapulmonary vasodilatation.

Where pulmonary disease is suspected, arterial blood gas estimation should be performed and the alveolar–arterial oxygen gradient compared to age-controlled normal values. If hypoxia is demonstrated, more common pulmonary diseases must be screened for and adequately treated in the first instance (Figure 20.8).

The preferred test to demonstrate intrapulmonary vasodilatation and shunting is transthoracic microbubble

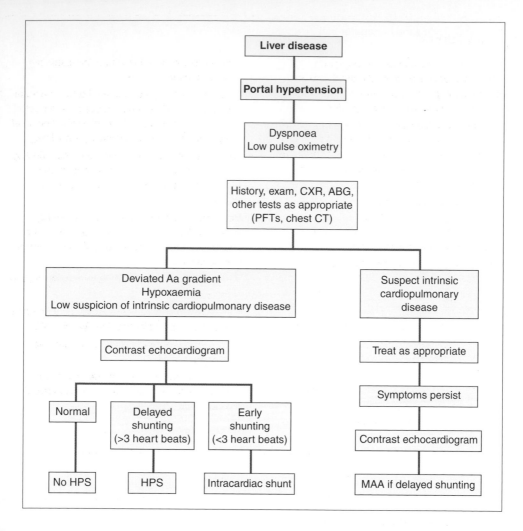

Figure 20.8 Diagnosis of hepatopulmonary syndrome (HPS). ABG, arterial blood gas; CT, computer tomography; CXR, chest X-ray; MAA, macroaggregated albumin scan; PFT, pulmonary function test.

contrast echocardiography. Echocardiography is performed by injecting agitated saline intravenously during normal transthoracic echocardiography, producing microbubbles that are visualised by ultrasonography. If an intracardiac shunt is present, contrast agent enters the left ventricle within three heart beats (early shunting). If intrapulmonary shunting characteristic of HPS is present, the left ventricle opacifies at least three heart beats after the right (delayed shunting).

In the presence of co-existing cardiac or pulmonary disease, establishing a diagnosis of HPS can be difficult. In the presence of cardiopulmonary disease, an estimate of the contribution of intrapulmonary shunting due to HPS, and its contribution to hypoxaemia, can be made using the macroaggregated albumin scan. In this test, radiolabelled aggregates of albumin

measuring approximately 20 μm in diameter are infused into the venous system. In the presence of significant intrapulmonary shunting, a fraction of the macroaggregated albumin passes through the lungs and into the systemic circulation. Scintigraphy then reveals uptake in other organs in addition to the lung, allowing the calculation of the shunt fraction.

Management

There are no effective medical therapies for HPS and liver transplantation is the only established effective treatment. Oxygen supplementation is the mainstay of supportive therapy for HPS patients with a PaO_2 <60 mmHg or with exercise-induced oxygen desaturation.

KEY POINTS

- The liver is responsible for removing and excreting substances (detoxification), processing and storing nutrients, synthesising proteins and production of bile to aid digestion.
- Jaundice is caused by either over-production of bilirubin (pre-hepatic) or a reduction in the eliminatory capacity of the liver. The latter occurs either within the liver (hepatic) or because of obstruction of bile outflow (post-hepatic).
- Portal hypertension can result from damage within the hepatic sinusoids (sinusoidal), proximal to the sinusoids (pre-sinusoidal) or distal to the sinusoids (post-sinusoidal)
- A high (>11 g/l) serum to ascites albumin gradient indicates that the ascites is due to portal hypertension.
- The diagnosis of spontaneous bacterial peritonitis is by paracentesis and identification of ascitic neutrophils >250/mm³.
  - The risk increases as the protein content of the fluid decreases.
  - Empiric therapy is with intravenous third-generation cephalosporin.
- The risk of bleeding from varices is predicted by their grade.

  - First-line treatment is with a non-selective beta-blocker.
  - Variceal banding can be used after a variceal bleed (secondary prophylaxis) or when beta-blockers are poorly tolerated or a patient is at high risk of bleeding (primary prophylaxis).
- Hepatic encephalopathy can be precipitated by direct neurotoxins, promoters of ammonia formation and factors altering blood–brain barrier function.
- Hepatorenal syndrome is acute, potentially reversible, oliguric renal failure resulting from intense intrarenal vasoconstriction in otherwise normal kidneys.
  - Management is aimed at correcting reversible factors.
  - Terlipressin and TIPSS improve renal function and may improve survival in Type 1 HRS.
  - Liver transplantation is the only definitive treatment for HRS.
- Hepatopulmonary syndrome develops when intrapulmonary vasodilatation impairs arterial oxygenation.

 SELF-ASSESSMENT QUESTION

(The answer to this question is given on p. 268)

A 52-year-old man is admitted to hospital because of increasing confusion, jaundice and ascites. He is a known alcoholic and has been previously shown to have a coarsened liver architecture on ultrasound and grade 1 varices at endoscopy. There is no clinical evidence of recent gastrointestinal haemorrhage.

Regarding the initial investigation and management of this man, which of the following statements is most true?

(a) Lactulose is currently preferred over Rifaximin for the treatment of his presumed hepatic encephalopathy.

(b) A diagnosis of spontaneous bacterial peritonitis is indicated by an ascites fluid lymphocyte count of more than 250/mm³.

(c) Empiric therapy for spontaneous bacterial peritonitis is best acheived with benzyl-penicillin.

(d) At endoscopy the patient continues to have grade 1 varices. He should now have prophylactic banding undertaken.

(e) A serum to ascites albumin gradient less than 11 g/L would be expected in this clinical situation.

21

Liver transplantation

Indications and contraindications

Orthotopic liver transplantation (OLT), when required, is indicated for most causes of acute or chronic liver disease. Cirrhosis accounts for > 80% of transplants performed in adults, hepatitis C and alcoholism being the two most common underlying diagnoses.

There are very few absolute contraindications to OLT:

- Anatomic abnormality precluding transplant.
- Malignancy outside the liver.
- Untreated sepsis.
- Advanced cardiopulmonary disease.
- Active alcohol and drug use.

However, conditions previously considered contraindications, such as HIV infection and older age, are now only relative considerations in many centres.

Preparation

Prior to pre-transplant assessment, the patient's requirements for transplantation need to be categorised in order to rationalise this limited resource. In **fulminant liver failure**, the King's College Criteria are used to predict outcome and the need for OLT (Box 21.1).

In patients with **cirrhosis**, referral for OLT should be considered once an index complication has occurred, as such events mark a relative reduction in survival rates in the cirrhotic patient. These complications ('decompensations' of chronic disease) include variceal bleeding, onset of ascites or hypoalbuminaemia and development of hepatorenal syndrome. The aim is to bring a patient to transplantation at a point where their expected survival is in the realm of 1–2 years, but before organ failure develops. Calculating the prognosis of patients with cirrhosis is currently defined using both disease-specific and generic clinical tools.

- The Child–Turcotte–Pugh score (see Table 2.4) is used most frequently to assess prognosis of cirrhotic patients, establishing three classes of severity (A, B and C).
- The Model for End-stage Liver Disease (MELD) score is in current use in the USA. It incorporates values for serum bilirubin, serum creatinine and INR for prothrombin time in a log-transformed equation to estimate likelihood of 3-month survival (Table 2.6). The formula is available at http://www.mayoclinic. org/meld/mayomodel6.html.
- A Child–Turcotte–Pugh Score of 7, a MELD score of 10 or any complication of portal hypertension is an appropriate indication for transplant evaluation.

Referral for pre-transplant assessment is then made in discussion with the transplant team. The pre-transplant assessment ensures that the patient will be able to tolerate the stress of the surgery, immunosuppression and highly demanding post-transplant care. It includes an extensive cardiopulmonary and psychosocial evaluation, screening for occult infection and neoplasia, as well as careful education of the patient and family.

Gastroenterology and Hepatology: Lecture Notes, Second Edition. Stephen Inns and Anton Emmanuel.
© 2017 John Wiley & Sons, Ltd. Published 2017 by John Wiley & Sons, Ltd.
Companion website: www.lecturenoteseries.com/gastroenterology

> ### Box 21.1 King's College Criteria for acute liver failure
>
> *Patients with paracetamol toxicity*
> - pH <7.3 or
> - PT >100 s and serum creatinine level > 300 µmol/l (>3.4 mg/dl) if in Grade III or IV encephalopathy
>
> *Other patients*
> Three of the following variables:
> - Age <10 years or >40 years
> - Cause:
>   - Non-A, non-B hepatitis
>   - Halothane hepatitis
>   - Idiosyncratic drug reaction
> - Duration of jaundice before encephalopathy >7 days
> - PT >50 s
> - Serum bilirubin >300 µmol/l (>17.6 mg/dl)

The operation

The operation to transplant a liver consists of three phases:

1 Removal of the donor liver.
2 Removal of the recipient's native liver.
3 Grafting of the transplant.
  - Two main types of incision are used: the 'Mercedes incision', which consists of bilateral subcostal incisions with a midline extension, and the inverted J incision.
  - A temporary shunt between the portal system and inferior vena cava is formed in order to reduce the haemodynamic changes that would occur if the hepatic vessels were simply clamped during removal of the native liver.
  - The liver is then isolated from the arterial and biliary systems, and removed.
  - All dissected vessels are prepared for subsequent anastomosis and the donor liver is finally grafted into the site of the native liver.

Postoperative care

Immunosuppression

Immunosuppression in OLT has three main phases: induction, maintenance and treatment of rejection episodes.

Induction

- Typically high-dose steroids along with introduction of a calcineurin inhibitor, either cyclosporin or tacrolimus.
- Common side-effects of the immunosuppressants used are listed in Table 21.1.
- Mycophenolate mofetil or azathioprine may be used as an adjuvant agent to allow lower doses of the calcineurin inhibitors.

Protection of renal function is especially important in the early post-transplant period. **Acute cellular rejection (ACR)** has decreased in incidence with the use of potent immunosuppressive agents, but it still affects 15–25% of liver transplant recipients, typically 5–14 days following transplantation (although it may present later). Treatment of ACR early in the post-transplant period is with intravenous corticosteroids tapered rapidly over several days. The addition of mycophenolate mofetil and higher levels of tacrolimus can treat ACR that is not responsive to steroids.

Maintenance

- In the majority of cases, immunosuppression is with a calcineurin inhibitor (cyclosporin or tacrolimus) started immediately postoperatively with corticosteroids.
- Steroids are slowly reduced and often withdrawn within 6–12 months of OLT, the exception being with autoimmune liver disease.

Chronic rejection occurs late in the post-OLT course and is characterised by vanishing bile ducts (ductopenia). It may respond to a higher dose of tacrolimus, but can lead to the need for retransplantation.

Early post-transplant care

- Admission to the intensive care unit postoperatively:
  - All patients have markedly abnormal aminotransferase, bilirubin and INR in the initial 48–72 hours, usually returning to normal within a few weeks. This is a result of insults to the graft (such as the ischaemia that occurs following harvesting), the preservation in transit and the subsequent reperfusion of the graft.
  - If the above indices are rising rather than falling in the early postoperative phase, hepatic artery thrombosis must be excluded by Doppler ultrasound. Primary non-function of the graft may occur and mandates urgent retransplantation.

Table 21.1 Mechanism of action and adverse effects of orthotopic liver transplantation immunosuppressive drugs.

Drug	Tacrolimus	Cyclosporin	Prednisone	Mycophenolate mofetil (MMF)	Azathioprine
Mechanism	Calcineurin inhibitors: bind to intracellular proteins, inhibiting the phosphatase activity of calcineurin, resulting in inhibition of gene transcription for the synthesis of lymphokines such as IL-2		Inhibits transcription of IL-1 and IL-6 Blocks antigen recognition Causes redistribution of lymphocytes	Inhibitor of inosine monophosphate dehydrogenase	Inhibitor of DNA and RNA synthesis
Use	Most commonly used immunosuppressants in induction and maintenance Methylprednisone IV is the mainstay of initial treatment of acute cellular reaction (ACR)			Used as adjuvant agents in order to allow lower doses of the calcineurin inhibitors (and hence reduce toxicity) MMF used in steroid-resistant ACR	
Toxicity	Nephrotoxicity Tremor Hypertension Headache GI symptoms Alopecia Diabetes	Nephrotoxicity Tremor Hypertension Headache Hirsutism Gingival hyperplasia	Osteoporosis Osteonecrosis Diabetes Hyperlipidaemia Hirsutism Hypertension Cushingoid habitus	Leukopenia Nausea and vomiting Diarrhoea	Haematological Pancreatitis Cholestatic jaundice Hepatitis Interstitial pneumonitis

GI, gastrointestinal.

- After 1 week:
  - ACR becomes an important and frequent cause of increases in the LFTs. It is confirmed by liver biopsy and treated as already described.
  - Nosocomial infectious complications may occur. Fungal infections are of particular concern and are associated with poor prognosis.
  - Toxic effects of the calcineurin inhibitors (early neurological dysfunction, renal impairment and hyperglycaemia) may become evident.
- Following discharge, patients remain under weekly monitoring for the first month. In this phase ACR continues to be a concern, prompting urgent liver biopsy if liver dysfunction recurs.
- Peak onset of action by the calcineurin inhibitors is at 1 month, which is when post-transplant and opportunistic infections can intervene:
  - These include cytomegalovirus, herpes simplex virus, *Pneumocystis carinii* pneumonia and toxoplasmosis. The use of prophylactic antimicrobials depends on the risk profile of the individual patient and donor in combination.
  - Early recurrence of HCV and HBV can occur at this time. In the case of HBV, prophylaxis with hepatitis B immunoglobulin (with or without antiviral treatment) is effective.

Long-term care

The long-term care of the liver transplant recipient increasingly involves the primary and secondary care teams. Post-OLT patients are at risk of conditions specifically related to immunosuppression, and the underlying liver condition. The common complications and their monitoring and management are summarised in Table 21.2.

Malignancies after OLT are more frequent than in the general population. This relates to high-risk behaviour before transplant, specifically cigarette and alcohol abuse, and chronic immunosuppression. However, neither the degree of immunosuppression nor the specific immunosuppressive regimen after OLT has been associated with an increased risk of cancer (Table 21.3).

Strategies to maximise donor pool

The number of donor livers available each year is far fewer than the number of patients listed for liver transplant. This results in significant morbidity and mortality in patients listed and awaiting transplantation. Novel surgical techniques under development to maximise donor organ access include split cadaveric liver and living donor transplantation.

Table 21.2 Pathogenesis and management of post–liver transplantation complications.

	Pathogenesis	Monitoring	Management
Hypertension	Calcineurin inhibitors (CNI): reversible, dose-dependent hypertension due to vasoconstriction of afferent renal arterioles Corticosteroids: partial mineralocorticoid agonism, expanding plasma volume	Regular medical review, including blood pressure measurement	Lifestyle modifications: • Weight loss • Sodium restriction • Smoking cessation • Exercise • Abstinence from alcohol Wean-off corticosteroids, or reduce CNI dose Medication if persistent: • First-line: calcium-channel blockers: amlodipine and nifedipine (nicardipine, verapamil and diltiazem, increase CNI levels) • Second-line: clonidine, beta-blockers, ACE inhibitors
Renal dysfunction	Pre-existing in substantial minority of cirrhotic patients Glomerular filtration rate (GFR) drops to 60% of baseline within 6 weeks of surgery Causes: • CNIs are major cause • Underlying kidney disease • Ischaemic injury • Diabetes mellitus • Hypertension • Other nephrotoxic drugs • HCV	Routine testing of renal function at review	Treat hypertension and diabetes aggressively Reduce CNI dose (addition of mycophenolate mofetil or sirolimus) Mortality of OLT recipients maintained on dialysis is high and renal transplantation should be considered

(Continued)

Table 21.2 (Continued)

	Pathogenesis	Monitoring	Management
Post-transplant diabetes mellitus	Affects 10–30% of OLT recipients in first postoperative year Abates with time as doses of corticosteroids and TAC are tapered Insulin resistance final common pathway Exacerbated by: • Corticosteroids • Obesity • CNIs (direct toxicity on pancreatic beta-cells) • HCV	Screening immediately post-transplant and regularly thereafter with fasting plasma glucose Once diagnosed: • Regular self-monitoring of blood glucose • Management of dyslipidaemia • Screen annually for diabetic complications	Steroid and TAC-sparing regimens in diabetes prior to OLT Lifestyle and immunosuppressive regimen modification Majority require treatment with an oral agent Oral combination therapy followed by oral agent and insulin instituted in a stepwise fashion if needed

Hyperlipidaemia	Prevalence 40–66%
	CNIs may cause hyperlipidaemia (CYA and, to a lesser extent, TAC)
	SIR contributes to hypertriglyceridaemia in association with diabetes
	Risk factors:
	• High cholesterol pre-OLT
	• Post-OLT renal dysfunction
	Metabolic syndrome: genetics, diet, obesity and diabetes
		Lipid panel:
		• Early after transplantation
		• After any change in immunosuppression
			Primary target = correction of LDL cholesterol
			Lifestyle changes (alone rarely result in sufficient improvement):
			• Smoking cessation
			• Exercise
			• Dietary modification
			Contributing medications:
			• Thiazide diuretics
			• Beta-blockers
			• Immunosuppressive agents
			Early post-OLT usually does not require medication and resolves with reduction in steroids
			Medical management if lifestyle management and alteration of medications unsuccessful:
			• Isolated hypercholesterolaemia or mixed hyperlipidaemia: HMG-CoA reductase inhibitors ('statins') treatment of choice
			(*Note*: metabolism of most statins is decreased by CYA)
			• Hypertriglyceridaemia:
			  ○ Less severe cases managed with fish oil supplements
			  ○ Refractory cases can be safely treated with a fibrate
			  ○ Consider changing SIR to CYA or TAC

Bone mineral density (BMD)	BMD in cirrhotic patients is low:	Bone densitometry prior to CLT if cirrhotic or other risk factor for osteoporosis
	• Hypogonadism • Malnutrition • Physical inactivity BMD declines after OLT: • Immunosuppressives cause increased resorption as well as decreased formation of bone • Bed rest • Corticosteroids Risk factors: • Most important is low BMD pre-OLT • Older age • Degree of immunosuppression • Graft dysfunction • Female sex • Lower BMI • Renal dysfunction • Postmenopausal state	Counselling about: • Adequate vitamin D and calcium intake • Weight-bearing exercise • Nutritional repletion • Alcohol use • Smoking cessation Consider postmenopausal women and men with evidence of hypogonadism for hormone replacement therapy Antiresorptive agents, such as bisphosphonates, are the treatment of choice when osteoporosis diagnosed or long-term steroids predicted

CYA, cyclosporin; HCV, hepatitis C virus; SIR, sirolimus; TAC, tacrolimus.

Table 21.3 Post–liver transplantation cancer complications.

Cancer type	Association with OLT	Recommended surveillance
Non-melanoma skin cancer	20-fold higher risk than population Most common malignancy in adult OLT recipients Squamous cell carcinomas outnumber basal cell carcinomas	Routine examinations by a dermatologist if: • Sun-damaged skin • Previous history of skin neoplasms • Countries with high ultraviolet light exposure
Colon cancer		Colonoscopic surveillance for all OLT recipients Interval of examination individualised: • 5-year examinations if no previous history of colonic neoplasia • More frequent examinations for higher-risk patients with previous polyps • Ulcerative colitis transplanted for primary sclerosing cholangitis: yearly surveillance
Carcinoma of the oropharynx and oesophagus		Consider routine upper endoscopy and oropharyngeal examination Any new symptom should prompt thorough examination Consider endoscopic surveillance of patients with Barrett's oesophagus
Lung cancer	Particularly increased in alcoholic liver disease (probably related to high rate of smoking)	Consider for screening chest imaging, such as with low-radiation dose chest CT scanning
Post-transplant lymphoproliferative disease	30–50 times risk in general population Usually driven by Epstein–Barr virus	
Recurrence and progression of malignant and premalignant conditions after OLT	Varies greatly with tumour type: • Gynaecological and testicular cancers seldom recur after OLT (<10%) • Prostate, colon and lymphomas recur in 10–20% • Breast, bladder and skin carcinoma recur in 20–50%	Dependent on individual cancer

CT, computer tomography.

KEY POINTS

- In adults >80% of transplants are for cirrhosis; hepatitis C and alcoholism are the two most common underlying diagnoses.

- In cirrhosis, transplant is considered once an index complication has occurred. These include variceal bleeding, onset of ascites or hypoalbuminaemia and development of hepatorenal syndrome.

- The Child–Turcotte–Pugh score or Model for End-stage Liver Disease (MELD) score is used to predict mortality and prioritise for transplantation.

- In fulminant liver failure, the King's College Criteria are used to predict mortality.

- Careful pre-transplant assessment ensures that the patient will be able to tolerate the stress of the surgery, immunosuppression and highly demanding post-transplant care.

- Immunosuppression in OLT has three main phases: induction, maintenance and treatment of rejection.

- Acute cellular rejection (ACR) develops in approximately 25% of liver transplant recipients and is generally treated with intravenous corticosteroids tapered rapidly over several days.

- Chronic rejection occurs late in the post-OLT course and is characterised by vanishing bile ducts. It may respond to a higher dose of tacrolimus, but can lead to the need for retransplantation.

 SELF-ASSESSMENT QUESTION

(The answer to this question is given on p. 268)

The patient in the assessment question in Chapter 20 is referred for assessment for liver transplantation.

Regarding assessment and transplantation, which of the following statements is most correct?

(a) The King's College Criteria should be used to ascertain his suitability for transplant.

(b) The Child-Turcotte-Pugh score combines serum bilirubin, serum creatinine and INR in a score that estimates likelihood of 3-month survival.

(c) Acute cellular rejection is demonstrated by disappearance of the bile ducts on liver biopsy.

(d) Acute cellular rejection occurs in up to 25% of transplants and is generally treated with intravenous corticosteroids.

(e) Hepatitis B virus infection is effectively cured by transplantation and does not recur in the transplanted liver.

22

Alcoholic liver disease

Epidemiology and causes

Alcohol misuse is a major public health problem, the World Health Organization estimates that 140 million people globally suffer from alcohol dependence. Alcoholic liver disease (ALD) encompasses a spectrum of diseases ranging from fatty liver to alcoholic hepatitis to cirrhosis. The main risk factors are the quantity and duration of alcohol ingestion. In addition, nutritional status and genetic and metabolic traits play a role. The main genetic factors are polymorphisms in the genes responsible for ethanol metabolism, aldehyde and alcohol dehydrogenases (ALDHs and ADHs, respectively) and cytochromes P450 (CYPs). The male-to-female ratio is 11:4. This is despite the fact that differences in body water composition mean that women are more susceptible than men to the harmful effects of alcohol.

The main pathogenic mechanism for liver damage is oxidative stress, arising from:

- Changes in the redox state of the hepatocytes.
- Elevation of hepatocyte iron.
- Reactive acetaldehyde derivatives.
- Mitochondrial damage.
- Reduced cellular antioxidants.
- Alterations in intracellular signalling.
- Action of inflammatory cytokines, adipokines and hormones (Figure 22.1).

The pathology of ALD is considered a continuum from fatty liver through alcoholic hepatitis on to cirrhosis, although in practice these features often overlap.

- **Fatty liver** is the initial, reversible, effect:
  - Consists of the accumulation of cytoplasmic macrovesicular triglyceride droplets that displace the nucleus.
  - Less often there are microvesicular accumulations, which do not displace the nucleus, representing mitochondrial damage.
- **Alcoholic hepatitis** is the next step:
  - Results from the combination of fatty liver and inflammation with necrosis of hepatocytes.
  - Hepatocytes develop a swollen and granular cytoplasm (termed 'balloon degeneration').
  - Deposition of fibrillar protein and clumping of organelles in the cytoplasm (termed 'Mallory', or alcoholic, hyaline bodies).
- **Cirrhosis** occurs when advanced liver disease disrupts the normal liver architecture:
  - Collagen fibrosis of the terminal venules compromises perfusion and contributes to portal hypertension.
  - Regeneration is typically limited to the production of small nodules (micronodular cirrhosis), although, particularly with abstinence, macronodular cirrhosis can occur.
  - Iron accumulation in the hepatocytes occurs in up to 10% of patients.

Gastroenterology and Hepatology: Lecture Notes, Second Edition. Stephen Inns and Anton Emmanuel.
© 2017 John Wiley & Sons, Ltd. Published 2017 by John Wiley & Sons, Ltd.
Companion website: www.lecturenoteseries.com/gastroenterology

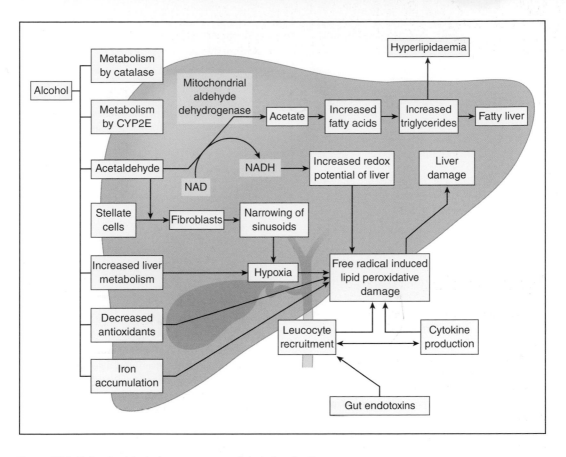

Figure 22.1 Pathophysiological consequences of alcohol on the liver.

Box 22.1 Features of Zieve's syndrome

Alcohol excess with:
- Alcoholic hepatitis
- Haemolysis
- Jaundice
- Abdominal pain
- Hyperlipidaemia

 Zieve's syndrome refers to a clinical state distinct from this progression of disease (Box 22.1).

Clinical features

Fatty liver

- Generally asymptomatic.
- Occasionally may cause anorexia, nausea and right upper quadrant pain (usually follows a prolonged, heavy alcoholic binge).

Alcoholic hepatitis

Wide range of symptoms from mild (limited, non-specific) to severe (fulminant); see Box 22.2.

- Moderate:
  - 2–3-week prodrome of fatigue, anorexia, nausea and weight loss.
  - Malnutrition is prominent.
  - Mild fever (<40 °C), jaundice and tender hepatomegaly.
- Severe:
  - Usually follows a period of drinking, and eating very poorly.
  - Gravely ill with fever, marked jaundice, ascites and evidence of a hyperdynamic circulation (marked palmar erythema is common), spider naevi, parotid enlargement and gynaecomastia.
  - Hypoglycaemia is common and can result in coma.
  - GI bleeding, usually due to a local gastric duodenal lesion, is common.

Box 22.2 Features of alcoholic hepatitis

- Tiredness, non-specific ill health
- Hepatomegaly, ascites
- Mild liver enzyme abnormalities
- Severity: encephalopathy or jaundice and elevated INR
- Histology: Mallory's hyaline, balloon degeneration, neutrophil infiltration
- Treatment: prednisolone for moderate–severe disease
- Alternative treatment: pentoxifylline, a phosphodi-esterase inhibitor that is thought to work through an anti-TNF mechanism

INR, international normalised ratio; TNF, tumour necrosis factor.

Box 22.3 CAGE questionnaire to identify alcohol misuse

This screening test is short and simple to administer. Two or more positive answers are correlated with alcohol dependence in 90% of cases. CAGE may not pick up problems in those who are fearful of negative consequences of disclosure (e.g. those looking for accommodation, or who are fearful of child protection issues) and those with mental health problems.
C – Have you ever thought you should CUT DOWN on your drinking?
A – Have you ever felt ANNOYED by others' criticism of your drinking?
G – Have you ever felt GUILTY about your drinking?
E – Do you have a morning EYE OPENER?

Cirrhosis

- Symptoms are those for any cause of cirrhosis (see Chapter 20).
- May be additional alcohol-related toxicities:
  - Peripheral neuropathy.
  - Wernicke's encephalopathy (ataxia, ophthalmo-plegia, confusion, impaired short-term memory).
  - Korsakoff's psychosis (amnesia, confabulation, apathy).
  - Hypogonadism and feminisation (in men).

Investigations

Diagnosis requires suspicion of alcohol as a cause of liver disease, remembering that patients may not always give an accurate alcohol history. CAGE and the Alcohol Use Disorders Identification Test (AUDIT, see http://www.who.int/substance_abuse/publications/alcohol/en/) are useful screening tools for the presence of an alcohol problem (Box 22.3).

No specific test exists for ALD. All *blood tests* suffer from the limitations of specificity:

- Serum gamma-glutamyl transferase (GGT) increases due to enzyme induction.
- Red-cell mean corpuscular volume (MCV): macrocytosis is a result of the effects of folate deficiency and alcohol on the bone marrow.
- Serum carbohydrate-deficient transferrin (CDT): relatively more specific for ALD than the other tests.
- Elevations of the aminotransferases are generally moderate (<300 IU/l) and do not reflect the degree of liver damage:

  - AST exceeds ALT (AST/ALT > 2).
  - Relatively low ALT is due to dietary deficiency of pyridoxal phosphate (vitamin B_6).
- Bilirubin and INR: severity of disease is related to the bilirubin (indicator of secretory function) and INR (synthetic function).
- All patients should have screening tests for treatable causes of liver disease, especially viral disease.

Liver biopsy is useful to confirm the diagnosis, stage the severity of the disease and rule out other liver conditions.

Management

- Abstinence is the mainstay of treatment.
- General supportive care:
  - Nutritious diet.
  - Vitamin (particularly B vitamin) supplementation, especially in the first few days of abstinence.
  - Withdrawal from alcohol is treated with benzodiazepines.
- Corticosteroid use is controversial. but may be beneficial for patients with severe alcoholic hepatitis complicated by encephalopathy. Maddrey's discriminative function is used to determine those who might benefit from corticosteroids (if score >32). It is calculated using the formula:

  (4.6 × (PT test – control)) + Serum bilirubin in mg/dl
- Trials of other drugs (propylthiouracil, colchicine) have not shown sustained benefit.

- Liver transplantation gives 5-year survival rates comparable to those after transplantation for non-alcoholic liver disease. However, about 50% of patients resume drinking after transplantation, so most programmes require 6 months of abstinence and assurance that good social networks are in place.

Prognosis

Once cirrhosis develops, patients who abstain have a 5-year survival rate of 60–70%, which falls to 40% in those who continue to drink. Negative prognostic indicators include:

- Low serum albumin.
- Increased INR/PT.
- Low haemoglobin.
- Encephalopathy.
- Persistent jaundice.
- Azotaemia.

Hepatocellular carcinoma occurs in 10% of stable cirrhotics, usually developing after a period of abstinence when macronodular cirrhosis is present.

 KEY POINTS

- Alcoholic liver disease occurs along a spectrum from fatty liver (the initial, reversible change) through alcoholic hepatitis to cirrhosis.
- Zieve's syndrome refers to a clinical state distinct from this progression of disease.
- The diagnosis of alcoholic liver disease requires suspicion of alcohol as a cause of liver disease.
  - CAGE and the Alcohol Use Disorders Identification Test (AUDIT) are useful screening tools.
- Abstinence is the mainstay of treatment.
- Corticosteroid use is controversial, but may be beneficial for patients with severe alcoholic hepatitis complicated by encephalopathy.

- Maddrey's discriminative function is used to help determine this.
- Once cirrhosis develops, patients who abstain have a 5-year survival rate of 60–70%. This falls to 40% in those who continue to drink.
- Liver transplantation gives 5-year survival rates comparable to those after transplantation for non-alcoholic liver disease.
  - However, about 50% of patients resume drinking after transplantation.
  - Most programmes require 6 months of abstinence and assurance that good social networks are in place.

23

Non-alcoholic fatty liver disease

Epidemiology and cause

Non-alcoholic fatty liver disease (NAFLD) is an umbrella term (Figure 23.1) encompassing simple steatosis (fatty liver) without liver inflammation, non-alcoholic steatohepatitis (NASH), where fatty infiltration results in inflammation of the liver and the risk of liver damage, and fibrosis and cirrhosis resulting from NASH.

NAFLD affects all age groups, including children, with an equal sex distribution. Its prevalence increases with increasing body weight, affecting 10–15% of normal individuals and up to 80% of the obese. NASH follows a similar pattern, affecting 3% of normal individuals and 20% of the morbidly obese (BMI >35 kg/m^2).

Most NAFLD is primary (idiopathic), but it can occur in association with rare disorders of lipid metabolism and insulin resistance, including:

- Abetalipoproteinaemia.
- Lipoatrophic diabetes.
- Mauriac and Weber–Christian syndrome.
- Iatrogenic:
  - Parenteral nutrition.
  - Acute starvation.
  - IV glucose therapy.
  - Abdominal surgery.
  - Drugs (amiodarone, tamoxifen, synthetic oestrogens and glucocorticoids).

NAFLD is principally associated with the metabolic syndrome and a 'two-hit' model of pathogenesis has been proposed:

- The first 'hit' consists of excessive triglyceride accumulation in the liver:
  - The driving factor is insulin resistance.
  - This primarily involves the muscles and adipose tissue and results in hyperinsulinaemia.
  - The liver remains insulin sensitive, resulting in increased hepatic uptake of free fatty acids (FFAs) and increased hepatic triglyceride synthesis.
  - This results in net hepatic fat accumulation. FFAs impair insulin signalling and cause further insulin resistance.
- Steatotic liver is then vulnerable to 'second hits', resulting in inflammation and liver damage:
  - Increased FFA oxidation produces hepatotoxic free oxygen radicals that contribute to oxidative stress and contribute to the 'second hit'.
  - Other contributors to the second hit include:
    - Pre-existing mitochondrial abnormalities.
    - Cytokine production (e.g. tumour necrosis factor-α).
    - Defects in peroxisome proliferator activating receptors (PPARs, which are involved in triggering the effects of insulin).
    - Resistance to leptin.

Clinical features

The symptoms of NAFLD, when there are any, are generally mild and non-specific (most commonly right upper quadrant abdominal pain). Most patients have no symptoms at all and the diagnosis is most commonly made incidentally. A detailed history

Gastroenterology and Hepatology: Lecture Notes, Second Edition. Stephen Inns and Anton Emmanuel.
© 2017 John Wiley & Sons, Ltd. Published 2017 by John Wiley & Sons, Ltd.
Companion website: www.lecturenoteseries.com/gastroenterology

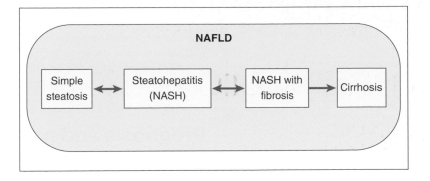

Figure 23.1 Spectrum of non-alcoholic fatty liver disease (NAFLD). NASH, non-alcoholic steatohepatitis.

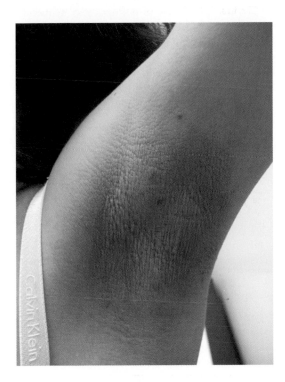

Figure 23.2 Acanthosis nigricans. Source: Badr D, Kurban M, Abbas O. Metformin in dermatology: an overview. J Eur Acad Dermatol Venereol. 2013;27(11):1329–1335. Reproduced with permission of John Wiley & Sons.

of alcohol consumption should be obtained. The findings on examination are those of the metabolic syndrome: commonly obesity (especially abdominal obesity), the complications of diabetes, hypertension and acanthosis nigricans (a dark pigmentation of the skin of the armpits and neck associated with insulin resistance; Figure 23.2). The liver usually feels normal; however, hepatomegaly may occur.

Investigations

Most commonly NAFLD is an accidental finding. There is no biochemical or imaging modality currently that can differentiate simple fatty liver from NASH.

The hallmark of NAFLD is macrovesicular steatosis in the absence of alcohol excess (<40 g of ethanol/week). In practice the diagnosis is made where there are persistently elevated LFTs, a negative alcohol history and other causes of fatty liver have been excluded. If weight loss results in a decrease or normalisation of the liver enzymes, the diagnosis of NAFLD is practically assured. Given the association with the metabolic syndrome, all patients should have fasting sugars and lipids measured.

The *transaminases* are mildly to moderately elevated but can fluctuate from month to month. Typically the ALT (alanine transaminase) is greater than the AST (aspartate aminotransferase), in contrast to alcoholic liver disease where the reverse is true.

Initial *imaging* is usually with ultrasound, which frequently shows a hyperechoic liver; however, this finding is neither sensitive nor specific.

Liver biopsy allows diagnosis, differentiation of simple steatosis from NASH and some assessment of disease severity and possibly prognosis. However, there remains no international consensus regarding when liver biopsy should be performed or the histopathological criteria that would firmly define NASH and differentiate between NAFLD entities. A scoring

Box 23.1 Components of the NAFLD Fibrosis Score

- Age
- Hyperglycaemia
- Body mass index (BMI)
- Platelet count
- Albumin
- AST/ALT ratio

system, the 'NAFLD Fibrosis Score', has been developed as a way of predicting fibrosis (hence potentially avoiding the need for biopsy in this common condition) and stratifying into outcome categories (Box 23.1).

Management

- Lifestyle modification is the main therapy. Short-term weight loss in combination with exercise leads to improvement in liver biochemical tests and to resolution of hepatic steatosis. The aim is for moderate weight loss, as overly rapid weight reduction could aggravate steatohepatitis. Multiple weight reduction therapies have been investigated, but bariatric surgery is perhaps the best therapeutic modality in the presence of severe obesity.

- Elevated cholesterol, triglycerides and blood sugar should be corrected.
- In diabetic patients, HbA_{1C} should be reduced to <7%.
- Pharmacological therapy is only considered when there is no change in the condition after lifestyle modification.

Prognosis and natural history

Patients with NAFLD have a slightly higher mortality than the general population. The natural history has not been clearly defined and estimates of the risk of NASH progressing to cirrhosis range between 8% and 15%. NASH progresses to cirrhosis less frequently than alcoholic steatohepatitis and has a better long-term survival. Even once NASH results in fibrosis, deterioration is not inevitable: fibrosis progresses in about a third, remains stable in a third and regresses in a third. The clinical and biochemical factors associated with risk of progression include:

- Increasing age.
- Obesity.
- Pronounced weight loss (especially if previously obese).
- Diabetes mellitus.
- AST/ALT ratio >1.
- ALT more than two times normal and raised triglycerides.

 KEY POINTS

- Non-alcoholic fatty liver disease (NAFLD) is an umbrella term encompassing simple steatosis, non-alcoholic steatohepatitis (NASH), and resultant fibrosis and cirrhosis.
- Prevalence increases with increasing body weight, affecting 10–15% of normal individuals and up to 80% of the obese.

- Typically the ALT is greater than the AST, in contrast to alcoholic liver disease where the reverse is true.
- Estimates of the risk of NASH progressing to cirrhosis range between 8% and 15%.

SELF-ASSESSMENT QUESTION

(The answer to this question is given on p. 268)

A 50-year-old man is found to have abnormal liver biochemistry when he presents to his GP for a routine health check: ALT 120, AST 40, ALP 110, GGT 100, bilirubin 20, albumin 35, INR 1.1. His BMI is 30 and he is known to have chronic hypertension, but is otherwise well. He admits to drinking 14 units of alcohol per week. Serology for viral liver disease and autoimmune markers of liver disease are negative.

Regarding the most likely cause of the liver test abnormalities in this man, which of the following statements is most true?

(a) The ALT:AST ratio of >2 suggests that alcoholic liver disease is more likely than NAFLD.

(b) The ALT:AST ratio of >2 suggests that NAFLD is more likely than alcoholic liver disease.

(c) Elevation of the GGT confirms that this is alcoholic hepatitis rather than NAFLD.

(d) The patient's report of drinking only 14 units of alcohol per week makes alcoholic liver disease very unlikely.

(e) A liver biopsy is essential in this case to differentiate alcoholic from non-alcoholic liver disease.

Viral hepatitides

Hepatitis A

Hepatitis A virus is highly infectious and spread by the faeco-oral route. Development of cell-line virus culture techniques has led to the development of vaccines.

Epidemiology

Hepatitis A has a worldwide distribution, with higher rates occurring in communities with low standards of sanitation. Outbreaks in industrialised countries have been seen to occur in daycare centres, in association with sewage-contaminated shellfish, in homosexual men and in intravenous (IV) drug abusers. There have been very rare reports of transmission by blood transfusion.

Cause

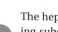

The hepatitis A virus (HAV) is very stable, withstanding substantial heat, drying, low pH and detergents. This means that it is able to survive in the environment (including in foods and drinking water) and the acid barrier of the stomach, and be excreted in the bile, leading to faecal shedding.

The mechanisms responsible for hepatocellular injury remain poorly characterised, but appear to be caused by the host's response to infection rather than a direct cytopathic effect of the virus. The long incubation phase of the virus is related to its ability to interfere with normal mechanisms for the recognition of viral infection and resultant synthesis of interferon (IFN)-β. With the onset of hepatocellular injury, HLA-restricted, virus-specific, cytotoxic CD8+ T cells begin to secrete IFN-γ, which stimulates the recruitment of additional, non-specific inflammatory cells, causing hepatocellular injury.

The secretion of neutralising antibodies occurs concurrent with the earliest evidence of serum aminotransferase elevation and hepatocellular injury. Neutralising antibodies are of primary importance in protection against HAV infection and disease.

Clinical features

Following an incubation period of 15–50 days (average 28–30 days), symptomatic individuals develop an acute febrile illness with jaundice, anorexia, nausea, abdominal discomfort, malaise and dark urine. Viral shedding is extensive throughout the incubation phase and continues for a further 1–3 weeks in adults, longer in young children. Most infections in infants and preschool children are very mild or asymptomatic. Symptoms are more common in adults, up to 70% having some symptoms, and with the severity tending to increase with age. While fulminant hepatitis can develop, it is rare. Chronic carrier states do not occur and permanent hepatic damage is extremely unlikely. However, patients with chronic liver disease are at particular risk of exacerbation with HAV and should be protected from infection.

Investigations

Diagnosis relies on the detection of serum antibodies to HAV (Figure 24.1). Immunoglobulin M (IgM)-specific antibody indicates recent infection, develops

Gastroenterology and Hepatology: Lecture Notes, Second Edition. Stephen Inns and Anton Emmanuel.
© 2017 John Wiley & Sons, Ltd. Published 2017 by John Wiley & Sons, Ltd.
Companion website: www.lecturenoteseries.com/gastroenterology

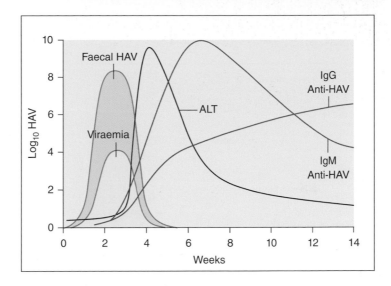

Figure 24.1 Natural history of hepatitis A. ALT, alanine aminotransferase; HAV, hepatitis A virus.

5–10 days after exposure and can persist for up to 6 months. Immunoglobulin G (IgG) antibody is detectable shortly after the appearance of IgM. Virus culture is not used in routine diagnosis.

Clinical features

- Management of the infected patient is largely symptomatic.
- Vaccination is effective both in preventing infection and in disease:
  ○ There is an ongoing role for the use of immunoglobulin in the control of outbreaks of the disease as long as it is given within 2 weeks of contact with the disease. Protection against HAV was first achieved using human normal IgG, providing passive immunity to the virus.
  ○ Use of immunoglobulin for vaccination has largely been replaced by the use of inactivated hepatitis A vaccines.
- While universal and targeted programmes for childhood immunisation have been introduced in some countries, in most industrialised countries vaccination is recommended only for groups at high risk of infection or in whom infection is more likely to cause serious illness. These groups include:
  ○ Patients infected with hepatitis B and C.
  ○ Travellers to countries with high rates of hepatitis A.
  ○ Certain occupational groups:
    – Employees of early childhood services.
    – Those involved in the care of the intellectually disabled.

– Healthcare workers exposed to faeces.
    – Sewerage and other workers exposed to faeces.
    – Military personnel.
  ○ Men who have sex with men.
  ○ Injecting drug users.
  ○ Recipients of blood products such as factor VIII.

Special attention should be paid to the group chronically infected with other hepatitis viruses, as superinfection with HAV in this group leads to increased morbidity and mortality. All patients should receive hepatitis A vaccine before liver decompensation occurs and, if this has not occurred prior to consideration for transplantation, as early as possible before liver transplantation.

Prognosis

The vast majority of infections are self-limiting. Mortality rates are as low as 4 deaths per 1000 cases for the general population, but do increase to 17.5 per 1000 in those aged over 50 and are higher in those with pre-existing liver disease.

Hepatitis E

Hepatitis E virus (HEV) is a distinct agent, unrelated to HAV, which causes epidemics of largely waterborne, enterically transmitted, acute hepatitis (Table 24.1).

Table 24.1 Hepatitis viruses.

	A	E	B	D	C
Family	Picornavirus	Hepevirus	Hepadnavirus	Deltavirus	Flavavirus
Size (nm)	27	32	42	40	30–60
Genome	ssRNA	ssRNA	dsDNA	ssRNA	ssRNA
Length (kb)	7.5	7.5	3.2	1.7	9.4
Transmission	Faeco-oral	Faeco-oral	Parenteral Sexual	Parenteral Sexual	Parenteral ?Sexual
Chronic infection (%)	None	None	3–7	2–70	80–90
Markers of infection	(HAV RNA) In practice HAV IgM is used as a marker of recent infection	HEV PCR	HBsAg HBeAg	HDV RNA	HCV RNA

ss, single stranded; ds, double stranded.

Epidemiology

The first extensively studied epidemic of HEV infection was in Delhi from 1955 to 1956. There were >29,000 icteric cases, with attack rates of 1–15% and an excess of cases among the 15–40-year-olds. Studies of other epidemics in Asia and the Indian subcontinent have since shown a high susceptibility in children also and a case fatality between 0.2% and 4%. In addition, there is a high risk of unexplained fulminant liver failure in pregnant women who are infected, especially in the third trimester. Intrauterine infection is common and associated with substantial prenatal morbidity and mortality. Outbreaks have been especially documented in countries of South-East Asia and Northern Africa.

Transmission:

- Primarily faeco-oral.
- Food-borne HEV infections increasingly detected.
- Vertical transmission in HEV-infected pregnant women is up to 50%.
- Parenteral transmission seems to be low.
- No evidence for sexual transmission.

Viraemia is usually brief, except in the immunosuppressed, where it can be protracted. It appears that HEV can cause zoonotic infection and that other mammalian hosts may constitute important reservoirs for the disease in humans.

Cause

HEV is the prototype member of the *Hepeviridae* family, and as such is given the genus *Orthohepivirus*. It was previously classified in the *Calciviridae* family. The virus was identified for the first time by immuno-electron micrograph in the faeces of an infected human. It has a spherical and non-enveloped virion, with surface spikes as well as cup-like indentations.

While an oral route of infection has been clearly demonstrated, the site of primary replication has not been identified, but is likely to be in the intestinal tract. The virus reaches the liver, presumably via the portal vein, and replicates in the cytoplasm of hepatocytes. It is able to survive the range of pH as it transits through the GI tract. While man is the natural host, it seems very likely that animals serve as a reservoir, with several claims of infection in domestic sheep and swine. Zoonotic transmission of HEV has also been demonstrated from deer to humans.

Clinical features

HEV infections manifest as epidemics of sporadic hepatitis in disease-endemic areas following an incubation period of 15–60 days (mean 40 days). As with other viral hepatitides, a spectrum of symptoms occurs:

- Asymptomatic (probably far more common than icteric disease).
- Acute viral febrile illness without any characteristic features. When infection is symptomatic it produces an acute self-limiting hepatitis, which runs a course of a few weeks. However, in some patients there may be a prolonged cholestatic course.

Symptomatic disease can be divided into two phases:

- **Pre-icteric phase**, lasting 1–10 days (average 3–4 days) with GI symptoms (epigastric pain, nausea and vomiting).

- **Icteric phase**, beginning abruptly with jaundice, dark urine and clay-coloured stools. Two-thirds of patients also report arthralgia. There is a:
  - Variable rise in serum bilirubin (predominately conjugated).
  - Marked elevation in aminotransferases that precedes symptoms by as long as 10 days and peaks at the end of the first week (degree of transaminase elevation does not correlate with disease severity).

An uncomplicated infection lasts 12–15 days with complete recovery within 1 month. Superinfection in chronic liver disease causes severe liver decompensation, a protracted course, and high morbidity and mortality. Chronicity of infection has not been documented apart from in cases with immunodeficiency.

Investigations (Figure 24.2)

- HEV RNA in stool can be detected in the pre-icteric phase, and then declines, disappearing by the peak of ALT.
- Anti-HEV IgM in serum can be identified at onset of symptoms, detectable for 2 weeks to 3 months.
- Anti-HEV IgG increases promptly after IgM, persisting for up to several years in 50% of patients.

Enzyme immunoassays (EIA) and immunochromatography are the most convenient detection methods. In residents of, or travellers to, endemic areas, testing for HEV infection should be included in the first line of diagnostic work-up for acute hepatitis.

Management

While vaccine development and testing are ongoing there is, as yet, no effective vaccine available. HEV infection control and prevention strategies aim at improving hygiene conditions in endemic areas and detecting contaminated sources. Improving sanitation and providing clean drinking water and proper sewage disposal can reduce infections.

Prognosis

Hepatitis E infection is self-limiting and no chronic cases have been reported. The overall case fatality is 4%, but this increases markedly to 20% in pregnant women overall, and is even greater in the second and third trimesters.

Hepatitis B

This hepatotropic DNA virus can cause chronic infection, leading to chronic hepatitis, cirrhosis and hepatocellular carcinoma (HCC) (Table 24.1).

Epidemiology

Hepatitis B virus (HBV) infection is one of the most common infections worldwide, with 400 million people estimated to be carriers. The mortality rate associated with HCC and other terminal complications of HBV infection is approximately 1 million people per year.

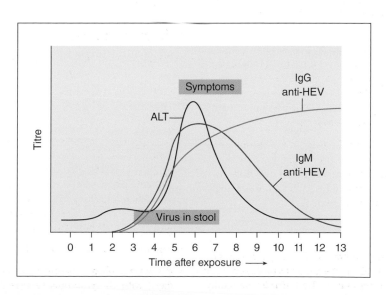

Figure 24.2 Serological and clinical course of hepatitis E virus infection.

The *risk factors* for HBV infection include:

- Transfusion.
- Needle sharing.
- Sexual transmission.
- Perinatal transmission.
- Men who have sex with men.
- Promiscuous heterosexuals.
- Immunosuppressed patients.
- Patients on haemodialysis.
- Transplantation.
- Healthcare transmission.

The prevalence of HBV infection varies widely and correlates with risk of infection, age of infection and mode of transmission (Table 24.2).

Eight genotypes are recognised (A–H). Each genotype:

- Is associated with a particular geographical prevalence.
- May also be of clinical importance:
  - Patients with genotype C infection develop advanced liver disease more frequently than those with B or D.
  - Rate of HBeAg seroconversion is lower in genotype C infection.
  - Genotype C infection is associated with risk of HCC.

Cause

The innate immune system does not appear to play a role in HBV disease pathogenesis or viral clearance. Instead:

- HBV remains undetected in the liver and continues to replicate non-cytopathically until the adaptive immune response is initiated.

- At the time of onset of hepatocellular damage, virus-specific CD4+ T helper cells are involved in facilitating the induction and maintenance of CD8+ cytotoxic T lymphocytes (which have a fundamental role in the pathogenesis of liver cell injury).
- This pathogen-specific response is supported by the influx of non-virus-specific inflammatory cells, including mononuclear and polymorphonuclear cells.
- Recent evidence also points to an important role for platelets in the modulation of liver damage.

Clinical features

The clinical manifestations of HBV vary greatly between the acute and chronic phases of the disease. In the *acute phase*, which occurs in the six months after infection, the majority of patients are asymptomatic or demonstrate only mild fatigue. In some cases, however, there may be subclinical or clinical icterus, or very infrequently fulminant hepatitis.

In the *chronic phase*, the clinical manifestations can range from asymptomatic liver test abnormalities to chronic hepatitis, cirrhosis and HCC. A number of factors determine whether an individual will clear an acute HBV infection or go on to develop chronic hepatitis:

- Age is the most important, with carrier rates of >90% in patients infected as a newborn, but <5% in those infected as adults.
- Immunological status, with immunocompromised patients (HIV, renal failure, post-transplant patients) having high rates of chronicity.
- Severity of acute disease determines progression to chronicity: those with less severe acute illness

Table 24.2 Epidemiology and modes of transmission of hepatitis B virus infection.

	High	Intermediate	Low
Carrier rate (%)	8	2–7	1
Geographical distribution	South-East Asia China Pacific islands Sub-Saharan Africa Alaska (Eskimos)	Mediterranean basin Eastern Europe Central Asia Japan Latin and South America Middle East	United States and Canada Western Europe Australia New Zealand
Predominant age at infection	Perinatal and early childhood	Early childhood	Adult
Predominant mode of infection	Maternal–infant Percutaneous	Percutaneous Sexual	Sexual Percutaneous

mount a less effective immune response and so are less likely to clear viral replication.

The disease is divided into three phases:

1 Replicative, during which aminotransferases are largely normal and there is little liver damage.
2 Inflammatory, where the aminotransferases become elevated, liver biopsy shows chronic hepatitis and viral replication declines.
3 Patients may enter the inactive phase where viral replication has stopped, the aminotransferases normalise and there is no ongoing liver inflammation.

Investigations

- To make a *diagnosis* of chronic HBV infection, the hepatitis B surface antigen (HBsAg) must be positive for six months; however, in practice the diagnosis is often suspected before this.
- Other markers are used to determine *immunity* and *infectivity*:
  ◦ Antibodies to HBsAg (anti-HBs) indicate immunity either following vaccination or clearance of an acute infection.
  ◦ Positivity for the HBV E-antigen (HBeAg), in the presence of HBV-DNA, indicates active replication.
  ◦ Level of HBV-DNA correlates with the amount of virus in the circulation and has prognostic implications.
  ◦ IgM antibodies to the HBV core protein (IgM anti-HBc) suggest recent exposure, except that patients with reactivation of infection may also be IgM anti-HBc positive.

Two special situations relating to chronic HBV infection are described in Boxes 24.1 and 24.2.

Box 24.1 Predicting risk of cirrhosis and hepatocellular carcinoma

Serum HBV DNA level is the strongest predictor of progression to cirrhosis and also contributes a dose-dependent effect on the risk of HCC. This risk is independent of ALT level and HBeAg status. Care must be taken in applying these results:

- More than one test is needed (as the level of HBV fluctuates greatly)
- In patients with perinatal or early childhood infection
- In those with a shorter duration of infection

Management

Prevention

Prevention is the cornerstone of management of HBV:

- Safe sex.
- Avoidance of sharing of IV drug use.
- Use of gloves.
- Careful cleaning of blood or body fluid spills.

Box 24.2 HBeAg-negative chronic hepatitis B

In chronic HBV infection, loss of the HBeAg is usually associated with development of the anti-HBe antibody and transition from the phase of high HBV replication to an inactive phase of infection. However, a variable proportion of patients continue to have, or re-develop, high serum HBV-DNA levels. This is termed HBeAg-negative chronic HBV infection and is a potentially severe and progressive form of liver disease.

The first discovered causes for this transformation were mutations in the precore region of the viral DNA, preventing translation of the e antigen by the core region. It generally occurs in geographical areas where HBV infection is transmitted vertically or even horizontally in very early life, and where the B and D genotypes of HBV prevail. HBeAg-negative chronic HBV infection may also develop with precore wild-type HBV strains, and in association with mutations in the basic core promoter region of the viral DNA.

Definitive diagnosis requires sequencing of the precore region, but this technique is confined to research settings. In practice the diagnosis is made by:

- HBsAg positive for at least 6 months
- Negative serum HBeAg and usually positive anti-HBe antibody for at least 6 months
- Increased serum ALT >2 × upper limit of normal (ULN) on one occasion or ALT >1.5 × ULN on at least 2 monthly determinations
- Detectable serum HBV DNA
- Exclusion of other causes of liver disease
- Moderate-to-severe necroinflammation on liver histology

Common non-HBV causes of liver damage in this setting include superinfections with hepatitis D or C viruses, alcohol excess, hepatotoxic drugs and rare metabolic diseases.

In HBeAg-negative chronic HBV infection, treatment responses to IFN and lamivudine have been disappointing, with frequent relapse at the end of treatment and higher rates of lamivudine resistance than in the treatment of wild-type virus strains.

- Disposal or adequate sterilisation of surgical instruments (including tattoo and piercing equipment).
- Careful disposal of sharps.
- Use of goggles where there is a risk of infected material splashing into the eye.
- Immunisation.

Immunisation is safe and effective. Many countries with a high endemic incidence of HBV have a policy of universal childhood vaccination. Elsewhere vaccination is recommended for:

- Those exposed to blood or blood products.
- Travellers who plan to spend long periods in high-prevalence areas or with pre-existing medical conditions that place them at a higher risk of requiring medical procedures abroad (including pregnancy).
- Haemophiliacs.
- Prisoners and prison officers.

All pregnant women should be screened for HBV and, if positive, the baby should receive hepatitis B vaccination and hepatitis B immunoglobulin soon after birth, and concurrent hepatitis B vaccination using an accelerated schedule. This strategy is 95% effective in preventing transmission. Hepatitis B positive mothers are generally encouraged to breastfeed. The risk of hepatitis B transmission is very low and comparable for both breast-fed and formula-fed infants.

Treatment

Current therapies for chronic HBV infection fall into two categories:

- IFN-α:
  - Used for a finite period with durable response in a subset of patients.
  - Disadvantages of administration by injection and adverse effects.
- Oral nucleoside and nucleotide analogue reverse-transcriptase inhibitors (e.g. entecavir and tenofovir).
  - Better tolerated but associated with resistance.
  - Expensive given they require administration for lengthy periods.

In addition, assays, including genotyping, HBV-DNA levels, genomic analysis, precore and core promoter mutations and resistance mutations, can be used to guide therapy. The overriding principle of therapy is that early, profound, sustained viral suppression improves response rates and reduces resistance.

Prognosis

While 95% of people who contract hepatitis B have a self-limiting illness, 5% go on to chronic infection. In the setting of chronic infection the serum level of HBV DNA is the major clinical feature related to liver disease progression. The relative risk of developing cirrhosis is significantly elevated for those with HBV DNA levels as low as 2000 IU/mL and is sixfold greater for those with HBV DNA ≥200,000 IU/mL at enrolment. Morbidity and mortality are linked to development of cirrhosis and hepatocellular carcinoma. Survival is reasonably good (about 85% probability at 5 years) in compensated cirrhosis, but very poor in decompensated cirrhosis.

Hepatitis D

Hepatitis D virus (HDV) is a subviral agent, dependent for its life cycle on HBV (Table 24.1). Co-infection or superinfection with this agent in HBV complicates the course of the disease.

Epidemiology

It is estimated that 20 million of the more than 400 million chronic HBV carriers worldwide also have chronic HDV. As both HBV and HDV are blood-borne, they share the same risk factors and may be contracted with the same or separate, exposures. When a naïve individual receives both viruses it is referred to as *co-infection*, whereas *superinfection* is when a person chronically infected with HBV then contracts HDV.

Cause

In humans, HDV cannot replicate without the presence of HBV, as it must make use of the three HBV envelope proteins. HBV particle assembly is very inefficient and most of the assembled particles are empty and do not contain the HBV nucleocapsid structure or genome. HDV assembly makes use of this excess production of envelope proteins, inserting the HDV genomic RNAs and other proteins into these empty particles.

Little information exists as to the exact mechanisms by which HDV enhances liver injury in HBV. However, it appears that HDV replication itself is not cytopathic; instead, immune mechanisms (both humoral and cellular) may be involved in the pathogenesis of liver injury.

Clinical features

Acute HDV superinfections carry a much greater risk of fulminating hepatitis and resultant liver failure than HBV alone. Chronic HDV infection is associated with more rapidly progressing liver damage.

Investigations (Figure 24.3)

The diagnosis of HDV should be considered in all patients diagnosed with HBV. It is particularly important to consider superinfection in patients with HBV undergoing a flare in disease activity.

- HDV produces two proteins, the small and large delta antigens (HDAg-S and HDAg-L). Even though these antigens are 90% identical, they have different effects in infection:
  - ○ HDAg-S is produced early and is required for viral replication.
  - ○ HDAg-L is produced later and is an inhibitor of viral replication, but is required for viral particle assembly.
- Total anti-HDV antibodies are used to make the diagnosis of infection.
- Reverse transcriptase-polymerase chain reaction (RT-PCR) is used to measure HDV RNA for monitoring chronic infection.

HDAg, IgM anti-HD antibodies and IgG anti-HD antibodies all disappear within months after clearance of viral replication, but persist in chronic infection.

Management

Vaccination against HBV also protects against HDV, and there has been a worldwide decrease in the incidence of HDV superinfection with the initiation of HBV vaccination programmes. Antivirals, such as lamivudine, do not reduce HDV titres.

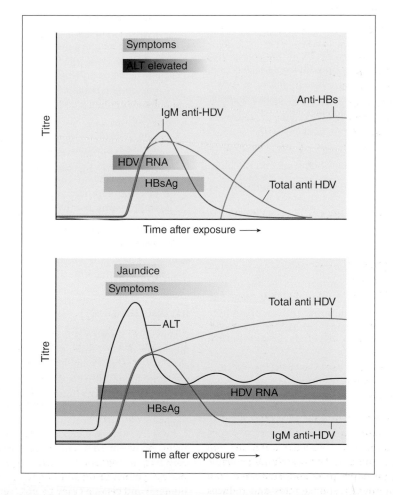

Figure 24.3 Serological and clinical course of hepatitis D co-infection (upper panel) and superinfection (lower panel).

Treatment of disease is limited to:

- Extensive IFN-α therapy, or
- In severe situations, liver transplantation.

Prognosis

The course of hepatitis D superinfection follows that of HBV infection but in an accelerated manner generally. Many patients with synchronous infection clear both viruses, but the risk of the development of fulminant hepatitis in this setting is much higher than with hepatitis B alone. Chronic superinfection is much commoner when hepatitis B is contracted in the setting of pre-existing chronic hepatitis B. In that case, given the current lack of effective treatment, many patients progress to cirrhosis over years, at a greater rate than is seen with hepatitis B chronic infection alone.

Hepatitis C

Hepatitis C virus (HCV) is the most common of the chronic blood-borne infections (Table 24.1). It is estimated that as many as 170 million people are infected worldwide. It has six genotypes, the relative preponderance of which varies globally.

Epidemiology

The risk factors for this blood-borne infection include:

- Blood transfusions (prior to institution of screening).
- IV drug use, tattoos, ear or body piercing.
- Sexual promiscuity.
- An HCV-positive partner.
- Incarceration.

Co-infection with HIV is common and the rate of HCV is high among the population with HIV. HCV has become one of the most important causes of morbidity and mortality in patients with HIV in the developed world.

Cause

Research into the mechanisms for liver damage in HCV infection has been greatly hampered by the lack of cell-line and animal models of disease. What is clear is:

- The innate immune system, the body's first line of defence, is insufficient to eliminate the virus.
- The acquired immune system is also attenuated, with T-cell failure, dysfunction and exhaustion.

- Hepatocyte apoptosis (programmed cell death) is enhanced, and this correlates with liver pathology and may contribute to fibrogenesis.

Clinical features

Acute infection is defined as the first 6 months following initial infection:

- Asymptomatic (the vast majority).
- Mild, non-specific complaints (fatigue, abdominal pain, anorexia, itching and flu-like symptoms), which lead to a diagnosis only in a minority.

Chronic infection is defined as >6 months of documented infection:

- Frequently remains asymptomatic until late in the disease when liver fibrosis develops.
- Those symptoms that are experienced are non-specific and varying.
- Liver function tests are variably elevated and fluctuant.
- Extrahepatic manifestations occur more commonly with chronic HCV infection than other forms of chronic hepatitis and include:
  ○ Cryoglobulinaemia.
  ○ Porphyria cutanea tarda.
  ○ Thyroiditis.
  ○ Sicca syndrome.
  ○ Thrombocytopenia.
  ○ Lichen planus.
  ○ Diabetes mellitus.
  ○ B-cell lymphoproliferative disorders.
  ○ Membranoproliferative glomerulonephritis.

75% of patients with acute infection go on to become chronically infected. The risk of cirrhosis is approximately 1% per year, so at 20 years 20% will have cirrhosis and in that time 5% will develop HCC.

Investigations

Given the absence of specific symptoms, the diagnosis of HCV infection needs to be actively considered by the clinician. The diagnosis is often made incidentally with the discovery of elevated liver tests and is occasionally diagnosed at screening, such as occurs with blood donation or contact tracing.

- Anti-HCV antibodies:
  ○ Pros:
    – Positive in 80% within 3 months of infection, >90% within 5 months and >97% by 6 months.
    – Have a strong positive predictive value.

◦ Cons:
  – Cannot determine ongoing infection.
  – May miss patients who have not yet developed antibodies or the rare patient who does not produce antibodies.
- RNA testing is necessary when antibody tests are negative, but the clinical suspicion is high. Virus is detectable in serum 1–3 weeks after infection:
  ◦ Most common modality is PCR.
  ◦ Titre assists in determining the probability of response to treatment, but not severity or likelihood of progression.

Management

Prevention

Prevention of hepatitis C centres on education and programmes to eliminate the risk factors for HCV infection, in particular avoidance of the sharing of IV needles during elicit drug use. Because of the variability and high rate of mutation of HCV, as well as difficulties with animal and cell-line models of disease, it has not been possible to develop an effective vaccine.

Treatment

The primary goal is viral eradication. This is defined by the sustained virological response (SVR), which is the absence of detectable serum HCV RNA 6 months following the completion of therapy. Combination therapy has been the norm for some time, traditionally with pegylated interferon alpha and ribavirin, but increasingly now with new interferon-free regimens. This has improved the acceptability, efficacy and side-effect profile of therapy, but has been associated with a marked increase in the cost of therapy.

- **Interferon and ribavirin combination therapy:**
  ◦ Pegylated IFN-α, which gives increased and sustained duration of activity due to longer serum half-life than conventional IFN-α.
  ◦ Ribavirin, the nucleoside antimetabolite.

Monitoring of serum RNA levels can allow rationalisation of treatment. Viral genotype is the greatest predictor of treatment response. Recently genetic factors in the host have also become important in tailoring therapy (see Box 24.3).

- **Genotype 1**: SVR is achievable in nearly half of patients:
  ◦ Lack of early viral response (EVR: defined as a minimum 2-log10 decrease in viral load during the first 12 weeks of therapy) is a strong predictor of not achieving SVR, enabling early treatment discontinuation.

◦ However, treatment of the (rarely diagnosed) acute infection is warranted, resulting in a >90% success rate with half the treatment time required for chronic infections.
- **Genotypes 2 and 3**: SVR is achievable in 80%:
  ◦ Often need lower doses of ribavirin and a shorter treatment duration than genotype 1.

There are significant adverse effects associated with the use of IFN-α and PEG-IFNs, including fatigue, flu-like symptoms, GI disturbances, haematological abnormalities, neuropsychiatric effects (particularly depression), thyroid dysfunction and dermatological effects, such as alopecia and pruritus. In addition, ribavirin is associated with haemolytic anaemia. Because treatment success is directly related to adherence to treatment, dose reductions and discontinuations should be avoided if possible, hence monitoring for, and management of, adverse effects is essential. Serotonin-reuptake inhibitors (SSRIs) are safe and effective for IFN-associated depression. Anaemia caused by ribavirin can be treated using erythropoietin.

Box 24.3 The use of IL28b genotype in the treatment of hepatitis C

Peginterferon alpha and ribavirin treatment for 48 weeks leads to a sustained virological response (SVR) in 40–50% of subjects infected with hepatitis C virus (HCV) genotype 1 or 4 (G1/4), while treatment for 24 weeks produces SVR in 70–80% of patients infected with HCV genotype 2 or 3. However, variability in response to treatment, especially between patients of different racial groups, suggested that human genetic variability might explain some of the differences in response rates between groups. Genome-wide association studies were thus employed to try to explain these differences, and SNPs (single nucleotide repeat polymorphisms) located near the gene for interleukin-28B (IL28B) were found to be strongly associated with the likelihood of achieving an SVR with peginterferon + ribavirin treatment. The genotypes for the IL28b gene can be divided into CC, which is associated with improved response to therapy, and non-CC (CT and TT).

Incorporating this test into a study of treatment naïve G1-infected subjects of European ancestry (the IDEAL study) showed that approximately 69% of those who carried the CC genotype achieved an SVR compared with 33% of those with the CT genotype and 27% with genotype TT. This result has been duplicated many times and has allowed treatment length, which was previously tailored to viral factors and the early response to therapy, to be tailored to IL28b genotype also.

- **Interferon-free regimens:** Treatment for HCV infection is changing rapidly. Key viral replication targets have been identified: the NS3 protease, NS5A and NS5B RNA polymerase (see Figure 24.4). Further targets for therapy will surely be explored at an increasing rate.

Potent antiviral inhibitors targeting these proteins initially provided the possibility of shorter-duration, interferon-sparing regimens with increased efficacy. However, such approaches are being replaced by interferon-free regimens with further improvements in efficacy and tolerability. The challenge has become keeping guidelines, treatment algorithms and licensing information up to date and available for clinicians. These treatments are costly and meeting demand for therapy of a common disease with these breakthrough therapies will create difficult resource decisions for policy makers. High cost might restrict access, thus restricting societal benefits.

Prognosis

Despite the advent of effective treatments for HCV, the mortality rate for this disease seems to be increasing in the developed world. Most of the deaths occur in middle-aged people (particularly those aged 50–59 years) and it seems likely that the increased rates are due to a cohort effect of increased rates of infection in the 1970s and 1980s. In order to slow this increase, strategies to detect cases of hepatitis C in the community and improve access to treatments will be key.

Other viral hepatitides

A number of other viruses can cause acute, and less commonly chronic, hepatitis:

- Epstein–Barr virus (EBV; the commonest).
- Cytomegalovirus (CMV).
- Varicella zoster virus.
- Herpes simplex virus.

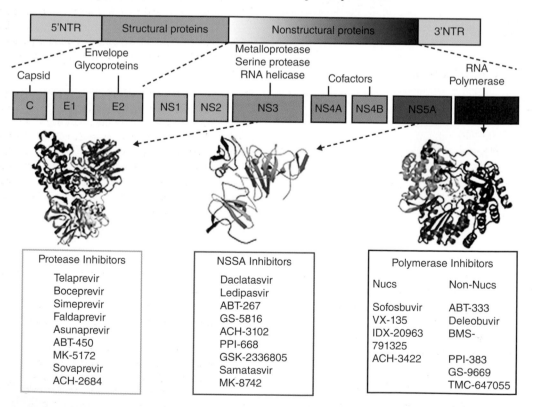

Figure 24.4 HCV genome and targets for drug discovery. The HCV RNA genome serves as a template for viral replication and as a viral messenger RNA for viral production. It is translated into a polyprotein that is cleaved by proteases. All the HCV enzymes – NS2-3 and NS3-4A proteases, NS3 helicase and NS5B RdRp – are essential for HCV replication and are therefore potential drug discovery targets. Source: Schinazi R, Halfon P, Marcellin P, Asselah T. The best interferon–free combinations. Liver Int., 2014;34:69–78. Reproduced with permission of John Wiley & Sons.

Epstein–Barr virus hepatitis

Epidemiology

Almost 95% of the population is seropositive for EBV infection by the end of childhood. Most infections are completely asymptomatic in childhood, but symptomatic disease tends to occur in adolescents and adults. EBV is more common in developed countries where the transmission rates during childhood are lower.

Cause

The exact mechanisms by which EBV causes liver damage remain unclear. It seems likely that the host's immune reaction, rather than the cytolytic effects of the virus, is responsible. The histology in EBV-induced hepatitis includes:

- Swelling and vacuolisation of the hepatocytes.
- Periportal infiltration by lymphocytes and monocytes.
- Mononuclear infiltration of the sinusoids.
- Bile ducts often mildly swollen, but obstruction is rare.

Clinical features

The term infectious mononucleosis describes the triad of:

- Fever,
- Sore throat,
- Adenopathy,

in combination with the finding of atypical mononuclear cells in the blood, as occurs with EBV infection.

Non-specific abdominal discomfort and nausea are seen in up to 15% of patients. Splenomegaly is detectable in up to 60%, but hepatomegaly in only about 15%. *Rare complications* include:

- Splenic rupture.
- Liver failure due to acute and/or chronic EBV infection (especially post-transplantation or in association with other immunodeficiency).
- Autoimmune hepatitis and HCC (controversially associated in Asian people).
- Lymphoproliferative disorders and lymphoma.

Investigations

Liver enzyme elevations are seen in 80–90% of those infected and are largely asymptomatic.

- Transaminases are elevated to 2–3 times the upper limit of normal. If elevations of >10 times are seen, it is less likely that the diagnosis is EBV. The liver function abnormalities usually occur in the second week of illness and resolve within 2–6 weeks.
- Alkaline phosphatase is elevated in 60%.
- Bilirubin is elevated in 45% (but jaundice occurs in <5%) and is self-limited. Jaundice may be cholestatic or haemolytic and an FBC and peripheral blood film should be performed to detect haemolysis.

The *diagnosis* of EBV infection revolves around recognition of the typical clinical symptoms in association with positive EBV IgM antibody, monospot and/or heterophile antibody tests (see Box 24.4). False-positive monospot tests occur in HIV, endocarditis and acute hepatitis A. Polymerase reaction testing is necessary where the suspicion is high but serological tests are unremarkable. Other potential viral aetiologies must be considered.

Box 24.4 Epstein–Barr virus tests

To diagnose infectious mononucleosis (IM), lymphocytes should represent >50% of leucocytes, 20% should be atypical and there should be positive serology. There are two types of serological test for EBV:

- Heterophile antibody tests
- Tests for antibodies to viral antigens

The *heterophile antibody tests*, Paul–Bunnel test and monospot test (if done on slides) detect antibodies that cause agglutination of the red blood cells from another species. False-negative results are more common in those under 14 years (especially under 5). Positive heterophile antibodies are seen during the first month of illness and decrease rapidly after week 4, but last >6 months after onset of infection.

Antibodies to several antigen complexes may be measured, including the early antigen, EBV nuclear antigen (EBNA) and viral capsid antigen (differentiation of IgG and IgM subclasses of this is often used). Interpretation of these results can be somewhat complex. The antibody profiles seen in each of the main clinical situations are:

- *Susceptibility to EBV infection*: if antibodies to the viral capsid antigen are not detected the patient is susceptible

- *Primary infection*:
  - IgM antibody to the viral capsid antigen is present and antibody to EBNA is absent, or
  - Elevated IgG antibody to the viral capsid antigen and negative antibody to EBNA after at least 4 weeks of illness, or
  - Elevated antibody to early antigen.
- *Past infection*: if antibodies to both the viral capsid antigen and EBNA are present, then past infection (from >4 months earlier) is indicated. Since 95% of adults have been infected with EBV, most will show antibodies to EBV from infection years earlier. High or elevated antibody levels may be present for years and are not diagnostic of recent infection.
- *Reactivation*: if antibodies to EBNA are present, an elevation of antibodies to early antigen suggests reactivation. However, positive antibody to the early antigen test does not automatically indicate that EBV caused a patient's current medical condition; healthy people with no symptoms can have antibodies to the EBV early antigen for years after their initial EBV infection. Reactivation often occurs subclinically.
- *Chronic EBV infection*: reliable laboratory evidence for continued active EBV infection is rare in patients who have been ill for >4 months. When the illness lasts >6 months, it should be investigated to see if other causes of chronic ill health or fatigue are present.

Management and prognosis

Treatment is supportive and the vast majority of cases resolve spontaneously. Steroids and antiviral medications have been used in severe disease, but remain of unproven benefit. Patients with splenomegaly should be advised to avoid abdominal trauma, and patients with elevated transaminases should avoid hepatotoxins until liver abnormalities resolve.

 KEY POINTS

- Hepatitis A virus:
  - Transferred by the faeco-oral route.
  - Management of the infected patient is largely symptomatic.
  - Vaccination is effective both in preventing infection and disease.
- Hepatitis E virus:
  - Causes epidemics of largely water-borne, enterically transmitted, acute hepatitis.
  - Prototype member of the *Hepeviridae* family.
  - No effective vaccine available.
- Hepatitis B hepatotropic DNA virus:
  - One of the most common infections worldwide with a mortality rate of 1 million people per year.
  - Clinical manifestations of HBV vary greatly between the acute and chronic phases.
  - Prevention is the cornerstone of management of HBV.
  - Immunisation is safe and effective.
  - Current therapies are either IFN-α or oral nucleoside and nucleotide analogue reverse-transcriptase inhibitors (e.g. entecavir and tenofovir).
- Hepatitis D is a subviral agent, dependent for its life cycle on HBV:
  - Co-infection or superinfection in HBV accelerates the progression of chronic disease and increases the risk of fulminating hepatitis and resultant liver failure.
  - Vaccination against HBV also protects against HDV.
- Hepatitis C virus:
  - 75% of patients with acute infection go on to become chronically infected.
  - After 20 years of infection 20% will have cirrhosis and 5% of those will develop HCC.
  - Prevention of hepatitis C centres on avoidance of the sharing of IV needles.
  - It has not been possible to develop an effective vaccine.
  - Treatment goal is viral eradication, defined by the sustained virological response (SVR).
  - Interferon and ribavirin combination therapy is giving way to interferon-free regimens using drugs that directly inhibit viral replication.

SELF-ASSESSMENT QUESTION

(The answer to this question is given on p. 269)

A 53-year-old man is referred by his GP after an ultrasound performed for vague abdominal pain revealed a cirrhotic-appearing liver. Initial bloods showed a mildly elevated ALT at 52, but no other abnormality. There is no family history of hepatitis and no travel history. He is Caucasian and has lived all his life in the UK.

Regarding the possible diagnosis of viral hepatitis, which of the following statements is most correct?

(a) Initial screening should include serology for hepatitis A, B and C.

(b) He is most likely to have contracted hepatitis B from his mother at birth.

(c) Hepatitis D causes water-borne outbreaks of acute hepatitis in developing countries and cannot be implicated in this patient.

(d) Hepatitis C is an RNA virus and sequencing of the genome has led to new treatment targets being identified.

(e) The absence of HBeAg rules out active infection with hepatitis B and means that he is at no risk of progression of his liver disease due to hepatitis B.

Drug-induced liver injury

Damage to the liver by medications is not uncommon and is the main reason for cessation of development of a drug or regulatory decisions to remove drugs from the market. In the majority of cases, drug-induced liver injury (DILI) is an unpredictable, idiosyncratic reaction. However, there are important exceptions that cause DILI by dose-dependent mechanisms. Liver injury takes three forms: hepatocellular injury, cholestasis and mixed. Treatment relies on prompt diagnosis and removal of the offending drug.

Causes

Hepatocellular injury may result from the drug or its metabolites. While most reactions are idiosyncratic, paracetamol and methotrexate are exceptions and cause direct hepatocellular toxicity. Idiosyncratic reactions may be either metabolic or immune mediated, or a combination of the two.

Given the variety of cellular mechanisms causing DILI, it cannot be viewed as a single disease. These mechanisms include:

- Disruption of the cell membrane.
- Production of immune targets by covalent binding of the drug to cell proteins.
- Inhibition of cellular pathways of drug metabolism.
- Abnormal bile flow due to disruption of subcellular actin filaments or interruption of transport pumps.
- Programmed cell death (apoptosis) mediated by tumour necrosis factor and Fas pathways.
- Inhibition of mitochondrial function causing accumulation of reactive oxygen species, lipid peroxidation, fat accumulation and cell death.

Pregnancy, concomitant medications and a history of drug reactions all increase susceptibility to DILI. The most important susceptibility factor is genetic variability. An example of this is differences in susceptibility related to polymorphisms in the *N*-acetyltransferase 2 gene, which result in so-called fast and slow acetylators, the latter being at increased risk of isoniazid toxicity.

Epidemiology

Approximately 20 new cases of DILI per 100,000 persons occur each year. Idiosyncratic DILI accounts for 11% of the cases of acute liver failure in the USA.

Clinical features

As DILI commonly simulates other common forms of acute and chronic liver disease, it is important that it is considered in every patient with liver dysfunction. The three commonest clinical scenarios (Table 25.1) are:

- Acute hepatitis.
- Cholestasis.
- A mixed condition resembling acute viral hepatitis.

The rarer forms are:

- Chronic hepatitis.
- Cirrhosis.
- Sinusoidal obstruction syndrome.
- Neoplasia.

Clues as to an allergic mechanism (fever, rash, peripheral eosinophilia) should not be overlooked. The time course may also help identify an allergic mechanism:

Gastroenterology and Hepatology: Lecture Notes, Second Edition. Stephen Inns and Anton Emmanuel.
© 2017 John Wiley & Sons, Ltd. Published 2017 by John Wiley & Sons, Ltd.
Companion website: www.lecturenoteseries.com/gastroenterology

Table 25.1 Causes of drug-induced liver injury.

	Hepatocellular (elevated ALT)	Mixed	Cholestatic (elevated ALP and bilirubin)
Antimicrobials	Isoniazid Ketoconazole Pyrazinamide Rifampin Fluconazole Isoniazid Tetracyclines Highly active antiretroviral therapy Trovafloxacin	Clindamycin Nitrofurantoin Sulphonamides Trimethoprim-sulphamethoxazole	Amoxycillin-clavulanic acid Erythromycins Ciprofloxacin Fluconazole Rifampin
Psychiatric medicines	Buproprion Fluoxetine Paroxetine Risperidone Sertraline Trazodone	Amitryptilline Trazodone	Chlorpromazine Phenothiazines Tricyclic antidepressants Mirtazapine
Analgesics	Paracetamol NSAIDs		
Cardiovascular medicines	Amiodarone Methyldopa Statins/HMG-CoA reductase inhibitors Lisinopril Losartan	Captopril Enalapril Verapamil	Clopidogrel Irbesartan
Others	Valproic acid Methotrexate Acarbose Allopurinol Baclofen Herbal medicines (Ma Huang, Kava, pyrrolizidine alkaloids in comfrey, germander and chaparral leaf) Omeprazole	Azathioprine Carbamazepine Cyproheptadine Flutamide Phenobarbitol Phenytoin	Anabolic steroids Oral contraceptives Oestrogens Terbinafine

ALP, alkaline phosphatase; ALT, alanine transaminase; NSAIDs, non-steroidal anti-inflammatory drugs.

typically there is a short latency period (1 month or less) and rapid symptom recurrence on rechallenge. In addition, there may be haematological features including neutropaenia, thrombocytopaenia and haemolytic anaemia. In rare cases, Steven–Johnson syndrome or toxic epidermal necrolysis strongly suggests an immunological mechanism.

In the case of hepatocellular injury, the clinical features are non-specific and not always associated with jaundice. Prognosis is largely dependent on the presence of jaundice. The rule of thumb is that the likelihood of mortality or liver transplantation is 10% in the presence of jaundice. Variables associated with a poor outcome include older age, female gender and AST (aspartate aminotransferase) levels.

Because the histological changes of DILI are not specific, the pattern of hepatotoxicity is defined by changes in the liver enzymes.

- Hepatocellular injury is defined by a rise in ALT more than two-fold that of the upper limit of normal ($2 \times$ ULN) or an ALT/AP ratio ≥ 5.
- Acute cholestatic injury is defined by an increase in the ALP $>2 \times$ ULN or an ALT/ALP ≤ 2. Older age is associated with an increased likelihood of DILI being expressed as cholestatic damage. There are two subtypes:
  - Pure cholestasis (resulting in jaundice, itching and an increase in conjugated bilirubin, ALP and GGT, with minimal alterations in the

transaminases; typically caused by anabolic or contraceptive steroids).
  ◦ Acute cholestatic hepatitis (resulting in abdominal pain and fever, and a picture similar to acute biliary obstruction; typically caused by amoxicillin-clavulanate, macrolide antibiotics and phenothiazine neuroleptics, among many others).
• Mixed DILI is a clinical and biological intermediate, predominated by either hepatocellular or cholestatic features. It is defined by an ALT:ALP ratio between 2 and 5.

Investigations

Due to a lack of specific clinical and pathological features, the diagnosis of DILI is largely subjective and based on the temporal associations between the initiation of therapy and onset of symptoms, and the rate of improvement after cessation of therapy. Alternative diagnoses must be carefully excluded. Patients must be closely questioned about the use of prescribed, over-the-counter and illicit drugs.

The latency period varies with each drug and is linked to the mechanism of damage. Intrinsic hepatotoxins may cause disease within a few hours; allergic reactions may have a latency of 1–5 weeks; and idiosyncratic reactions take between 1 and 12 weeks to manifest. With some drugs (amoxicillin-clavulanate, midecamycin, oxacin and trovafloxacin) there is a delay of 3 or 4 weeks between cessation of treatment and presentation. The reasons for this are unclear, but might represent a late immune reaction due to retention of the drug in the body.

When patients are taking a number of medications, discerning the probable culprit can be very difficult. In the first instance, suspicion should be directed at the latest introduced drug and known hepatotoxins. The main causative agents in DILI are antibiotics, NSAIDs, antiseizure medications and herbal preparations.

Rapid improvements after withdrawal of the offending agent suggest a toxic aetiology:

• A decrease of 50% liver enzymes in the first 8 days following cessation is said to indicate that a hepatotoxic mechanism is 'highly likely'.
• Course is 'suggestive' of hepatotoxicity if the same improvement occurs within 30 days.
• The only way to confidently confirm idiosyncratic drug-induced hepatotoxicity is to demonstrate at least a doubling of the ALT (in hepatocellular toxicity) or ALP (in cholestatic injury) on rechallenge with the implicated drug. However, intentional rechallenge is contraindicated in hypersensitivity reactions due to the risk of a more severe reaction, and in idiosyncratic

reactions the amount of drug needed to induce a reaction cannot be known. Hence, rechallenge cannot be used for purely diagnostic reasons and should only be attempted when continuation of the drug is essential.

Liver biopsy may be useful:

• Where there is a suspicion of an underlying liver disease.
• In the rare cases where there is chronic toxic hepatocellular injury.
• If the suspected offending agent needs to be continued for therapeutic reasons and hence it is important to quantify the degree of liver injury generated.

In hepatocellular DILI, the histology is variable:

• With necrosis and inflammation, and often an abundance of eosinophils in the inflammatory infiltrate.
• Acute cholestasis causes hepatocyte cholestasis and dilated biliary canaliculi with bile plugs, but little or no inflammation and necrosis.
• Mixed injury often results in a granulomatous reaction seen on biopsy.

Management

Generally there is no effective treatment for DILI other than stopping the implicated drug and providing supportive care. The main exceptions are the use of *N*-acetylcysteine after paracetamol overdose and intravenous carnitine for valproate-induced mitochondrial damage.

Prognosis

The majority of patients with symptomatic acute DILI recover completely. Even patients with clinically significant liver injury such as jaundice also have a generally favourable prognosis. In one study 91% of DILI patients with jaundice recovered, and only 9% died or underwent liver transplant surgery. However, the prognosis of patients with severe DILI who progress to acute liver failure with concomitant coagulopathy (i.e. INR >1.5) and encephalopathy is usually poor.

Paracetamol overdose
Epidemiology

In the UK paracetamol overdose is the commonest form of intentional self-harm, with 70,000 cases per year, and it is the leading cause of acute liver failure.

Serious or fatal adverse effects in adults occur at a dose of around 150 mg/kg.

Cause

Paracetamol is inactivated by liver conjugation to two metabolites: the glucuronide and the sulphate. It is then renally excreted. In overdose conjugation is inundated and metabolism is by an alternative pathway, creating N-acetyl-p-benzoquinone imine (NABQI), which is then inactivated by glutathione. However, glutathione is easily run down, preventing inactivation of NABQI and resulting in reaction with nucleophilic aspects of the cell, causing necrosis of the liver and kidney tubules. Increased toxicity occurs with:

- Drug-induced induction of the cytochrome P450 system:
  ○ Rifampicin.
  ○ Carbamazepine.
  ○ Phenytoin.
- Low glutathione reserves due to:
  ○ Genetic variation.
  ○ HIV positivity.
  ○ Malnutrition.
  ○ Ethanol excess.
  ○ Liver disease.

Clinical features

Patients are generally asymptomatic in the first 24 hours after ingestion or have non-specific abdominal symptoms (such as nausea and vomiting). Hepatic necrosis begins after 24 hours, resulting in right upper quadrant pain, jaundice and elevated transaminases. Examination reveals little until acute liver failure ensues.

Investigations

- Paracetamol level sampled 4 h after ingestion (or at presentation if after this time or if ingestion was staggered), usually with a salicylate level. In the case of staggered overdose, the level cannot guide treatment and is used only to confirm ingestion.
- Baseline FBC, U&E, creatinine and LFTs.
- Prothombin time is the best indicator of severity of liver failure.
- Blood glucose is measured, as hypoglycaemia is common.
- Arterial blood gas is analysed, as acidosis can occur early.

Management

- Charcoal:
  ○ If there has been significant overdose (150 mg/kg or 12 g, whichever is the smaller).
  ○ When ingestion is within 1 h of presentation or is unknown.
- Urine output and blood glucose are monitored hourly. U&E, LFTs and INR should be checked 12-hourly.
- 4-h paracetamol level guides therapy. Risk is assessed using a nomogram:
  ○ Patients at high risk (i.e. those at risk of enzyme induction or glutathione depletion) are assessed using the 'high-risk' threshold.
  ○ N-acetylcysteine (NAC) is given to patients (Box 25.1):
    – With levels above the treatment line.
    – Immediately at presentation if the overdose is >150 mg/kg (or 12 g in an adult) or the overdose is staggered or the patient presents >15 h after ingestion.
- When there is significant hepatotoxicity, early referral to a specialist unit must be considered (see Chapter 9).

Prognosis

Fortunately, prognosis is generally better in acetaminophen-induced liver failure patients treated with N-acetylcysteine than in acute liver failure patients with idiosyncratic DILI (i.e. 60–80% versus 20–40%, respectively, transplant-free survival).

Box 25.1 N-acetylcysteine (NAC)

- NAC has beneficial effects by a number of protective mechanisms:
  ○ Precursor for glutathione
  ○ Supplying thiols
  ○ Antioxidant effects
- Its protective effect is greatest within 12 h of ingestion
- Allergy occurs in <5% of patients:
  ○ Infusion rate should be slowed if reaction occurs
  ○ Pretreatment with IV hydrocortisone and chlorphenamine if known allergy to NAC
- Methionine is an oral alternative, but absorption is unreliable and it must be given early

KEY POINTS

- The majority of cases consist of an unpredictable, idiosyncratic reaction, but there are important exceptions that cause DILI by dose-dependent mechanisms.
- Liver injury takes three forms: hepatocellular injury, cholestasis and mixed.
  - Injury may result from the drug or its metabolites and be metabolic or immune mediated, or a combination of the two.
  - Pregnancy, concomitant medications and a history of drug reactions all increase susceptibility to DILI.
  - However, the most important susceptibility factor is genetic variability.
- Time course is important:
  - Intrinsic hepatotoxins may cause disease within a few hours.

- Allergic reactions may have a latency of 1–5 weeks.
  - Idiosyncratic reactions take between 1 and 12 weeks to manifest.
- With some drugs (amoxicillin-clavulanate, midecamycin, oxacin and trovafloxacin) there is a delay of 3 or 4 weeks between cessation of treatment and presentation.
- Generally there is no effective treatment for DILI other than stopping the implicated drug and providing supportive care.
- The main exceptions are the use of N-acetylcysteine after paracetamol overdose and intravenous carnitine for valproate-induced mitochondrial damage.

 SELF-ASSESSMENT QUESTION

(The answer to this question is given on p. 269)

A 45-year-old woman presents to her GP feeling non-specifically unwell. Routine testing reveals isolated abnormalities of the liver biochemistry: ALT 35 IU/L (0–30), ALP 235 IU/L (20–110), bilirubin 30 Umol/L (0–20), albumin 35 g/L (34–50), Hb 130, platelets 200, WCC 5.5, INR 1.2. She has a history of Crohn's disease and has been treated with 150 mg of azathioprine daily (body weight 71 kg) for 10 years. She has liver biochemistry performed every 6 months as monitoring for this and the last tests, performed 4 months ago, were normal. The disease has been clinically inactive for the last 3 years. She received a 7-day course of amoxicillin with clavulanate for a sinus infection 4 weeks ago. She is on no other regular medicines and has no other health problems.

Regarding the liver test abnormalities, which of the following statements is most true?

(a) Azathioprine commonly causes unpredictable liver test abnormalities in a cholestatic pattern, which frequently develop many years after the drug is started.

(b) Drug-induced liver disease caused by antibiotic use tends to develop during use of the medicine or immediately after its cessation.

(c) Because azathioprine is a potent cause of liver test abnormalities, it should be stopped in this situation whether or not it is the cause of of the liver test abnormality.

(d) Amoxycillin clavulanate is a not-uncommon cause of a mixed pattern of liver test abnormality developing 3 to 4 weeks after cessation of therapy.

(e) Amoxycillin clavulanate is metabolised via the same enzymatic pathway as azathioprine and an interaction between these drugs can result in azathioprine-related liver injury.

Autoimmune hepatitis

A rare autoimmune condition, autoimmune hepatitis (AIH) is diagnosed by the presence of a constellation of clinical, laboratory and pathological features. The disease usually responds to corticosteroid treatment, although relapses on stopping therapy are common. The immune biliary conditions primary biliary cirrhosis (PBC) and sclerosing cholangitis (PSC) are considered in Chapter 19.

Epidemiology and cause

AIH is a condition of unknown cause, which particularly affects young females of any age. However, both sexes and all ethnicities may be affected. AIH has an incidence of 1–2 per 100,000 per year, and a prevalence of 10–20/100,000. It is associated with concurrent immune disease. It is relatively common for AIH to recur or develop *de novo* after liver transplantation, and the diagnosis must be considered in all transplanted patients with allograft dysfunction.

While the exact pathogenesis is unknown, there are identified aetiological triggers, in particular drugs (Table 26.1). The principal effector cells of the autoimmune process in AIH are the CD4+ and CD8+ T lymphocytes. The regulatory CD4+ CD25+ T cells are decreased in number and function and so fail to modulate CD8+ T-cell proliferation and cytokine production, thus facilitating liver injury. This activity can be modulated by genetic factors, in particular the HLA haplotype. The association between AIH and the class II antigens of the major histocompatibility complex (MHC) varies between ethnic and geographical groups. Corticosteroids reconstitute the T-regulatory

cell function and attenuate the cell-mediated cytotoxic response in AIH.

Clinical features

- Clinical presentation of AIH is often acute, and rarely fulminant, and may mimic acute viral or toxic hepatitis.
- There are also indolent, asymptomatic forms of the disease:
  - The commonest complaints are of fatigue, amenorrhea and those associated with an accompanying rheumatological disorder such as arthritis or thyroid disease.
  - Physical findings include jaundice (in severe disease), spider naevi, palmar erythema and hepatosplenomegaly.

Concurrent immune diseases may obscure the underlying liver disease. The associated immune conditions include systemic sclerosis, polymyositis, neuritis multiplex and polyglandular autoimmune syndrome type III.

Investigations

- **Blood testing**:
  - Autoantibodies are the hallmark of AIH, particularly antinuclear factor and smooth-muscle antibodies. The disease is often subclassified into Type 1 and Type 2, the latter demonstrating

Gastroenterology and Hepatology: Lecture Notes, Second Edition. Stephen Inns and Anton Emmanuel.
© 2017 John Wiley & Sons, Ltd. Published 2017 by John Wiley & Sons, Ltd.
Companion website: www.lecturenoteseries.com/gastroenterology

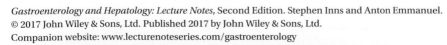

Table 26.1 Drugs implicated in the aetiogenesis of autoimmune hepatitis (AIH).

First implicated drug	DialosePlus® (dioctylsodium sulphosuccinate, carboxymethyl cellulose, oxyphenisatinacetate) First report of AIH in 1971; over 100 cases since then, removed from market	
Type 1 AIH-like liver disease	Multiple reports: • Oxyphenisatin • Nitrofurantoin • Minocycline • Alpha-methyldopa • Clometacine Few reports – herbal compounds: • Dai-saiko-to • 3,4-methylenedioxy-metamphetamine ('Ecstasy') • Morindacitrifolia (Nonijuice)	Few reports – conventional drugs: • Papaverine • Diclofenac • Doxycycline • Phenprocoumon • Fenofibrate • HMG-CoA reductase inhibitors (artorvastatin, rosuvastatin, simvastatin) • Rifampin + infliximab • Pyrazinamide • Interferon
Type 2 AIH-like liver disease	Dihydralazine Tienilic acid Halothane Black cohosh (*Actaea racemosa*)	

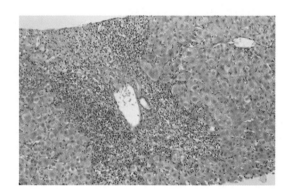

Figure 26.1 Interface hepatitis. Mononuclear inflammatory infiltrate disrupts the limiting plate of the portal tract and extends into parenchymal tissue (haematoxylin and eosin stain, original magnification × 100). Source: Czaja AJ. Clinical features, differential diagnosis and treatment of autoimmune hepatitis in the elderly. Drug Aging. 2008;25(3):219–240, p. 226. Reproduced by permission of Springer Science + Business Media.

antibodies to liver/kidney microsome (anti-LKM 1 hepatitis).

○ Hypergammaglobulinaemia, with pronounced elevation of IgG levels, is invariable. Serum Ig levels can be useful in monitoring response to treatment and are predictive of future flares.

○ Reduced serum albumin is common.

• **Liver biopsy**: essential both for diagnosis and assessment of severity, as well as to exclude other

liver disease. Characteristically this shows an interface hepatitis (Figure 26.1) which may coexist with cirrhosis.

The important differential diagnosis is with PBC, which differs from AIH by:

• Immunohistochemistry demonstration of nuclear envelope protein, gp210.

• Less marked serum aminotransferase elevations, absence of antinuclear antibodies.

• Histological changes of greater bile duct injury than interface hepatitis.

Management

If untreated, AIH may progress rapidly to cirrhosis within 3–5 years.

• Mainstay of treatment is high-dose corticosteroids (prednisone 40–60 mg/day) for 4–6 weeks, then tapered to a maintenance level (e.g. 5–10 mg/day):

○ The aim is to keep the liver enzymes within normal values.

○ This may not prevent fibrosis, but is lifesaving in this otherwise fatal condition.

○ On stopping corticosteroids many patients relapse, and treatment failure and drug toxicities are all too common.

- Often azathioprine is added for its steroid-sparing effect. With this strategy the frequency of relapse can be reduced from 93% to 60%.
- Other immunosuppressives, including tacrolimus, mycophenolate mofetil and rapamycin, have been used empirically as frontline and salvage treatments for problematic patients.
- In those not responsive to, or who relapse on, conventional therapy, liver transplantation is highly successful.

Prognosis

Prognosis is determined by the disease's response to corticosteroids. Responsiveness is similar in all age groups. Disease onset during pregnancy carries a relatively high risk of an adverse outcome and high rates of postpartum exacerbation.

 KEY POINTS

- Diagnosed by the presence of a constellation of clinical, laboratory and pathological features.
- Aetiological triggers, in particular drugs, have been demonstrated.
- Clinical presentation is often acute, and rarely fulminant, and may mimic acute viral or toxic hepatitis.
- Autoantibodies are the hallmark of AIH:
  - Particularly antinuclear factor and smooth-muscle antibodies.
- Type 1 AIH differentiated from Type 2 by liver/kidney microsome antibody.
- Liver biopsy is essential both for diagnosis and assessment of severity, as well as to exclude other liver disease.
  - Characteristically this shows an interface hepatitis.
- Mainstay of treatment is high-dose corticosteroids.
- Often azathioprine is added for its steroid-sparing effect.

 SELF-ASSESSMENT QUESTION

(The answer to this question is given on p. 269)

A 42-year-old woman is found to have abnormal liver tests after she presented to her GP with a 3-month history of feeling non-specifically unwell and fatigued: ALT 120, ALP 135, GGT 300, bilirubin 25, albumin 30, INR 1.0. The only other significant history was of the use of nitrofurantoin 4 months ago for a short-lived urinary tract infection. All other routine bloods were normal. A complete liver screen is performed and the only abnormalities found are serum globulins 67 g/L, antinuclear antibody 1:1280, smooth muscle antibody titre 1:160 (positive), antimitochondrial antibody negative, liver kidney microsomal antibody 1 negative.

Regarding the likely diagnosis in this woman, which of the following statements is most true?

(a) A history of nitrofurantion use would make an antibiotic reaction more likely than autoimmune hepatitis.

(b) Azathioprine would be contraindicated in this situation because of its hepatotoxic effects.

(c) The markedly positive ANA makes primary biliary cirrhosis the most likely immune disease of the liver.

(d) In a young woman with negative liver kidney microsomal antibodies, the most likely diagnosis is Type 2 autoimmune hepatitis.

(e) Liver biopsy is likely to show interface hepatitis with or without hepatic fibrosis.

27

Liver tumours and lesions

Classification of liver lesions revolves around whether the lesion is likely to be benign or malignant. The degree of certainty of this will determine the need for further imaging or biopsy. Table 27.1 summarises the details of each of the main liver lesions.

Epidemiology and causes

The incidence of liver cancer varies widely throughout the world. Liver cancer is the sixth most common cancer worldwide, with an estimated 750,000 new cases diagnosed each year (6% of the total). Liver cancer incidence rates are highest in Eastern Asia and lowest in South-Central Asia and Northern Europe, with more than a ten-fold variation between countries. In the UK, the lifetime risk of developing liver cancer is 1 in 120 for men and 1 in 215 for women. Around half of all cases are liver cell cancers; these comprise hepatocellular carcinomas, hepatoblastomas, angiosarcomas of liver, other sarcomas of liver and other specified carcinomas of liver. Intrahepatic bile duct carcinomas make up a further 40% of the total, and the remaining 9% are of unspecified type.

Clinical features

The vast majority of liver lesions are asymptomatic and are discovered incidentally when imaging is performed for another reason. In this situation, the history and examination are directed at discovering risk factors for, and features of, underlying hepatic disease or systemic conditions associated with liver lesions. The two clear exceptions are when:

- Patient is undergoing surveillance for hepatocellular carcinoma (HCC).
- Liver mass was discovered because it is palpable.

These situations obviously incur a different range of likely diagnoses and are frequently associated with more sinister pathologies.

Investigations
Serology

- FBC and biochemistry, primarily aimed at detecting underlying liver dysfunction or associated pathology.
- Raised levels of alpha-fetoprotein (AFP) are indicative of HCC in the right clinical setting. Other tumour markers, while not specific or sensitive, may guide diagnostic decision making.

Radiology

- Ultrasound remains the initial study of choice:
  - Advantages include safety, minimal necessary pre-examination preparation and relatively low cost.
  - Preferred modality for serial imaging of lesions to monitor for progression.
- Next modality of investigation, if needed, depends on the differential diagnosis based on the ultrasound features: CT and MRI most commonly.

Gastroenterology and Hepatology: Lecture Notes, Second Edition. Stephen Inns and Anton Emmanuel.
© 2017 John Wiley & Sons, Ltd. Published 2017 by John Wiley & Sons, Ltd.
Companion website: www.lecturenoteseries.com/gastroenterology

Table 27.1 Cardinal features of the commonest liver tumours.

		Clinical features	Radiological features	Diagnosis	Treatment	Prognosis
Benign liver tumours	Hepatocellular adenoma	Women of childbearing age Associated with oral contraceptives Mostly asymptomatic Large lesions may cause RUQ discomfort Rarely, peritonitis and shock due to rupture and intraperitoneal haemorrhage	Usually involving the right lobe Often hypervascular but with hypovascular areas	Biopsy usually needed for confirmation and to rule out malignant transformation	Adenomas due to contraceptive use often regress if the drug is stopped Resection of larger, symptomatic tumours only	Very rarely undergo malignant transformation
	Focal nodular hyperplasia	Female predominance May resemble macronodular cirrhosis Multiple tumours in 20% Not related to the oral contraceptive	Stellate fibrous septae ('stellate scar') Presence of Kupffer cells shows as an area of increased uptake on radionuclear scanning MRI: lesions usually hypointense to liver on T_1 and T_2 (scar may be hyperintense on T_2)	Diagnosis usually based on contrast MRI or CT Biopsy may be necessary Solid tumours have a fibrous core and include other cell types (atypical hepatocytes, Kupffer cells and inflammatory cells)	Treatment is rarely needed (especially if asymptomatic)	Haemorrhage in only 2–3% (most common complication)
	Haemangioma	Found in 0.5–7% of the general population Usually asymptomatic More common in women	Ultrasound: increased echogenicity CT: decreased density, enhances from periphery	Radiological	Does not require any treatment	Rupture is rare, even in large tumours No malignant potential
Hepatic cysts	Benign hepatic cysts	Idiopathic: rarely associated with polycystic kidneys, usually asymptomatic and have no clinical significance	Isolated cysts are commonly detected incidentally on abdominal ultrasound or CT	Radiological	Not necessary	Rare congenital condition, polycystic liver commonly associated with polycystic disease of the kidneys True cystic tumours rare

(Continued)

Table 27.1 (Continued)

	Clinical features	Radiological features	Diagnosis	Treatment	Prognosis
Hydatid cysts	Tapeworm of the genus Echinococcus Endemic areas: Mediterranean, Middle East, South America, Iceland, Australia, New Zealand, Southern Africa	Ultrasound may demonstrate classical daughter cysts and 'hydatid sand' CT highly sensitive and specific	Parasite serology and radiological features Biopsy avoided	Surgical treatment of larger and superficial cysts Medical treatment: albendazole or mebendazole 3–6 months Emerging use of puncture, aspiration, injection, and re-aspiration technique	Morbidity is usually secondary to free rupture of the echinococcal cyst (with or without anaphylaxis), infection of cyst, biliary obstruction, cirrhosis
Caroli's disease (Figure 27.1)	Rare autosomal recessive disease Usually detected in childhood or early adulthood Associated with medullary sponge kidney (renal tubular ectasia) in 80%	Characterised by segmental cystic dilation of intrahepatic bile ducts	MRCP or ERCP	Treatment for complications	No associated cirrhosis or portal hypertension Predisposed to calculus formation Prone to recurrent cholangitis and resultant liver abscesses Increased risk of cholangiocarcinoma
Malignant liver tumours	**Primary liver cancer (HCC)** Male predominance Usually cirrhotic Risk greatest in: • Chronic hepatitis B (cirrhotic and non-cirrhotic) • Hepatitis C • Haemochromatosis • Cirrhosis from α-1-antitrypsin deficiency Worldwide incidence 1 million cases per year Risk of HCC in cirrhosis 1–6% per year	CT: isodense lesion surrounded by a low-density contrast-enhancing ring Associated with portal vein thrombosis	Serum α-fetoprotein levels (AFP) are > 500 µg/l in 70–80% of cases Biopsy often not needed when characteristic radiology and cirrhosis	Treatment is disappointing Resection often complicated by the presence of underlying cirrhosis, multiple lesions and micrometastases Liver transplantation may be considered for multiple lesions and cirrhosis	Up to 70% of patients already have metastatic disease at the time of diagnosis Mean survival from time of diagnosis is 6–12 months

Metastatic liver cancer	Accounts for 95% of all hepatic malignancies in 50% of malignancies in cirrhotic liver Majority associated with end-stage disease Colonic adenocarcinoma commonest cause of potentially curable solitary metastases	CT: lesions generally hypovascular and hypoattenuating when imaged during portal venous phase Intraoperative ultrasound useful for detecting liver metastases at surgery	Characteristic radiology and known primary usually sufficient Biopsy may help to determine diagnosis and treatment if primary lesion not found	Approximately 20% colorectal liver metastases are resectable Neoadjuvant systemic chemotherapy may increase number resectable	'Curative' resection 5-year survival rate of 25–38% Non-operative therapy only provides a median survival rate of 9 months
Fibrolamellar carcinoma	Distinct variant of HCC Young adults No association with pre-existing cirrhosis, viral hepatitis or other known risk factors	Lobulated heterogeneous mass with a central scar in an otherwise normal liver	Characteristic morphology of malignant hepatocytes enmeshed in lamellar fibrous tissue AFP levels are rarely elevated	Initial treatment usually involves resection of the primary tumour or liver transplantation, with en bloc resection of metastatic lymphadenopathy	Prognosis is better than for HCC Many patients survive several years after tumour resection Tumour recurrence common and almost always involves the liver
Cholangiocarcinoma	Second most common primary liver tumour Male predominance Predisposing: primary sclerosing cholangitis, choledochal cysts	Features helpful in differentiating from other primary tumours: • Homogeneously echogenic or high attenuation • Presence of calcification • Invasion of portal or hepatic veins uncommon	Histology necessary May require exploratory laparotomy for adequate biopsy Endoscopic ultrasound may be useful for imaging and biopsy	Approximately 30% are resectable at time of diagnosis	Overall survival rate after resection dependent upon tumour staging, tumour-free surgical margins and lymph node status
Hepatoblastoma	Affects children, almost all < 3 years old	Right lobe (75%), both lobes or multicentric (33%)	Increased AFP in 67–90%	Surgical resection only curative option Control of metastatic disease with adjuvant chemotherapy 30% resectable at presentation	Metastases at diagnosis in 10%

AFP, alpha-fetoprotein; CT, computed tomography; ECRP, endoscopic retrograde cholangic-pancreatography; HCC, hepatocellular carcinoma; MRCP, magnetic resonance cholangiopancreatography; MRI, magnetic resonance imaging; RUQ, right upper quadrant.

Biopsy

After the discovery of a liver lesion, liver biopsy might be required to determine either:

- Diagnosis, including the presence or absence of malignancy, or
- Presence or absence of underlying liver disease and cirrhosis.

Biopsy is avoided if HCC or hydatid is strongly suspected, to avoid the risk of 'seeding' the tumour along the biopsy tract.

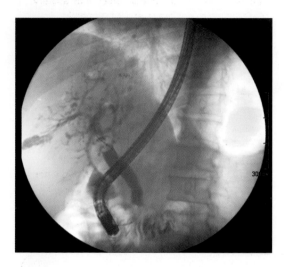

Figure 27.1 ERCP picture showing Caroli's disease.

Management and prognosis

The vast majority of benign liver lesions require no active treatment. The main exceptions are when a large lesion close to the capsule of the liver is causing pain or when central lesions cause biliary obstruction. Treatment of malignant lesions depends on the condition and the underlying liver disease.

Metastatic liver cancer

Many malignant conditions metastasise to the liver as a late feature of terminal disease. Only colorectal adenocarcinoma (commonest) and neuroendocrine tumours present as solitary metastases to the liver and are potentially curable. Approximately 20% of patients with colorectal liver metastases have disease that is resectable at the time of diagnosis. Curative resection gives 5-year survival rates of 25–38%; non-operative therapy only provides a median survival rate of 9 months. Neoadjuvant systemic chemotherapy may increase the proportion of patients with resectable disease.

Hepatocellular carcinoma

Treatment of HCC localised to the liver depends on the presence or absence of cirrhosis. Survival is usually not >6 months in patients with a large tumour mass and Child C cirrhosis. Patients with small HCCs (<5 cm diameter) and stable liver function

(a)

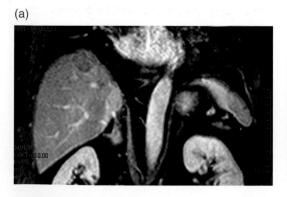

(b)

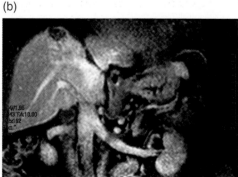

Figure 27.2 MRI of HCC before (a) and after (b) treatment with radiofrequency ablation. The contrast enhancing lesion seen in the dome of the liver in image A was treated with radiofrequency ablation. At a 3-month follow-up scan the lesion had lost its contrast enhancement. The enhancement and size of the lesion had not changed at MRI 2 years after original therapy.

have a better prognosis, but survival rates are still only 21% at 3 years. Surgical resection is recommended for patients without cirrhosis or with limited segmental or lobar HCC and preserved hepatic function. Local treatments, such as radiofrequency ablation, can be used to treat lesions that are not amenable to surgical resection (see Figure 27.2). Transplantation is mainly recommended when the tumour is small, extrahepatic disease is non-existent and hepatic reserve is poor.

 KEY POINTS

- Liver cancer is the sixth most common cancer worldwide.
  - Rates are highest in Eastern Asia and lowest in South-Central Asia and Northern Europe.
- Half of all hepatic cancer cases are liver cell cancers.
  - Liver cell cancers comprise hepatocellular carcinomas, hepatoblastomas, angiosarcomas of liver, other sarcomas of liver and other specified carcinomas of liver.
  - Intrahepatic bile duct carcinomas make up a further 40% of the total.
  - The remaining 9% are of unspecified type.
- The vast majority of liver cancer cases are discovered incidentally.
- Raised levels of alpha-fetoprotein (AFP) are indicative of HCC in the right clinical setting.
- Ultrasound remains the initial study of choice.

- Liver biopsy is avoided if HCC or hydatid is strongly suspected, to avoid the risk of 'seeding'.
- Only colorectal adenocarcinoma (commonest) and neuroendocrine tumours present as solitary metastases to the liver and are potentially curable.
- Hepatocellular carcinoma treatment depends on the presence or absence of cirrhosis:
  - Surgical resection is recommended for patients without cirrhosis or with limited segmental or lobar HCC.
  - Local treatments, such as radiofrequency ablation, can be used to treat lesions that are not amenable to surgical resection.
  - Transplantation is mainly recommended when the tumour is small, extrahepatic disease is non-existent and hepatic reserve is poor.

 SELF-ASSESSMENT QUESTION

(The answer to this question is given on p. 269)

A 42-year-old woman presents to her GP with pain typical of biliary colic. An ultrasound is conducted that confirms cholelithiasis, but also shows a 2 cm lesion in the right lobe of the liver, with no other abnormality of the liver and no evidence of cirrhosis, portal cavernous transformation or ascites. Initial investigation shows that, previously unknown to her, she is hepatitis B virus (HBV) S antigen positive and has a HBV DNA of 10,000 copies per mL. ALT 65, bilirubin 20, INR 1.1, platelets 255. She is otherwise well with no significant past medical history and her only medication is the combined oral contraceptive.

Regarding the incidentally diagnosed liver lesion, which of the following statements is most true?

(a) The absence of cirrhosis both clinically and on ultrasound means that HBV-related hepatocellular carcinoma is very unlikely.

(b) A biopsy is needed to confirm the diagnosis.

(c) Hepatocellular adenoma is a lesion associated with oral contraceptive use and often regresses if the oral contraceptive is stopped.

(d) Haemangiomas of the liver are an uncommon incidental finding on liver imaging and always require resection because of the high risk of haemorrhage.

(e) Isolated (single-lesion) liver metastases from adenocarcinoma of the colon are very uncommon and no effective treatment exists for them.

28

Vascular liver diseases

Obstruction of the venous system of the liver causes a spectrum of disease ranging from acute hepatic failure to passive hepatic congestion. It can be divided into three categories:

- Budd–Chiari syndrome.
- Veno-occlusive disease.
- Congestive hepatopathy.

In addition, reduction of oxygen delivery to hepatocytes (by obstruction of the arterial system or systemic hypotension or hypoxia), with/without concomitant congestion, can cause profound hepatic dysfunction.

Embryology

The liver arises from a diverticulum on the ventral surface of the gut and gives off two solid buds of cells that grow into columns or cylinders, termed the hepatic cylinders. These then branch and anastomose to form a close meshwork. This network invades the vitelline and umbilical veins, and breaks up these vessels into a series of capillary-like vessels, termed sinusoids, which ramify in the meshes of the cellular network and ultimately form the venous capillaries of the liver.

Vascular anatomy of the liver

The vessels of the liver are the hepatic artery, portal vein and hepatic veins. Blood running to the liver travels in the hepatic artery and portal vein. These ascend to the porta, between the layers of the lesser omentum, in combination with the bile duct (Figure 28.1). The bile duct lies to the right, the hepatic artery to the left and the portal vein behind and between the other two (Figure 28.2). The hepatic veins convey the blood away from the liver and are formed as the sublobular veins unite to form progressively larger conduits. The hepatic veins converge to form three large trunks draining into the inferior vena cava.

The substance of the liver is composed of lobules. Each lobule consists of a mass of hepatic cells, arranged in irregular radiating columns between which are the blood channels (sinusoids). These convey the blood from the circumference to the centre of the lobule, ending in the intralobular vein, which in turn empties into a sublobular vein. The portal vein and hepatic artery, after entering the liver at the porta, run through the portal canals and repeatedly branch, eventually giving interlobular branches, which form a plexus outside each lobule. All the blood carried to the liver by the portal vein and hepatic artery finds its way into the interlobular plexus. From this plexus, lobular branches enter the lobule and end in the network of sinusoids between the cells.

Budd–Chiari syndrome

Budd–Chiari syndrome (BCS) is an uncommon and potentially life-threatening condition caused by the obstruction of hepatic venous outflow at any level from the small hepatic veins to the junction of the inferior vena cava (IVC) with the right atrium. Its

Gastroenterology and Hepatology: Lecture Notes, Second Edition. Stephen Inns and Anton Emmanuel.
© 2017 John Wiley & Sons, Ltd. Published 2017 by John Wiley & Sons, Ltd.
Companion website: www.lecturenoteseries.com/gastroenterology

(a)

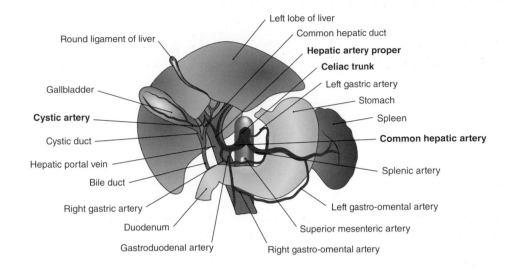

(b)

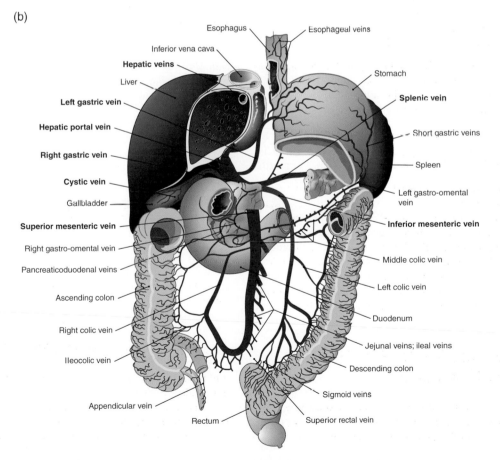

Figure 28.1 Normal arterial (a) and venous (b) anatomy of the liver. Source: Paulsen F. ed. 2013. Sobotta atlas of human anatomy, Vol. 2, 15th edn. Munich: Urban & Fischer Verlag. Reproduced by permission of Elsevier.

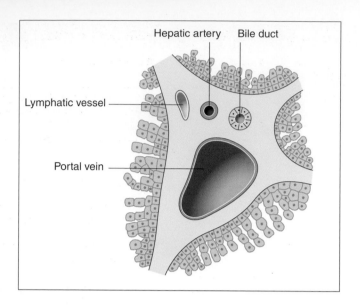

Figure 28.2 Cross-section of a portal canal.

presentation is variable depending on the degree and rapidity of onset of obstruction.

Epidemiology and causes

BCS is an uncommon disorder that occurs in 1 in 100,000 of the general population worldwide. It is more common in women, and in the third or fourth decade. It has multiple aetiologies:

- Primary:
  - Intraluminal thrombosis (commonest cause):
    - Primary myeloproliferative disorders (especially polycythaemia vera > essential thrombocythaemia, myelofibrosis).
    - Inherited deficiencies of protein C, protein S and antithrombin III (factor V Leiden mutation underlies the majority of pregnancy- and oral contraceptive–related cases).
    - Paroxysmal nocturnal haemoglobinuria.
  - Vascular webs.
- Secondary:
  - To intraluminal invasion (by parasites or malignant tumour).
  - To extraluminal compression (by abscess, cyst or solid tumour).

The pathological features of BCS result from the increased sinusoidal pressure that occurs with hepatic venous obstruction. This in turn results in portal hypertension, causing portal perfusion to decrease, potentially

resulting in portal vein thrombosis (PVT; a complication that substantially worsens prognosis). Reduced venous perfusion and congestion result in hypoxic damage to the liver parenchymal cells, releasing free radicals. These cause oxidative injury to the hepatocytes and the development of centrilobular hepatocyte necrosis. Centrilobular fibrosis and nodular regenerative hyperplasia ensue and, ultimately, cirrhosis may occur. However, if sinusoidal pressure is reduced (by portosystemic shunt formation or the development of a portal venous collateral system), liver function improves.

Clinical features

BCS demonstrates a wide spectrum of clinical features, ranging from asymptomatic disease to fulminant liver failure, depending on the location, extent and rapidity of onset of the obstructive process, and whether there is portal vein occlusion. Ascites, hepatomegaly and abdominal pain commonly occur. The disease can be classified into asymptomatic, fulminant, acute, subacute or chronic groups. However, the correlation between the history, duration of occlusion and prognosis is unclear (Table 28.1).

The natural history of BCS is poorly understood because most patients receive some form of treatment along the way. The introduction of anticoagulation and the earlier recognition of asymptomatic disease have resulted in a decrease in mortality.

Table 28.1 Clinical features and classification of Budd–Chiari syndrome (BCS).

Clinical classification	Proportion of BCS	Presentation	Clinical features
Asymptomatic	5–20%	Incidental discovery of abnormal LFTs	Absence of symptoms due to large collaterals (intrahepatic and portosystemic) or the patency of one large hepatic vein
Acute	20%	Symptoms develop over a few weeks	Severe RUQ pain, hepatomegaly, jaundice and intractable ascites
Fulminant	Uncommon	Onset of encephalopathy within 8 weeks of symptom onset	Follows rapid complete occlusion of all major hepatic veins Acute-onset encephalopathy, renal failure, coagulopathy and marked aminotransferase elevations Acute development of oesophagogastric varices, tender hepatosplenomegaly
Subacute and chronic	>60%	Onset insidious over >6 months	Subacute: • Minimal ascites, with hepatosplenomegaly and vague RUQ discomfort • Jaundice absent or mild • Ascites and hepatic necrosis minimal (because hepatic sinusoids have been decompressed by a portal and hepatic vein collateral circulation) Chronic: • Presenting with complications of cirrhosis: variceal bleeding, encephalopathy, renal failure, coagulopathy, hepatopulmonary syndrome

LFTs, liver function tests; RUQ, right upper quadrant.

Differential diagnosis

BCS is frequently misdiagnosed initially. Cholecystitis is considered due to the combination of abdominal pain and ultrasonographically visible thickening of the gallbladder wall. It is not unusual for these patients to come to cholecystectomy. BCS must be considered in any patient at risk of thrombophilia who presents with ascites, upper abdominal pain or abnormalities on LFTs.

Inferior vena cava (IVC) compression or thrombosis causes less severe disease, clinically recognisable by the development of leg oedema or venous collaterals over the trunk and back. It follows a chronic course, with repeated acute episodes eventually resulting in congestive cirrhosis. IVC obstruction is associated with good short-term prognosis, but there is limited long-term data.

Cardiac conditions (tricuspid regurgitation, constrictive pericarditis, right atrial myxoma) can be ruled out by careful cardiovascular examination. The absence of a hepatojugular reflux on abdominal pressure rules out a cardiac cause of ascites.

Investigations

Diagnosis of BCS requires a high level of suspicion and should be considered in anyone presenting with ascites, hepatomegaly and right upper quadrant (RUQ) pain. Laboratory findings are non-specific. Ascitic albumin varies at different stages of the disease; however, the serum–ascitic fluid albumin gradient is high, usually with a total protein >25 g/l.

Diagnosis is dependent on *imaging*:

• Real-time or colour and pulsed Doppler ultrasound is the initial investigation of choice, with a sensitivity and specificity of nearly 85%. It can demonstrate hepatic vein obstruction or abnormal flow in large intrahepatic or subcapsular venous collaterals.
• Contrast-enhanced CT is less useful for visualisation of hepatic veins and the IVC; however, it does allow assessment for parenchymal disease, ascites and splenomegaly.
• MRI with gadolinium enhancement allows excellent visualisation of the hepatic veins and IVC but, unlike Doppler, it does not demonstrate the direction of

hepatic venous blood flow. It is most useful in cases where ultrasound is non-contributory but clinical suspicion is high.

- Venography is not essential for the diagnosis of BCS, but does give useful information about the extent of the thrombosis and the caval pressures. It guides decision making when considering surgical treatment of BCS.

Pathology shows variable degrees of parenchymal damage dependent on the location and extent of venous congestion. Ischaemic necrosis and fibrosis in perivenular areas are characteristic. Concomitant PVT results in periportal fibrosis. In chronic BCS, collateralisation compensates for this and there may be caudate hypertrophic cirrhosis with atrophy in the rest of the liver.

Management

The goals of treatment are to:

- Alleviate obstruction.
- Prevent extension of thrombosis.
- Preserve hepatic function by decreasing centrilobular congestion.

Medical management

Medical therapy alone can only be considered when there is no ongoing hepatic necrosis (as indicated by the relative absence of symptoms, normal LFTs and easily controlled ascites). These patients should be carefully monitored for progression using serial upper GI endoscopies and liver biopsies. The focus is to:

- Control the ascites (low-sodium diet, diuretics or paracentesis with IV albumin cover).
- Prevent thrombosis extension (anticoagulation, or thrombolysis in the small number of cases where it is appropriate).
- Treat complications.
- Investigate and treat underlying cause.

Angiographic and surgical management

Restoration of hepatic blood flow may be achieved by the use of:

- Thrombolytic therapy:
  - Indicated in the acute situation where angiography suggests fresh thrombus.
  - Thrombolytic agent (urokinase or tissue plasminogen activator) can be given systemically or, preferably, directly into the obstructed hepatic vein.

- Percutaneous angioplasty:
  - To caval webs or short hepatic vein stenoses.
  - Excellent short-term patency, falling to 50% by 2 years.
  - Can be improved to 90% with use of intraluminal stents.
- Transjugular intrahepatic portosystemic shunt (TIPS):
  - Provides an alternative venous outflow tract to decompress the liver.
  - Useful as a bridge to liver transplantation and in acute situations, such as variceal bleeding and fulminant hepatic failure, where thrombolysis and angioplasty have been unsuccessful.
  - May function by allowing time for venous collaterals to form, so while long-term occlusion occurs in 50%, these patients do not generally worsen.
- Portosystemic shunt surgery:
  - Creates hepatofugal flow in the portal vein.
  - Recommended in subacute disease when the underlying cause has a favourable long-term outcome.

Liver transplantation

Liver transplantation is the treatment of choice in the presence of cirrhosis, fulminant hepatic failure or biochemical evidence of advanced liver dysfunction. The long-term survival after transplantation in BCS is 50–95%. While liver transplantation effectively cures most inherited thrombophilias, because of the frequent multifactorial aetiology of BCS, life-long anticoagulation is needed in most post-transplant patients.

Prognosis

Five-year survival is 60% in patients with concomitant PVT and 85% in isolated BCS. Prognosis is associated with the presence of ascites, encephalopathy, prothrombin time and serum bilirubin levels. Histology on liver biopsy is *not* accurate in determining prognosis, perhaps because of the uneven distribution of hepatic lesions in BCS.

Hepatic veno-occlusive disease

Epidemiology

Veno-occlusive disease (VOD) typically occurs after haematopoietic stem cell transplantation (HSCT), but also after ingestion of pyrrolizidine alkaloids. The reported incidence after HSCT varies from 5–50%, due to differences in chemotherapeutic regimens. The reported mortality of VOD varies greatly, from 3–67% depending on disease severity.

Causes

The histological features of VOD are:

- Loss of sinusoidal endothelial cell (SEC) fenestrae.
- Appearance of gaps in the SEC barrier.
- Narrowing of the sublobular and central veins due to subendothelial oedema.
- In advanced disease the sinusoidal and venous lumina become obliterated.

One of the main hypotheses for the pathogenesis of VOD is that depletion of liver glutathione reserves diminishes the liver's ability to detoxify acrolein (which is an inactive but hepatotoxic metabolite of cyclophosphamide). It is unclear whether coagulation plays a primary role or is a secondary event. It is also possible that immunological mechanisms have a pathogenic role.

Clinical features

Signs and symptoms develop within three weeks of exposure in the case of HSCT and are primarily those of tender hepatomegaly, fluid retention, ascites and jaundice. Liver enzyme changes may occur a few days later (hyperbilirubinaemia, sometimes in association with increased ALT and ALP).

In the majority, the first, and often only, symptom is RUQ pain.

Risk factors for the development of VOD include:

- Advanced age.
- Presence of liver injury prior to HSCT.
- Previous HSCT.
- Clotting cascade mutations (Factor V Leiden and prothrombin G20210A).
- Type and dose of the conditioning regimens prior to and during HSCT:
  ○ Cyclophosphamide is used in combination with busulphan.
  ○ Total body irradiation.
  ○ Carmustine and etoposide.

Investigations

- Liver biopsy is the diagnostic gold standard for VOD:
  ○ However, patients are frequently thrombocytopenic, making biopsy risky when taken by percutaneous, laparoscopic or even transvenous (transjugular or femoral) means.
  ○ Thus the diagnosis is primarily clinical. The Seattle and Baltimore clinical criteria are commonly applied and correlate well with biopsy-proven diagnosis.
  ○ Transvenous biopsy does also allow measurement of the wedge hepatic venous pressures, providing useful additional diagnostic information.
- Ultrasound is useful, primarily for excluding other disorders.
- Plasma plasminogen activator inhibitor-1 (PAI-1) levels have proven 100% sensitive and specific for VOD diagnosis in the group of post-HSCT patients with bilirubin levels >60 µmol/l (>3 mg/dl).

Important differential diagnoses for liver dysfunction post-HSCT include:

- Acute graft-versus-host disease (GVHD):
  ○ Tends to occur later and only after intestinal and cutaneous manifestations become obvious.
  ○ Does not cause hepatomegaly or ascites.
- Sepsis-related cholestasis:
  ○ Does not cause hepatomegaly or ascites.
- Cyclosporin-induced cholestasis.

Management

Prevention

As there is no established effective therapy, prevention of VOD is the priority. This includes modifying the conditioning regimen in patients at increased risk of VOD and (possibly) use of ursodeoxycholic acid as prophylaxis. Heparin infusion may be useful, but carries an increased risk of bleeding. Low-molecular-weight heparin is safer and easier; it may have a preventive role but evidence is lacking.

Treatment

Once VOD is established, the treatment for most patients is simply diuretics and sodium restriction. Repeated paracenteses may be required. Hepatotoxic drugs should be avoided and infections treated promptly. Perhaps the most promising new development is defibrotide, a polydisperse oligonucleotide derived from porcine intestinal mucosa, with antithrombotic and protective properties on the microvasculature but minimal haemorrhagic risk. Orthotopic liver transplantation is a possible last resort, but is difficult and high risk in patients undergoing HSCT.

Prognosis

The lack of an effective treatment means that the outcome from VOD remains poor. In one paediatric study 5-year survival was 62%. Predictors of mortality included donors other than autologous or matched sibling, hepatic and cutaneous graft-versus-host disease, maximal weight gain >9%, pleural effusion, and the bilirubin level.

Congestive hepatopathy and cardiac cirrhosis

Epidemiology and causes

While mild degrees of hepatic dysfunction in the presence of congestive cardiac failure are common, the development of cardiac cirrhosis is rare. When it does occur, the chief causes are:

- Ischaemic heart disease (31%).
- Cardiomyopathy (23%).
- Valvular heart disease (23%).
- Restrictive lung disease (15%).
- Pericardial disease (8%).

The classical pathological description is that of 'nutmeg liver' (Figure 28.3), with contrasting areas of red caused by *sinusoidal congestion* and bleeding in the *necrotic* regions surrounding the enlarged hepatic veins, and yellow due to the normal or *fatty liver* tissue. These macroscopic changes are also evident histologi-

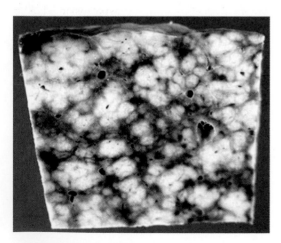

Figure 28.3 Nutmeg liver. Source: Mahtab M-A. 2012. Liver: a complete book on hepato-pancreato-biliary diseases. Kidlington: Elsevier Health Sciences, Fig. 48.5. Reproduced with permission of Elsevier.

cally. The degree of cholestasis is variable, with occasional bile thrombi in the canaliculi. In the presence of chronic heart failure, *fibrosis* develops in the perivenular region, leading ultimately to bridging fibrosis between central veins. Cardiac fibrosis is distinct from primary liver cirrhosis in which fibrous bands tend to link adjacent portal areas. If the underlying cardiac disease is treated successfully, the early histological changes resolve, and even fibrosis may regress.

The pathogenesis of these changes relates to the reaction of the hepatic stroma evoked by increased venous pressure, hypoxia or hepatocellular necrosis. Thrombosis in the hepatic and portal veins is also contributory.

Clinical features

- Liver dysfunction in congestive cardiac failure is generally mild and asymptomatic, and is usually detected incidentally.
- With more severe congestion, mild jaundice, RUQ discomfort (due to stretching of the liver capsule) and ascites develop.
- Where severe jaundice and elevated aminotransferases develop, this is due to acute hepatic ischaemia resulting from marked reductions in cardiac output.
- Reported cases of fulminant hepatic failure have resulted from the combination of both hepatic congestion and ischaemia.

Symptoms of exertional dyspnoea, orthopnoea and angina may help in diagnosis. Examination may reveal tender hepatomegaly with a firm and smooth liver edge. Splenomegaly is uncommon and when it occurs, like ascites, is due to increased transmitted central venous pressure. The detection of jugular venous distension and hepatojugular reflux are helpful pointers to an underlying cardiac cause. The liver may be pulsatile, particularly in the presence of tricuspid regurgitation. Oesophageal varices may also be present. The mortality rate is determined by the severity of the underlying cardiac disease and not the liver disease.

Investigations

The diagnosis is not always obvious and right-sided heart failure must be considered in all patients with hepatomegaly with or without jaundice. The diagnosis is suggested by the triad of:

- Right heart failure.
- Hepatomegaly.
- Ascites (with high protein content in the presence of a high serum to ascites albumin gradient, along

with refractoriness of ascites to diuretic treatment, which contrasts with resolution of peripheral oedema with diuretics).

Initial investigation includes:

- Liver biochemistry:
  - Hyperbilirubinaemia is mostly unconjugated and is seen in up to 70% of cases.
  - Bilirubin level increases with prolonged and repeated bouts of congestive heart failure and correlates with the right atrial pressure (but not cardiac output).
  - Alkaline phosphatase is only mildly elevated and aminotransferase elevations are mild unless cardiac output is impaired.
  - Hepatic synthetic function is usually preserved with a normal plasma albumin and prothrombin time.
  - Improvement in liver biochemistry with treatment of cardiac disease supports the diagnosis.
- Viral hepatitis serology.
- Abdominal ultrasound with Doppler studies of the liver (the discovery of dilatation of all three main hepatic veins on ultrasound mandates vigorous investigation for a cardiac cause).
- Liver biopsy may be useful in equivocal cases.
- ECG and echocardiogram.

Management

Management centres on treatment of the underlying heart disease. Jaundice and ascites usually respond well to diuresis. Repeated paracentesis may be necessary in the presence of refractory ascites. There is no need to regularly replace the albumin lost during paracentesis because synthetic function is preserved in congestive hepatopathy. It should be noted that liver disease rarely contributes to the morbidity or mortality in these patients, and serious complications, such as variceal bleeding and HCC, rarely develop.

Prognosis

The exact effect of congestive hepatopathy on the mortality of congestive heart failure has not been determined. Treatment of the heart failure remains the priority.

Ischaemic/hypoxic hepatitis

Liver cell injury resulting from subcritical supply of oxygen to hepatocytes is traditionally classified as:

- Inadequate blood supply due to reduced hepatic arterial flow and/or passive venous congestion (e.g. heart failure) termed ischaemic hepatitis, or

- Hypoxic insult (e.g. respiratory failure), termed hypoxic hepatitis.

While the pathogenesis is multifactorial, the final common pathway is hepatocellular dysfunction secondary to critically low levels of oxygen for metabolic processes, and these will be considered together in this section under the term hypoxic hepatitis (HH).

Epidemiology and causes

Hypoxic injury to the liver is a reversible subclinical condition affecting at least 1% of critically ill patients and accounting for >50% of dramatic serum aminotransferase activity (24–48 hours following the hypoxic insult) identified in hospital admissions.

The main aetiologies for HH include:

- Primary heart disease (78%).
- Congestive heart failure (65%).
- Acute myocardial infarction (17%).
- Chronic respiratory failure (12%).
- Circulatory shock and sepsis (15%) (sepsis alone, in the absence of shock, does not cause hepatic enzyme elevation).

The aetiology of the marked liver enzyme rise seen in HH is presumed to be hypoxic injury to the hepatocyte mitochondria and endoplasmic reticulum, especially to the centrilobular region. While hypotension/shock is a common antecedent to the onset of liver injury, severe hypotension/shock per se is unnecessary for the development of HH, which occurs frequently without hypotension due to forward (i.e. ischaemia) and backward (i.e. passive congestion) flow abnormalities, producing hypoxic injury through the common pathway of *hypoperfusion*, especially in the setting of systemic factors resulting in increased oxygen consumption or decreased oxygen availability.

The histological findings include central hepatic vein congestion with centrilobular hepatic necrosis, fragmentation of liver bulks, polymorphonuclear cell infiltration, abnormal hepatocyte complexes, pyknosis and disintegration of hepatocyte nuclei. Hyperplasia, inflammation and regeneration, which are characteristic of many other forms of hepatitis, are absent.

Clinical features

Frequently the liver injury is subclinical, with only non-specific nausea and vomiting. The liver may be tender and enlarged.

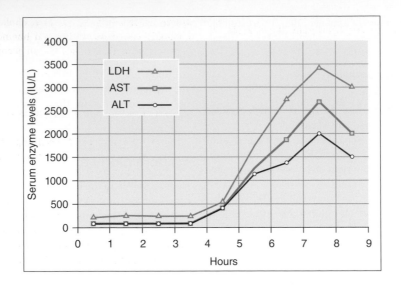

Figure 28.4 Degree of hepatic enzyme elevation over time after hypotensive injury.

Risk factors for HH may be present (acute and chronic heart failure, respiratory failure, sepsis, prolonged hypotension, toxin ingestion and heat stroke).

Investigations

The diagnosis is based on clinical and biochemical criteria, generally without the need for procedural intervention. There is a profound transient serum enzyme elevation in conjunction with abnormal renal function and abnormalities in PT and APTT activity (Figure 28.4). There are no biochemical differences that distinguish between patients with injury caused predominantly by hypotension versus non-hypotensive, non-hypovolaemic patients with hypoxic hepatopathy.

Management

Management is purely supportive and focuses on correcting the underlying conditions leading to hypotension, and hypoxic and hepatic hypoperfusion, including congestion.

Prognosis

The prognosis depends on that of the underlying disease, being largely independent of the liver injury. That said, the occurrence of hypoxic hepatopathy is a harbinger of a potentially poor prognosis, since the mortality rate varies from 25–73%.

Portal vein thrombosis

Epidemiology and causes

The exact frequency of PVT is unknown. It occurs most commonly as a complication of cirrhosis, particularly in decompensated disease, and in up to 35% of cirrhotic patients with hepatocellular carcinoma (HCC). The combination of multiple aetiological factors is important in the pathogenesis (Box 28.1), a cause being identifiable in most cases, classifiable as general thrombophilic factors (in 60% of cases) and local factors (in 40%). These include systemic factors such as inherited prothrombotic disorders, acquired haematological diseases and sepsis, in particular *Bacteroides fragilis* infection.

PVT can be divided into four anatomical categories:

- Thrombus confined to the portal vein beyond confluence with the superior mesenteric vein (SMV).
- Extension into the SMV but patent mesenteric vessels.
- Diffuse splanchnic venous involvement with large collaterals.
- Splanchnic involvement but extensive fine collaterals.

This system is most useful in determining operability, but may also be helpful in determining prognosis, as thrombus involving the SMV is associated with a higher risk of bowel infarction and a lower risk of variceal bleeding than is isolated PVT.

<table>
<tr><td>

Box 28.1 Causes of portal vein thrombosis

Idiopathic causes
Causes secondary to tumour
- Hepatocellular carcinoma
- Cholangiocarcinoma
- Pancreatic carcinoma
- Gastric carcinoma

Trauma
Intra-abdominal sepsis/inflammation
- Perinatal omphalitis
- Appendicitis
- Diverticulitis
- Ascending cholangitis
- Intra-abdominal abscess
- Pancreatitis

Haematological disorders
- Myeloproliferative disorders
- Clotting disorders (hypercoagulable syndromes)

Iatrogenic
- Umbilical vein catheterisation
- Oestrogen therapy

Severe dehydration
Cirrhosis
Portal hypertension

</td></tr>
</table>

'Cavernous transformation of the portal vein' results from the development of multiple small vessels in and around the recanalising or occluded main portal vein, giving a leash of fine or markedly enlarged serpiginous vessels in place of the portal vein.

Clinical features

While somewhat arbitrary and often difficult, it is useful to distinguish between acute and chronic PVT. *Acute* onset is suggested by the absence of clinical, endoscopic and radiological evidence of portal hypertension, typically thrombosis occurring <60 days prior to assessment. *Chronic* thrombosis presents with the complications of portal hypertension, including GI bleeding, splenomegaly and hypersplenism. Ascites is rare, except in the elderly, unless there is comorbid liver disease. While the causes of acute and chronic PVT are similar, sepsis is a more common cause of chronic thrombosis.

Problems in the extrahepatic biliary tree are frequently seen, the mechanisms for which include biliary compression by choledochal or periportal varices, external compression by portal cavernoma formation, pericholedochal fibrosis or ischaemic stricturing. In addition, jaundice, cholangitis, choledocholithiasis, cholecystitis and haemobilia due to rupture of choledochal varices can occur.

Investigations

- Initial investigation of choice is colour Doppler ultrasound.
- Contrast-enhanced CT scanning is particularly useful for demonstrating portosystemic collaterals or the development of a cavernoma, which suggest well-established PVT.
- Where an underlying local cause is found, investigation for other co-factors is not required. However, where no local cause is found, systemic causes, including myeloproliferative disorders and prothrombotic conditions, should be sought.

Management

Treatment aims either to reverse or prevent the advancement of thrombosis and to treat the complications. Treatment recommendations are hampered by a lack of randomised controlled studies. Variceal bleeding is managed in standard fashion: endoscopic therapy and/or medical therapy, including non-selective beta-blockers and nitrates.

In PVT thrombolysis and/or anticoagulation may result in recanalisation of the thrombosed portal system. Thrombolysis should be considered in acute PVT and anticoagulation considered for chronic thrombosis where there is no evidence of cirrhosis. No consensus exists as to the duration or degree of anticoagulation and generally a similar strategy to deep vein thromboses in the lower limb is applied: a finite course of treatment where a reversible cause is found, but long-term anticoagulation where the underlying cause is not reversible.

Where splenomegaly causes hypersplenism, splenectomy may be of benefit. Symptomatic bile duct abnormalities are best treated endoscopically.

Prognosis

The natural history of PVT is uncertain and reported mortality varies from 0–76%. Variceal bleeding is the presenting problem in approximately 30% of cases and is the most common complication of PVT. Concomitant disease, in particular bowel infarction, contributes greatly to the prognosis and is a more important cause of death than variceal bleeding.

KEY POINTS

- Obstruction of the venous system causes disease ranging from acute hepatic failure to passive hepatic congestion. It can be divided into three categories:
  - Budd–Chiari syndrome:
    - Obstruction of hepatic venous outflow.
    - Classified into asymptomatic, fulminant, acute, subacute or chronic groups.
    - Real-time or colour and pulsed Doppler ultrasound is the initial investigation of choice.
    - Liver transplantation is the treatment of choice in the presence of cirrhosis, fulminant hepatic failure or biochemical evidence of advanced liver dysfunction.
  - Veno-occlusive disease:
    - Typically occurs after haematopoietic stem cell transplantation.
    - Also after ingestion of pyrrolizidine alkaloids.
    - Liver biopsy is the diagnostic gold standard for VOD.
    - No established effective therapy, so prevention of VOD is the priority.
  - Congestive hepatopathy:
    - Classical pathological description is that of 'nutmeg liver'.
    - Mortality rate is determined by the severity of the underlying cardiac disease and not the liver disease.
  - Diagnosis is suggested by the triad of right heart failure, hepatomegaly and ascites.
  - Management centres on treatment of the underlying heart disease.
- Ischaemic/hypoxic hepatitis:
  - Caused by inadequate blood supply or hypoxic insult to the liver.
  - Frequently the liver injury is subclinical.
  - Diagnosis is based on clinical and biochemical criteria.
  - Management is purely supportive.
- Portal vein thrombosis occurs most commonly as a complication of cirrhosis:
  - Treatment aims either to reverse or prevent the advancement of thrombosis and to treat the complications.
  - Variceal bleeding is managed in standard fashion.
  - Thrombolysis and/or anticoagulation may result in recanalisation of the thrombosed portal system:
    - Thrombolysis should be considered in acute PVT.
    - Anticoagulation should be considered for chronic thrombosis where there is no evidence of cirrhosis.

 SELF-ASSESSMENT QUESTION

(The answer to this question is given on p. 269)

A 71-year-old man is brought to hospital after being found collapsed in a public place. Bystanders performed CPR and, on arrival, ambulance staff found him to be in ventricular fibrillation and performed DC cardioversion with the return of sinus rhythm. He is known to have ischaemic heart disease and has had previous admissions with unstable angina, but has never suffered myocardial infarction. He is admitted to ICU for monitoring, but is conscious and breathing spontaneously. On day 2 of the admission he is found to have a tender RUQ, examination is otherwise normal and there is no shifting dullness on abdominal examination. Liver tests show marked abnormalities of the transaminases: ALT 1530, AST 2155, bilirubin 78, ALP 235, INR 1.7, albumin 28. Liver tests taken at the time of admission were normal.

Regarding the liver test abnormalities, which of the following statements is most true?

(a) The most likely reason for the liver test abnormalities in this man with cardiac disease is congestive hepatopathy.

(b) Ischaemic/hypoxic hepatitis accounts for the majority of massive elevations of aminotransferase activity indentified during hospital admissions.

(c) Budd–Chiari syndrome commonly presents with fulminant hepatitis such as is seen in this case.

(d) Acute portal vein thrombosis frequently results in liver test abnormalities of the magnitude seen in this case and should be managed with thrombolysis and anticoagulation.

(e) Hepatic veno-occlusive disease develops spontaneously in patients with pre-existing cardiac disease.

Pregnancy-related liver disease

Liver disease in pregnancy may take the form of problems that occur more frequently in pregnancy (e.g. gallstones) or run a more serious course (e.g. acute hepatitis E); coincident liver disease that may affect management or have implications after delivery (e.g. chronic hepatitis B and C); or liver diseases specific to pregnancy. The latter are the most common cause of liver dysfunction in pregnancy and it is these that are considered in this chapter.

In recognising pregnancy-related liver disease, the clinician must be aware of the normal physiological changes affecting the liver in pregnancy. Generally speaking, palmar erythema, spider angiomas, low serum albumin levels and high serum alkaline phosphatase levels are benign changes in the liver during pregnancy. High levels of serum liver aminotransferase or bilirubin signal a problem.

HELLP syndrome

Epidemiology and cause

The HELLP syndrome complicates 0.1% of pregnancies, and is associated with poor maternal and neonatal outcomes. The exact cause of HELLP syndrome is unknown, but it is hypothesised that defective placental vascular remodelling results in placental hypoxia and release of placental factors that further placental and endothelial cell dysfunction. This in turn activates the coagulation cascade, with resultant multiorgan microvascular injury, including hepatic necrosis and dysfunction. Other theories have also been proposed,

including maternal immune rejection and genetic disorders of fatty acid oxidative metabolism.

Risk factors for HELLP syndrome include:

- Maternal age older than 34 years.
- Multiparity.
- White race.
- History of poor pregnancy outcome.

Clinical features

The HELLP syndrome may be thought of as a severe form of pre-eclampsia. Pre-eclampsia itself is a condition, occurring after 20 weeks' gestation, consisting of a triad of hypertension, proteinuria and oedema. The lungs and brain are the most vulnerable organs in pre-eclampsia. It often causes abnormal LFTs (modest elevation of serum transaminases and occasionally mild hyperbilirubinaemia), but does not usually seriously affect the liver.

The HELLP syndrome, in contrast to pre-eclampsia, is associated with significant hepatic dysfunction. A syndrome of Haemolysis, Elevated Liver enzymes and Low Platelets on a background of pre-eclampsia or eclampsia defines it (Box 29.1). Patients may present from 20 weeks' gestation, but the syndrome usually occurs between 27 and 36 weeks. Presentation is non-specific – abdominal pain, nausea and sometimes headache.

Investigations

- Nadir platelet count and peak transaminase levels are a reflection of disease severity.
- While the haemoglobin level may be normal initially, haemolysis occurs, with the deformed red

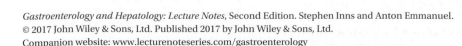

Gastroenterology and Hepatology: Lecture Notes, Second Edition. Stephen Inns and Anton Emmanuel.
© 2017 John Wiley & Sons, Ltd. Published 2017 by John Wiley & Sons, Ltd.
Companion website: www.lecturenoteseries.com/gastroenterology

> **Box 29.1 Hellp Syndrome**
>
> **H**aemolysis
>
> **E**levated **L**iver enzymes
>
> **L**ow **P**latelets.

cells of microangiopathy visible on blood film, and often a marked decrease in the haemoglobin.
- Renal dysfunction is common.
- Clotting must be monitored, but remains normal except in advanced disease with the onset of disseminated intravascular coagulation.

Management

- Treatment is by delivery as soon as is practicable, balancing maternal health and foetal outcome. In uncomplicated disease, once 34 weeks' gestation is reached, this decision is not difficult. However, in complicated disease or early gestation the balance is not straightforward.
- Where organ failure occurs, immediate delivery is dangerous and must be preceded by transfer to intensive care and rapid correction of fluid imbalance, hypertension, hypoxia, seizures and coagulopathy:
  - Dexamethasone promotes maturity of the foetal lungs and ameliorates HELLP.
  - Most serious complications stem not from liver disease but the other effects of this severe form of pre-eclampsia, although rarely subcapsular haematoma and resultant liver rupture are fatal.
- Medical treatment in an attempt to ameliorate disease and gain gestational time (plasma volume expansion, vasodilatation, low-dose aspirin, corticosteroids) is advocated, but has not been subjected to controlled trials.

Prognosis

While with aggressive management and improved disease recognition maternal mortality has fallen below 1%, perinatal mortality is still 10–20%.

Acute fatty liver of pregnancy

Epidemiology and cause

Acute fatty liver of pregnancy (AFLP) results in hepatic failure, and maternal and foetal mortality. Originally considered rare, it is now recognised that

AFLP occurs relatively commonly in a less severe form, which is associated with better outcomes. Incidence is estimated at 1 in 1000 deliveries. There are no clear geographical or racial predispositions to AFLP. Risk factors for disease include older maternal age, primiparity, multiple pregnancies, pre-eclampsia, male foetus and previous AFLP.

The pathophysiology is one of microvesicular fat deposition. In a minority of cases this can be attributed directly to an inherited defect of fatty acid oxidation, but the majority of affected mothers do not have such a deficiency and the cause of AFLP remains unknown.

The characteristic histological features are swollen foamy hepatocytes due to microvesicular fat. The architecture is not disturbed and neither inflammation nor necrosis is prominent, but some cholestasis is common.

Clinical features

- AFLP occurs at 32–36 weeks' gestation, presenting non-specifically (nausea, abdominal pain).
- Polyuria and polydipsia are common, sometimes diabetes insipidus.
- Jaundice and encephalopathy only occur late.
- Pancreatitis is frequently associated, but because the symptoms are similar to AFLP the diagnosis is difficult.
- There are no specific examination features and examination is often normal.

Investigations

The features are of acute impairment of hepatic function in late pregnancy. Biopsy is often contraindicated in the face of severe disease, but when performed shows characteristic histological features (see earlier).

Typical laboratory findings are:

- Neutrophilia (present in almost all cases), a platelet count that is initially normal but drops with disease progression, and a normal haemoglobin.
- Transaminases are moderately elevated and renal dysfunction is common.
- Antithrombin III activity is profoundly and consistently decreased.
- Hyperammonaemia, coagulopathy and hypoglycaemia are early features that assist in differentiating AFLP from HELLP (the main differential diagnosis: the presence of polyuria and polydipsia, and early absence of anaemia, are also useful in this regard).

- Radiological imaging is not particularly helpful, as microvesicular steatosis is not easily detected.

Management

Early delivery is the mainstay of treatment. The safest way of achieving this is emergency caesarean section in combination with ICU management of coagulopathy, renal dysfunction, acidosis and sepsis. Occasionally, liver transplantation is required. It should be noted that AFLP may recur in subsequent pregnancies.

Prognosis

Maternal death is uncommon and the rate of perinatal death is <10%.

Obstetric cholestasis

Epidemiology and cause

There has been an apparent increase in the incidence of obstetric cholestasis (OC) or intrahepatic cholestasis of pregnancy. This is at least in large part an artefact of better case ascertainment with the increasing investigation of the symptom of pruritis in pregnancy. The pathophysiology is of pure cholestasis without hepatic inflammation or necrosis.

No single cause is responsible for all cases. Important factors influencing the incidence of the disease include:

- Ethnicity (Asians being at greater risk).
- Environment (possible association with low selenium levels).
- Hormonal effects, as demonstrated by the increased incidence in late pregnancy and multiple pregnancies, and precipitation by exogenous progestogens.
- Genetic influences, with a strong familial tendency and the discovery of specific gene mutations in a minority of cases.

Clinical features

- Patients present with generalised pruritis, which particularly involves the palms and soles and is worst at night. This tends to occur at 30–36 weeks' gestation, but can start as early as the first trimester.
- Jaundice is not common, occurring in <10%, and when it occurs it indicates more severe cholestasis.
- Family history is common (up to 30%).
- Urinary infection often precipitates, or is associated with, OC.

Investigations

- It must be noted that **the laboratory findings of OC are not those normally expected with cholestasis**. The observed **elevation of serum transaminases** (up to 10 times normal) may be explained by increased membrane permeability. It does not necessarily occur at the onset of pruritis, and transaminase elevation in an otherwise well woman with pruritis in pregnancy is virtually diagnostic of OC.
- ALP is not useful, as it is mildly elevated in late pregnancy normally. GGT is raised in only 30% of cases.
- Serum bile acids are more sensitive and specific.
- Bilirubin may be slightly elevated in about 10% of cases.
- Imaging is not usually contributory.

Management

The main effect of this disease is not on the mother but on the foetus, with increased rates of prematurity, foetal distress and stillbirth. Peak bile acid levels may influence foetal outcome.

Treatment traditionally consists of the following:

- Ursodeoxycholic acid (UDCA) is the treatment of choice. It reduces maternal bile acid levels and affects pruritis. As yet there is no evidence that it affects perinatal mortality; given the very low mortality rate of <1%, a very large number would be required for such a trial.
- Antihistamines and cholestyramine may have a slight effect.
- Delivery is recommended at 36–38 weeks' gestation, as the risk of stillbirth increases beyond 36 weeks.

The features of OC resolve rapidly after delivery, usually within a few days. If abnormalities persist, the diagnosis should be reconsidered.

Prognosis

Older studies reported perinatal mortality as high as 10%; however, with current active management this appears now to be <1%. There is a high (50–75%) rate of repeat OC in future pregnancies.

Hyperemesis gravidarum

Nausea and vomiting are common in early pregnancy. In contrast, hyperemesis, defined as severe intractable vomiting requiring admission, occurs in

<1%. It is commoner in younger, obese, multiparous women and twin pregnancies.

The onset of disease is at 4–10 weeks' gestation. LFTs are deranged by up to 50%, with transaminase elevation between 2 and 10 times normal. Jaundice is uncommon. Invasive tests are not warranted.

Most cases settle with rehydration, electrolyte replacement and glucose. Symptoms typically resolve after 20 weeks' gestation. If improvement is slow, parenteral hydrocortisone sometimes leads to rapid resolution. Maternal and foetal outcomes are not influenced, providing that dehydration is avoided.

 KEY POINTS

- Palmar erythema, spider angiomas, low serum albumin levels and high serum alkaline phosphatase levels are benign changes during pregnancy.
- High levels of serum liver aminotransferase or bilirubin signal a problem.
- HELLP syndrome complicates 0.1% of pregnancies:
  - Haemolysis, Elevated Liver enzymes and Low Platelets on a background of pre-eclampsia.
  - Treatment is by delivery as soon as is practicable.
  - Dexamethasone promotes maturity of the foetal lungs and ameliorates HELLP.
  - Most serious complications stem not from liver disease but the other effects of this severe form of pre-eclampsia.
- Acute fatty liver of pregnancy:
  - Characteristic histological features are swollen foamy hepatocytes due to microvesicular fat.

- Occurs at 32–36 weeks' gestation, presenting non-specifically.
- Early delivery is the mainstay of treatment.
- Occasionally, liver transplantation is required.
- Obstetric cholestasis:
  - Pathophysiology is of pure cholestasis without hepatic inflammation or necrosis.
  - Presents with generalised pruritis at 30–36 weeks' gestation.
  - Laboratory findings are elevation of serum transaminases (up to 10 times normal) rather than those normally expected with cholestasis.
  - Ursodeoxycholic acid (UDCA) is the treatment of choice.
- Hyperemesis gravidarum:
  - Defined as severe intractable vomiting requiring admission.
  - Occurs in <1% of pregnancies. Onset of disease is at 4–10 weeks' gestation.
  - LFTs are deranged by up to 50%.
  - Most cases settle with rehydration, electrolyte replacement and glucose.

 SELF-ASSESSMENT QUESTION

(The answer to this question is given on p. 270)

A 29-year-old woman who is 31 weeks pregnant presents to her lead maternity carer feeling non-specifically unwell with increasing swelling of her ankles. This is her first pregnancy and her health prior to, and up to this point in, the pregnancy has been very good. Examination reveals palmar erythema and spider naevi as well as a pregnant abdomen with a normal fundal height for dates. Heart rate 90/min, BP 152/96. albumin 20, ALP 140, ALT 75, INR 1.1, platelets 110, Hb 9.6, creatinine 134, fasting blood sugar 6.3.

Regarding the patient's clinical situation, which of the following statements is most true?

(a) The presence of spider naevi and palmar erythema as well as reduced platelets and albumin indicate underlying chronic liver disease with probable cirrhosis.

(b) Elevation of the ALP suggests that the diagnosis is intrahepatic cholestasis of pregnancy.

(c) The absence of hypoglycaemia is most consistent with acute fatty liver of pregnancy.

(d) It is likely that the blood film will show deformed red cells.

(e) Steroid administration is contraindicated in this clinical situation.

Hereditary and congenital liver diseases

The exponential growth in genetic and molecular techniques over the last decade has led to improved understanding of the genetic and molecular mechanisms of inherited liver diseases. This has in turn led to genetic testing, allowing the diagnosis of genetic abnormalities before or soon after the onset of clinical disease. A description follows of the more common genetic conditions affecting the liver, and some of the important congenital conditions that do not appear to have a genetic basis.

Hereditary haemochromatosis

Epidemiology

Heriditary haemochromatosis (HHC) is the commonest genetic disease in Caucasians, with a prevalence of between 1 in 300 and 1 in 400. The fact that the carrier frequency is as high as 1 in 9 in some populations would predict a much higher disease prevalence, emphasising the complex genotype–phenotype association.

Causes

Systemic iron overload is the hallmark of HHC. Iron deposits at sufficient concentrations can cause clinically relevant damage to the liver, pancreas, heart, joints and pituitary. Mutations of the HHC gene (*HFE*) cause a defect in iron handling that leads to iron overload. However, the exact mechanism of this remains poorly understood despite description of the underlying genetic defect.

HFE codes for a major histocompatibility complex (MHC) class I protein that is expressed on many cells, including duodenal crypts. This MHC protein interacts with the transferrin receptor to facilitate iron uptake into cells and defects in it alter this interaction.

Haemachromatosis may result from a variety of causes other than heredity (Box 30.1).

Genetics

HHC is an autosomal dominant inherited condition, but genotype–phenotype correlations in HHC are highly variable, related to poorly understood genetic factors. However, female gender (and thus menstruation), conditions causing iron loss, and age are implicated in modifying the phenotype.

While the molecular mechanism has yet to be elucidated, the genetic defect is now well described: 80–90% of clinically diagnosed HHC patients are homozygous for a single G-to-A mutation in *HFE* that results in a cysteine-to-tyrosine substitution at position 282 (C282Y) of the gene product. Thus, this mutation accounts for the vast majority of disease. A second, less common mutation (H63D) has been discovered; however, its role in causing clinically relevant iron overload is not clear, as it is present in patients and controls at similar frequencies. While homozygotes for H63D do not exhibit significant iron overload, compound heterozygotes (i.e. C282Y/H63D) do have modest increased total body iron stores and progress to hepatic fibrosis or cirrhosis is rare.

Gastroenterology and Hepatology: Lecture Notes, Second Edition. Stephen Inns and Anton Emmanuel.
© 2017 John Wiley & Sons, Ltd. Published 2017 by John Wiley & Sons, Ltd.
Companion website: www.lecturenoteseries.com/gastroenterology

---

Box 30.1 Causes of haemochromatosis

Genetic disorders
- Hereditary haemochromatosis (*HFE*, non-*HFE* and juvenile)
- Autosomal dominant haemochromatosis

Haematological disorders
- Thalassaemia major
- Sideroblastic anaemia

Others
- Increased dietary iron (African iron overload)
- Parenteral iron (e.g. multiple transfusions)
- End-stage alcoholic cirrhosis
- Neonatal haemochromatosis

Clinical features

These largely relate to iron deposition and depend on organ involvement.

- **General features**:
  - Lethargy.
  - Abdominal pain, episodic, can be severe (unclear cause, see later).
- **Hepatic features**:
  - Hepatomegaly.
  - Hepatic function is often well preserved and liver function tests may be normal despite high hepatic iron content and fibrosis.
  - Features of chronic liver disease may be present in advanced disease.
- **Extrahepatic manifestations**:
  - *Diabetes mellitus* occurs in relation to deposition of haemosiderin, predominantly in pancreatic acinar cells, with resultant dense fibrosis. This damage occurs at a threshold tissue iron concentration similar to that of liver fibrosis. Diabetes develops in 30–60% of cases with advanced liver disease;
  - *Cardiac manifestations* are not uncommon and may be the presenting pathology in 5–15% of symptomatic patients. ECG abnormalities are seen in about 30% of patients. The most common cardiac complications are congestive heart failure, typically a dilated cardiomyopathy, and arrhythmias. If instituted early, phlebotomy results in improvement in cardiac manifestations.
  - Iron overload results in a variable destructive *arthropathy*. This is not improved by venesection and may progress despite maintenance of normal iron stores.
  - Pituitary gonadotrophs selectively express the transferrin receptor, leading to accumulation of

intracellular ferritin. *Hypogonadotropic hypogonadism* can thus occur early in the natural history of the disease.
- **Porphyria cutanea tarda** (PCT) is associated with iron overload, and may occur in association with haemochromatosis (see Table 30.4).

Patients with iron overload are at increased risk of ***Yersinia enterocolitica* infection**. This organism is not commonly pathogenic in the absence of iron overload, because it does not possess a high-affinity iron-chelating system and is not able to obtain sufficient iron from the internal environment of the normal human body. It is speculated that at least some of the episodes of acute abdominal pain in HHC are related to infection with this organism.

Investigations

Clinicians should have a high index of suspicion for this common genetic condition.

- **Blood tests**:
  - Transferrin saturation.
  - Serum ferritin concentration (a very sensitive test for elevation of total body iron stores).
  - High serum iron.
  - High total iron-binding capacity.
- **Genetic testing**:
  - Has replaced liver biopsy as the next test in suspected iron overload.
  - Both the C282Y and H63D mutations should be tested for – compound heterozygous states may act as a cofactor leading to fibrosis in conditions such as porphyria cutanea tarda, hepatitis C and steatohepatitis.
- **Liver biopsy**:
  - Useful in quantifying iron overload.
  - Useful in assessing hepatic fibrosis.
  - The hepatic iron index is calculated by dividing the hepatic iron concentration (in μmol/g dry weight) by the age of the patients (in years). Values >1.9 are consistent with HHC.

Screening

Screening for HHC can be considered in three population groups:

1 Relatives of a proband with the disease (mandatory for all first-degree relatives and advisable to extend screening to second-degree relatives).
2 People undergoing a health check (probably cost-effective).
3 General population.

Screening should consist of a history and physical examination, measurement of transferrin saturation and serum ferritin. Assay for the C282Y mutation is undertaken in groups 2 and 3 if the transferrin saturation is >45% or the serum ferritin is elevated (because of the cost of genetic testing).

Screening for hepatocellular carcinoma

When cirrhosis is present, HHC patients have a 200-fold increased risk of hepatocellular carcinoma (HCC). HCC is the commonest cause of death in such patients. Patients who have developed HCC may present with unexplained weight loss, fever, nodular enlargement of the liver, variceal haemorrhage, ascites, jaundice and abdominal pain.

Patients who develop HCC usually have advanced hepatic fibrosis and cirrhosis. For this reason, screening is reserved for patients with cirrhosis. Serum alpha-fetoprotein and serial ultrasound are used in a similar manner as in other forms of cirrhosis (see Chapter 27).

Management

Venesection is the mainstay of treatment. This should occur at weekly intervals until the haemoglobin concentration falls to 10.5 g/dl and does not recover immediately. *Monitoring of serum ferritin* shows a progressive decline during initial treatment, the aim being to keep the value within the low normal range (50–100 pg/l). Maintenance venesection is lifelong, approximately four times per year, but this needs to be individualised. Iron deficiency must be avoided (ferritin kept >20 pg/l).

In the presence of cardiac insufficiency, treatment is still with venesection, as it is the most efficient, safest and cheapest alternative, but may need to be in smaller amounts and less frequently. The iron-chelating agent desferrioxamine can be used when there is anaemia from other causes, but at best removes only 10–20 mg of iron/day.

Prognosis

Prognosis is dependent on the presence of cirrhosis or diabetes. In the absence of these, life expectancy is normal provided that maintenance venesection is adhered to. Liver transplantation should be considered where there is end-stage liver disease or small HCCs. However, liver transplantation for HHC has been disappointing at least in part due to the degree of iron loading in these patients, as iron-loaded patients are at risk of infection as well as cardiac failure and arrhythmia.

Wilson's disease

Cause

Wilson's disease is an autosomal recessive disorder caused by a defect in hepatic copper excretion, resulting in copper overload and copper deposition in various organs, including the liver, brain, kidneys and cornea, with resultant hepatic, neurological, psychiatric, haematological, renal, eye and other abnormalities.

In this condition copper is not incorporated into its carrier protein, caeruloplasmin, within hepatocytes. It is therefore not adequately excreted into bile and accumulates in the liver. Eventually it is released into blood and deposited in other tissues. Liver disease is attributed to oxidative stress resulting from the pro-oxidant properties of copper. There are high concentrations of copper in the hepatocellular mitochondria in hepatic copper overload and it may be that mitochondrial damage plays a role in the pathogenesis.

Genetics and epidemiology

The prevalence of Wilson's disease is 1 in 30,000 and the carrier frequency is 1 in 90. The abnormal *ATP7B* (conventionally called *WND*) gene is on chromosome 13. It encodes an intracellular membrane-spanning ATPase transporter with six copper-binding sites, which has a role in incorporating copper into caeruloplasmin.

Clinical features

Wilson's disease is highly variable and may present as:

- Acute hepatitis.
- Chronic liver disease.
- Fulminant liver disease.
- Progressive neurological disorder (often without clinically evident hepatic dysfunction).
- Psychiatric illness.

Patients usually become symptomatic between the ages of 6 and 45 years, but may be diagnosed younger or older.

- **Hepatic presentation:** liver disease presentation is more common in children and adolescents. The features are often non-specific, with fatigue, abdominal pain and anorexia:
  - Simple acute hepatitis: a self-limited clinical illness indistinguishable from autoimmune hepatitis, with:
    - Elevated serum aminotransferases.
    - Greatly increased serum IgG.

- Detectable non-organ-specific autoantibodies, including antinuclear antibody and antismooth muscle (antiactin) antibody.
  - Repeated episodes of short-lived jaundice: largely asymptomatic, related to haemolysis.
  - Severe established chronic liver disease. Typically, this occurs in late-stage patients with:
    - Acute Coombs-negative intravascular haemolysis.
    - Renal failure.
    - Kayser–Fleischer rings on slit-lamp examination.
    - Greatly elevated urinary copper excretion.
  - These patients do not respond to chelation treatment and require urgent liver transplantation. HCC rarely develops in Wilson's disease.
- **Neurological presentation:** a predominantly neurological presentation usually occurs in older teenagers or adults. There are two predominant patterns of involvement:
  - Movement disorders, including tremors, poor coordination and loss of fine motor control.
  - Rigid dystonia with mask-like facies, rigidity and gait disturbance.
  - Pseudobulbar involvement is more common in older patients and may result in dysarthria, drooling and swallowing problems. Seizures may occur.
- **Psychiatric presentation:** a purely psychiatric presentation occurs in 20% of patients and the symptoms are highly variable. Depression is common and neuroses, including phobias and compulsive behaviours, are reported. Pure psychosis is uncommon. Intellectual deterioration may also occur.
- **Other manifestations:**
  - Fatigue, malaise, arthropathy and rashes.
  - Renal dysfunction.
  - Vitamin D–resistant rickets with severe renal dysfunction.
  - Haemolysis related to copper release into the bloodstream.
  - Cholelithiasis may occur with repeated haemolysis.
  - Pancreatitis.
  - Endocrine: hypoparathyroidism, amenorrhoea, testicular dysfunction, repeated spontaneous abortion.
  - Kayser–Fleischer rings due to copper accumulation in Decemet's membrane in the posterior cornea.
  - Sunburst cataracts, in approximately 20% of patients.
  - Cardiomyopathy and cardiac arrhythmias (rare).
  - Rhabdomyolysis (very rare).

Investigations

Essential to the diagnosis of this rare condition is a high index of suspicion in the appropriate clinical setting. All patients being investigated for suspected autoimmune hepatitis should be tested for Wilson's disease because of the similarities in clinical features between the two.

Blood tests

The hallmark of Wilson's disease is a low caeruloplasmin. This carrier protein binds most of the copper in plasma (>90%). The normal adult serum concentration of caeruloplasmin is 200–600 mg/l and in most patients with Wilson's disease this is greatly reduced (typically <50 mg/l).

False negatives may occur:

- Difficulties with laboratory assays.
- Hepatic inflammation (as caeruloplasmin is elevated in inflammatory conditions).
- Pregnancy.
- Exogenous oestrogen.

False positives may occur:

- Decompensated cirrhosis of any cause or acute liver failure.
- Protein-losing enteropathy.
- Nephritic syndrome.
- Malnutrition.
- Heterozygotes for Wilson's disease (10% of whom have low levels).

Other tests

- Urinary copper excretion increases (24-h urinary collections are typically >100 µg/24 h).
- Liver biopsy determines hepatic copper concentration (a value >250 µg/g dry weight is considered diagnostic, values <40 µg/g make Wilson's disease unlikely).
- Genetic testing is complex, with almost 300 mutations in the *ATP7B* gene, and most patients are compound heterozygotes. Where biochemical findings are equivocal, demonstration of two abnormal alleles is necessary for diagnosis. Mutational analysis can allow presymptomatic diagnosis of the siblings of affected individuals, including those whose biochemical testing is negative (thus permitting early chelation therapy).

Management

The mainstay of treatment is chelation therapy. First-line treatment consists of penicillamine, which greatly increases urinary excretion of copper and induces tissue metallothioneins. Its use is limited by common mild side-effects (skin rashes, loss of taste, GI upset, diarrhoea, arthralgias). Severe side-effects are rarer (proteinuria, leucopaenia or thrombocytopenia, and rarely aplastic anaemia). 30% of patients with Wilson's disease develop some side-effect of penicillamine, leading to a change of treatment. Deterioration in neurological status occurs initially after starting penicillamine in up to 50% of patients who present with mainly neurological symptoms. Most, but not all, recover with continued use. Pyridoxine 25 mg/day is given in conjunction with penicillamine.

Second-line treatment for patients intolerant of penicillamine is with Trien (trientine). Side-effects are rare apart from occasional gastritis, iron-deficiency (due to chelation of dietary iron) and sideroblastic anaemia. Neurological worsening is much less common than with penicillamine. Finally, zinc can be used as chelation and, apart from gastritis, has few adverse effects.

With all treatment modalities, compliance and efficacy should be checked by measuring 24-h urinary copper excretion every 6–12 months; FBC and urinalysis should be monitored regularly. Some reduction of dietary copper is probably also beneficial.

Prognosis

With effective and early treatment, most patients are well and live normally.

Alpha-1-antitrypsin deficiency

Cause

Alpha-1-antitrypsin is a protease inhibitor that controls tissue degradation by inhibiting a large number of proteases, including trypsin, plasmin, thrombin, neutrophil elastase and proteinase 3. It is predominantly produced in the liver, with some production in the monocytes and bronchoalveolar macrophages also. Deficiency of alpha-1-antitrypsin is one of the commonest hereditary disorders in Caucasians.

Liver disease in this condition is mediated by accumulation of aggregated alpha-1-antitrypsin within the hepatocyte endoplasmic reticulum, visible as periodic acid-Schiff (PAS)-positive inclusion bodies on liver histology. The liver cell injury of alpha-1-antitrypsin deficiency is directly related to this accumulation, and not to a deficiency of elastase inhibitory capacity.

This is evidenced by the fact that individuals with a genetic mutation that aborts alpha-1-antitrypsin production (hence no detectable alpha-1-antitrypsin in their plasma), and lack of the PAS-positive inclusion bodies, do not develop liver disease.

By contrast, lung injury is a result of loss of protease inhibition; chronic obstructive respiratory disease (CORD) due to emphysema is the most prevalent clinical disorder associated with alpha-1-antitrypsin deficiency. Emphysema is due to loss of the normal antiproteolytic defences against elastase. The resultant degradation of elastic fibres with loss of elastic recoil in the lung and air-flow obstruction lead to emphysema, markedly exacerbated by smoking, as the elastase burden is increased by recruitment of both neutrophils and macrophages.

There is an association between small-vessel systemic necrotising vasculitis and severe alpha-1-antitrypsin deficiency. It seems likely that the association is due to a loss of the protective effects of alpha-1-antitrypsin in small-vessel vasculitis rather than a direct causative effect.

Genetics

A single gene located on chromosome 14 encodes alpha-1-antitrypsin. There are at least 75 different identified allelic variants and inheritance is codominant; thus each parental allele contributes its own gene product in the individual. Given the complexity of the genotypic abnormalities, a phenotypic classification system is used that is based on the isoelectric properties (on protein electrophoresis) of the protease inhibitor (Pi) produced. Letters near the beginning of the alphabet identify variants that result in faster-moving proteins, the slowest-moving allele being designated PiZ. The important genetic variants and their clinical consequences are summarised in Table 30.1.

Epidemiology

Alpha-1-antitrypsin deficiency occurs worldwide, but its prevalence varies by population. This disorder affects about 1 in 1500 to 3500 individuals with European ancestry. It is uncommon in people of Asian descent.

Clinical features of liver disease

Childhood-onset liver disease

Alpha-1-antitrypsin deficiency is the most common genetic cause of liver disease in infants and children and the most common metabolic error for which liver transplantation is indicated. The majority (70%) of

Table 30.1 Genetic variants of alpha-1-antitrypsin deficiency.

Variant	% Normal serum alpha-1-antitrypsin levels	Clinical features
PiZZ	15–20%	20–40% cirrhosis in adulthood Onset of COPD-related dyspnoea aged 30–40 in smokers and 10–15 years later in non-smokers Associated with small-vessel vasculitides
PiSZ	30–40%	Probable association with end-stage liver disease in combination with several aetiologies (in particular hepatitis C virus and alcohol-related liver disease) Increased risk of COPD Associated with small-vessel vasculitides
PiMZ	50–60%	Probable association with end-stage liver disease in combination with several aetiologies No predisposition to early development of COPD Associated with small-vessel vasculitides
PiSS	60%	Normal
PiMM	Normal	Normal

COPD, chronic obstructive pulmonary disease.

neonates with homozygous (PiZZ) alpha-1-antitrypsin deficiency have abnormal LFTs and a significant minority (10–20%) develop clinically important liver disease. They present with the 'neonatal hepatitis syndrome':

- Pruritus.
- Hepatomegaly.
- Conjugated hyperbilirubinaemia.
- Increased serum aminotransferase.
- Cholestasis can be marked and the disease can be confused with hepatic biliary atresia.

Alpha-1-antitrypsin states (PiMZ and PiSZ) cause partly self-limiting, predominantly subclinical liver involvement in 10–20% of affected children and adolescents.

The disease usually resolves spontaneously within 6 months, although mild biochemical abnormalities persist in a proportion. In a small minority (<5%), the liver disease does not subside, progressing to cirrhosis and liver failure.

Adult-onset liver disease

The phenotypic expression of alpha-1-antitrypsin deficiency-related liver disease in adults is variable. There is a high risk of cirrhosis and HCC in adults with severe alpha-1-antitrypsin deficiency (PiZZ). Approximately 40% and 15% of alpha-1-antitrypsin-deficient adults develop cirrhosis and HCC respectively. Patients may or may not have a history of neonatal liver disease.

Prognosis is poor in patients with cirrhosis, partly due to concomitant emphysema.

In adults, intermediate deficiency has been associated with chronic liver disease in combination with concomitant liver pathology, in particular with hepatitis C virus and alcohol-related liver disease. The mechanism for this may be that the concomitant condition promotes retention of the abnormal protein in the hepatocyte endoplasmic reticulum.

Investigations

- Alpha-1-antitrypsin deficiency can be diagnosed by a marked reduction or absence of the alpha-1-globulin band in an agarose gel electrophoresis.
- Serum or plasma concentrations can be measured, but are not accurately indicative of the phenotype because of the large variability in serum levels.
- Phenotype is usually assessed using isoelectric focusing (IEF) to ascertain the isoelectric band focusing patterns of the Pi variants. Enzyme-linked immunosorbent assay (ELISA) and DNA-based methods can be used, particularly for screening large populations. At least the first-degree relatives of patients found to have alpha-1-antitrypsin deficiency should be screened in order to detect the 25% of siblings who will be homozygotes at an early asymptomatic stage (although the only preventative measure likely to prolong survival is smoking cessation).

Management

Monitoring

- All patients diagnosed with alpha-1-antitrypsin deficiency should be regularly assessed with tests of liver function. If cirrhosis is established, screening for HCC may be appropriate.
- Monitoring for renal disease and vasculitis in both heterozygotes and homozygotes.
- Chest X-ray and pulmonary function assessment (especially in smokers).

Specific

Attempts to increase serum levels of alpha-1-antitrypsin may affect the progression of pulmonary disease, but will have no beneficial effect on liver disease, as the pathogenic abnormality is related to intrahepatocytic accumulation of abnormal protein rather than reduced Pi activity.

- The androgen danazol and the oestrogen antagonist tamoxifen increase synthesis of alpha-1-antitrypsin slightly, but not sufficiently to have a beneficial effect.
- Purified human alpha-1-antitrypsin can be given by infusion. Its use is mainly in patients with progressive emphysema and vasculitis.
- While the primary pulmonary defect is emphysema, there may be a reversible obstructive component that responds to bronchodilator treatment.
- Orthotopic liver transplantation is curative for both liver disease and the alpha-1-antitrypsin deficiency state, as the recipient assumes the donor's phenotype. It is reserved for advanced liver disease in the absence of HCC and where preoperative evaluation of lung function is satisfactory. With this careful selection, survival rates in children are close to 90% at 1 year and 80% at 5 years. Survival in adults is lower, due partly to concomitant emphysema.
- Somatic gene therapy uses a virus as a 'vector' to insert the normal gene into affected cells. At present, somatic gene therapy is not an available alternative, but it is being tested in animals and human trials may follow.

Prognosis

Prognosis varies according to the alpha-1-antitrypsin deficiency genotype, smoking status and the presence of comorbid liver disease. One study showed that PiZZ patients had a standardised mortality ratio of 4.8. In those who had never smoked this was reduced to 2.3. Most of the mortality is related to pulmonary disease, with liver disease accounting for only 12% of deaths.

Alagille's syndrome

Cause

Alagille's syndrome (AS) is an inherited disease causing cholestasis in conjunction with cardiovascular, facial, ocular, skeletal and neurodevelopmental abnormalities. It is also known as arteriohepatic dysplasia. Cholestasis is a result of a marked paucity of interlobular bile ducts. The mechanisms by which these abnormalities come about are unknown, but the genetic defect has been described.

Genetics and epidemiology

AS is an autosomal dominant disease, but in up to 15% of cases it is due to a new mutation. There is a large variability in expression of the disease, even within affected families. The incidence of AS in mixed Caucasian populations is 1 in 100,000 live births with no gender differences. The genetic defect is a mutation of the *JAG1* gene on chromosome 12. It encodes a protein belonging to the family of Notch ligands, which are regulatory receptors of the signalling pathway controlling cell fate decisions in a number of developmental processes.

Clinical features

- AS characteristically presents as prolonged neonatal cholestasis (jaundice, pale stools, dark urine). In this setting it must be differentiated from biliary atresia in particular.
- Presentation in older children is with features of chronic liver disease, pruritus and xanthomata.
- It is common for adults to go undiagnosed until a related index case is diagnosed, but questioning may reveal a history of pruritus as a child.

HCC has been reported in AS with and without cirrhosis.

Extrahepatic features

- Facial appearance:
  - Triangular face, broad forehead, saddle-shaped nose, widely spaced deep-set eyes, pointed chin.
- Vascular abnormalities (85–100%):
  - Commonly peripheral pulmonary stenoses of no clinical significance.
  - Occasionally pulmonary vascular hypoplasia or severe pulmonary artery stenosis.
- Severe vascular lesions often occur with other congenital heart anomalies:

- Tetralogy of Fallot, truncus arteriosus, septal defects, systemic vascular abnormalities, narrowing of the abdominal aorta.
- Increased risk of intracranial haemorrhage (particularly in young adults):
  - Related to abnormalities in clotting secondary to chronic liver disease or structural abnormalities in intracranial vessels.
- Other manifestations:
  - Spinal problems:
    - Butterfly vertebrae.
    - Occult spina bifida.
  - Characteristic eye changes in up to 90%:
    - Prominent line in the anterior chamber (Schwalbe's line).
    - Ocular problems secondary to chronic cholestasis.
  - Renal abnormalities.
  - Neurodevelopmental delay.
  - Malnutrition and failure to thrive.

Investigations

Because of the variability of expression of the disease, diagnosis remains phenotypic and is based on the occurrence of cholestasis with histological paucity of interlobular bile ducts, plus two of four extrahepatic features (characteristic facies, cardiac murmur, vertebral anomalies, posterior embryotoxon).

Evaluation of all possible manifestations of the disease is mandatory (nutritional assessment, liver biochemistry and biopsy, cardiovascular testing, renal function, slit-lamp eye examination, spinal X-rays, serum bile acids, cholesterol and triglycerides).

A complete genetic evaluation is required, including family pedigree (with examination of family members), molecular genetic studies, cytogenetic studies and genetic counselling.

Management

- Management of the consequences of chronic cholestasis is of the utmost importance:
  - Careful provision of adequate calories, protein and fat-soluble vitamins (A, D, E and K).
  - Management of mineral deficiencies.
- Severe hyperlipidaemia is associated with early atherosclerosis and can be managed to a degree with cholestyramine and ursodeoxycholic acid (UDCA).
- Treatment of pruritus is with antihistamines, but if intractable may respond to biliary diversion and occasionally liver transplantation.

Prognosis

The natural history of AS is variable, with a 74% 10-year survival. Complex cardiovascular anomalies are the major cause of early mortality, hepatic complications the cause of late morbidity and mortality.

Hereditary hyperbilirubinaemias

In an infant or child presenting with jaundice due to hyperbilirubinaemia, the differential diagnosis is broad. Determination of the concentrations and proportions of conjugated and unconjugated bilirubin is important (Figure 30.1). Once other forms of liver disease have been excluded, and particularly in the presence of a family history of hyperbilirubinaemia, the hereditary hyperbiluribinaemias should be considered (Table 30.2).

While conjugated hyperbilirubinaemia is almost always a consequence of underlying liver disease, and is harmless in itself, unconjugated bilirubin causes neurotoxicity by inhibiting RNA, carbohydrate and protein synthesis in the brain when it is persistently elevated.

Physiology of bilirubin metabolism

Degradation of haemoglobin, and other haem proteins, produces bilirubin. This is tightly but reversibly bound to plasma proteins, in particular albumin. On reaching the hepatocyte membrane, bilirubin dissociates from albumin and enters the hepatocyte via a membrane carrier-mediated process. In the cell it is bound to glutathione S-transferase, which acts as the intracellular store for bilirubin. In the endoplasmic reticulum, bilirubin is conjugated by bilirubin uridine-diphosphate glucuronosyltransferase (B-UGT) for efficient elimination in bile. There are two main families of B-UGT, both of which derive from a gene complex on chromosome 2. The vast majority of bilirubin conjugates are excreted in the bile as bilirubin diglucuronide (80%) and bilirubin monoglucuronide (15%). Unconjugated bilirubin accounts only for 1–2% of bilirubin excreted into the bile.

Autoimmune polyglandular syndromes

The autoimmune polyglandular syndromes (APS) are autoimmune syndromes with symptoms affecting gland-bearing tissues, and as such the gut is often

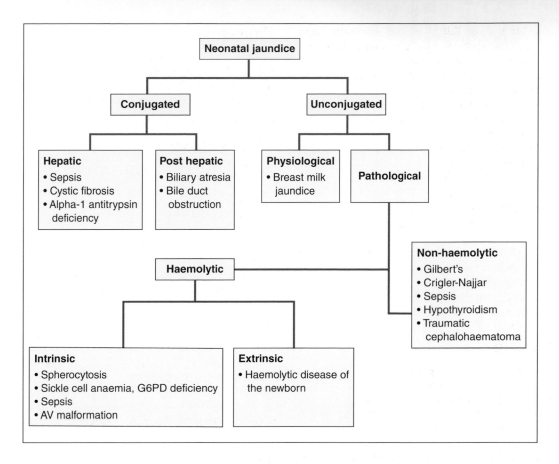

Figure 30.1 Causes of neonatal jaundice.

involved (Table 30.3). A single gene defect is responsible for APS type 1. Diagnosis is based on the pattern of glandular disease. APS type 1 is associated with a low but recognised incidence of GI disease.

The porphyrias

Epidemiology

The porphyrias are rare. The prevalence of all types of porphyria taken together has been estimated to be approximately 1 in 25,000 in the United States. The worldwide prevalence has been estimated to be somewhere between 1 in 500 to 1 in 50,000 people.

Causes

The porphyrias are disorders of haem biosynthesis, characterised as either hepatic or erythropoietic (depending on the site of excess porphyrin production). They are mostly autosomal dominant inherited partial enzyme deficiencies. The key role of environmental factors in causing symptoms explains why penetrance is poor: alcohol, iron excess, oestrogens and hepatitis C infection are the commonest environmental triggers.

Clinical features

The porphyrias usually present after puberty. Two presentations are described (Table 30.4).

- Photosensitive *skin* features:
  - Pain.
  - Erythema, bullae.
  - Hirsutism and hyperpigmentation.
- Acute relapsing–remitting *neurological* features (triggered by anticonvulsants, oral contraception, alcohol, fasting):
  - Acute abdominal pain.
  - Autonomic symptoms (hypertensive headaches, constipation).
  - Peripheral neuropathy.
  - Psychiatric manifestations.
  - Inappropriate ADH secretion.

Table 30.2 Clinical features of the familial hyperbilirubinaemias.

	Cause	Clinical features	Diagnosis	Treatment
Familial unconjugated hyperbilirubinaemia syndromes				
Crigler-Najjar I (CNS-I)	Autosomal recessive Consanguinity common Several genetic mutations identified Deficiency of both UGT1 and UGT2 Massive bilirubin deposition in tissues including: • Kidney • Endocardium • Intestinal mucosa • Brain	Severe, chronic unconjugated hyperbilirubinaemia: • Onset after birth • Bilirubin between 342 and 599 μmol/l Lesser degrees of hyperbilirubinaemia may not develop neurological symptoms until second decade Cerebellar symptoms may predominate	No detectable B-UGT1 activity on assay of hepatic tissue Phenobarbital challenge: • CNS-II decrease bilirubin levels by >30% • CNS-I have no response	Definitive treatments • OLT curative (survival similar to that of OLT for other indications) Alternatives to OLT: • Auxiliary liver transplantation • Hepatocyte transplantation • Gene therapy Temporary treatments: • Phototherapy • Exchange transfusion (CNS-I does not respond to phenobarbital) • Tin-containing compounds (inhibit haem oxygenase, thus decreasing haem degradation and bilirubin production) NB: Only 1–2% functioning hepatocytes necessary for bilirubin conjugation
Crigler-Najjar II (CNS-II)	Autosomal recessive Genetics less well defined	Hyperbilirubinaemia less severe: • Rarely exceeding 342 μmol/l • Increased to >342 μmol/l during illness Icterus: • Present in 50% within the first year of life • Can occur as late as 30 years • Non-specific neurological symptoms as late as 50 years	Activity of B-UGTI reduced to <10% Bilirubin monoglucuronide in bile: • Collected by small bowel intubation • In CNS-I it is absent • Not significant enough to allow differentiation with certainty	Adequately treated with phenobarbital Phototherapy may be needed as an adjunct Mechanisms for the action of phenobarbital include: • Induction of binding proteins and mobilisation of bilirubin • Enhanced B-UGTI transcription and activity • Atrophic effect on the endoplasmic reticulum

Gilbert's syndrome	Reduction in hepatic bilirubin clearance to approximately one-third normal	Mild, chronic unconjugated hyperbilirubinaemia:	Other hepatic and haematological diseases excluded by history, physical examination and laboratory studies	Only treatment necessary is reassurance and education
	Proposed mechanisms:	• Absence of haemolysis	If no abnormalities develop after 12–18 months of follow-up, diagnosis almost certain	
	• Defective uptake into the hepatocyte,	• No hepatic injury	Provocative testing:	
	• Intracellular binding	Common (prevalence 3–12%):	• Caloric deprivation (400 kcal/day) for 48–72 h, followed by a subsequent rise in plasma unconjugated bilirubin levels	
	• Conjugation	• Most often adolescents and young adults	• Nicotinic acid tolerance test	
	Hereditary basis	• Males > females		
	• Inherited either as an autosomal dominant or autosomal recessive	Approx. one-third asymptomatic except for jaundice		
	Likely Gilbert's syndrome represents a heterogeneous group of disorders	Non-specific symptoms		
		• Fatigue		
		• Weakness		
		• Abdominal discomfort		
		• Malaise		
		• All felt to be incidental		
		Degree of hyperbilirubinaemia fluctuates:		
		• Usually 52 μmol/l		
		• May reach levels as high as 137 μmol/l		
		Triggered by		
		• Physical stress		
		• Fatigue		
		• Intercurrent illness		
		• Alcohol intake		

(Continued)

Table 30.2 (Continued)

	Cause	Clinical features	Diagnosis	Treatment
Familial conjugated hyperbilirubinaemia syndromes				
Dubin–Johnson syndrome	Autosomal recessive Worldwide distribution Male = female Dubin–Johnson Syndrome more common than Rotor syndrome Mechanism: • Defective hepatic secretion into the bile • Caused by the absence of the *MRP* (multidrug resistance protein) gene	Mild, predominantly conjugated hyperbilirubinaemia: • 34–120 μmol/l, • >50% conjugated. • Level of bilirubin • Fluctuates • Oral contraceptives and pregnancy exacerbate hyperbilirubinaemia Vague, non-specific abdominal complaints probably incidental Hepatosplenomegaly rarely	Cholescintigraphy: • ⁹⁹ᵐTc-HIDA scan • Intense prolonged visualisation of the liver • Delayed visualisation of gallbladder and bile ducts Differentiation of Dubin–Johnson syndrome from Rotor syndrome and other hepatobiliary diseases: • Urine coproporphyrin patterns after d-ALA administration	Benign disorders, without need for treatment
Rotor syndrome	Autosomal recessive Worldwide distribution Male = female Mechanism: Decreased intracellular storage of bilirubin Excretion of bilirubin is moderately decreased	Asymptomatic except for jaundice	• Bromsulphalein (BSP) clearance Oral cholecystography (gallbladder visualised in Rotor syndrome, but not Dubin–Johnson syndrome)	

OLT, Orthotopic liver transplantation; B-UGT1, bilirubin uridine-diphosphate glucuronosyltransferase 1.

Table 30.3 Clinical features of the autoimmune polyglandular syndromes.

	Cause	Clinical features and diagnosis

Autoimmune polyglandular syndrome type I (APS1) *also known as* Autoimmune polyendocrinopathy-candidiasis-ectodermal- dystrophy (APECED)	Autoimmune disease Mendelian inheritance:
	• Defects in a single gene
	• 100% penetrance
	• Gene on chromosome 21
	• Named autoimmune regulator 1 (*AIRE-1*) or *APECED* gene
	Lack of HLA dependence
	Male = female
	High prevalence in Iranian Jews, Finnish and Sardinian people
		First clinical manifestation typically in first decade of life
		Progressively new disease components may manifest even in the fifth decade
		Other associated immune disorders are frequently found
		Three groups of disease components:
		1 Mucocutaneous candidiasis
		2 Autoimmune tissue destruction, predominantly of endocrine glands:
		  • Hypoparathyroiditis (89%)
		  • Adrenocortical insufficiency (70%)
		3 Ectodermal dystrophy
		  • Dystrophy of the nails
		  • Enamel hypoplasia
		  • Alopecia
		  • Keratopathy
		Associated GI disease:
		  • Intestinal malabsorption in about 18% of patients
		  • Autoimmune hepatitis in about 12% of patients
		Diagnosis: two of the following three (however, if APS1 in a brother or a sister, one disease component is sufficient):
		  • Addison disease
		  • Hypoparathyroidism
		  • Chronic mucocutaneous candidiasis

Autoimmune polyglandular syndrome type 2	Autosomal dominant mode of transmission Polygenic Female preponderance Linkage to HLA-DR3 and DR4 Far more common than APS1	Adult onset of disease Associated autoimmune manifestations: • Vitiligo • Gonadal failure • Alopecia • Pernicious anaemia Diagnosis: • Addison disease, autoimmune thyroid disease and/or insulin-dependent diabetes mellitus (Schmidt's syndrome) • Occurring in a single patient not affected by hypoparathyroidism or candidiasis
Autoimmune polyglandular syndrome type 3	Heterogeneous	Autoimmune thyroid disease and the presence of at least one second autoimmune disorder in the absence of Addison disease

Table 30.4 Clinical features and investigation findings of the porphyrias.

Condition	Symptoms	Blood findings	Urine findings	Stool findings
Plumboporphyria	Neurological	Protoporphyrin IX	ALA, coproporphyrin III	
Acute intermittent porphyria (AIP)	Neurological		ALA, porphobilinogen	
Congenital erythropoietic porphyria (CEP)	Skin	Uroporphyrin I	Uroporphyrin I	Coproporphyrin I
Porphyria cutanea tarda (PCT)	Skin		Uroporphyrin I	Isocoproporphyrin
Hereditary coproporphyria	Neurological and skin		ALA, porphobilinogen, coproporphyrin III	Coproporphyrin III
Variegate porphyria	Neurological and skin		ALA, porphobilinogen, coproporphyrin III	Protoporphyrin IX
Erythropoietic porphyria	Skin	Protoporphyrin IX		Protoporphyrin IX

ALA, amino laevulonic acid.

Investigations

Table 30.4 illustrates the blood, urine and stool features of the porphyrias. Additionally, the identification of the genes of the haem biosynthesis pathway has allowed genetic screening of family members, although there are a large number of mutations for each porphyria.

Management

- **Cutaneous forms**:
  - Avoid skin exposure and trauma, use of barrier creams.
  - In porphyria cutanea tarda, venesection or chloroquine can be helpful.
- **Neurological forms**:
  - Avoidance of triggers.
  - Intravenous glucose (calories reduce abnormal enzyme activity, helping terminate attacks).
  - Administration of haem (reduces metabolite excretion and accelerates recovery).
- **Hepatic consequences and liver transplant as a treatment**:
  - Erythropoietic protoporphyria is associated with progression to cirrhosis in some patients. Liver transplant has been used successfully in that situation.
  - Treatment-resistant acute intermittent porphyria and variegate porphyria have been successfully treated with liver transplant.
  - Porphyria cutanea tarda is often associated with underlying liver disease, particularly hepatitis C.

Prognosis

The natural history of the porphyrias is not well understood. At least in acute intermittent porphyria, there is evidence that an increased mortality relates to the acute porphyric attacks. In one study the mortality rate was three times that of the general population. In some studies of the neurological porphyrias, an increased rate of suicide has been found.

Glycogen storage diseases

The glycogen storage diseases represent a broad range of clinical entities brought about by disruption of the normal mechanisms of glycogenolysis and gluconeogenesis (Table 30.5). Treatment focuses on avoiding hypoglycaemia and managing the hepatic and extrahepatic consequences of these diseases.

Biliary atresia

Epidemiology

The rate of biliary atresia is less than 1 in 10,000 live births. There does seem to be a seasonal variation in the rates of disease, with rates three times higher in December to March compared with April to July in one US study. The incidence is highest in Asian populations. Infants with low birth weight also had a higher rate of biliary atresia. Despite its rareness, biliary atresia is the leading cause of extrahepatic obstructive jaundice in the newborn and is the single most frequent indication for liver transplantation in children.

Pathogenesis

Biliary atresia is a very rare congenital condition of unknown cause in which there is obliteration or discontinuity of the extrahepatic biliary system.

Clinical features

Biliary atresia is indistinguishable from other causes of neonatal jaundice. As well as jaundice, patients may exhibit pale stools, dark urine, failure to thrive, splenomegaly and hepatomegaly. In any neonate with prolonged jaundice that is resistant to phototherapy and/or exchange transfusions, a search for secondary causes should ensue. Kernicterus does not develop as the liver is still able to conjugate bilirubin, which is unable to cross the blood–brain barrier.

Biliary atresia is divided into two distinct groups:

- Isolated biliary atresia (postnatal form), which accounts for 65–90% of cases.
- Associated situs inversus or polysplenia/asplenia with or without other congenital anomalies (foetal/embryonic form), comprising 10–35% of cases.

In addition there are three distinct types of atresia (Box 30.2).

Box 30.2 Types of biliary atresia

- Type I involves obliteration of the common duct; the proximal ducts are patent
- Type II is characterised by atresia of the hepatic duct, with cystic structures found in the porta hepatis
- Type III (>90% of patients) involves atresia of the right and left hepatic ducts to the level of the porta hepatis

Table 30.5 Clinical features of the glycogen storage diseases.

	Clinical features	Treatment

Type 1 glycogen storage disease	Impaired glucose-6-phosphatase system activity:
	• Excessive accumulation of glycogen and fat
	• inadequate hepatic glucose production via glycogenolysis and gluconeogenesis
	Classic presentation:
	• Neonatal period with hypoglycaemia and lactic acidosis or 3–4 months of age with hepatomegaly and/or hypoglycaemic seizures
	• Doll-like faces with excess adipose tissue in cheeks
	• Short stature
	• Protuberant abdomen
	• Kidneys often symmetrically enlarged
	• Liver transaminases normal or only slightly elevated
	• Hypoglycaemia and lacticacidaemia can occur after a short fast
	• Hyperuricaemia often present
	• Intermittent diarrhoea
	• Bruising and expistaxis – prolonged bleeding time as a result of impaired platelet aggregation and adhesion
	• Significant elevation of triglycerides:
	  ○ Cholesterol and phospholipids elevated, but less prominently
	  ○ Skin xanthomas
	  ○ Retinal changes associated with hyperlipidaemia
	NB: Some patients do not show all the classic symptoms and/or have only relatively mild symptoms. In rare cases asymptomatic
	Liver histology:
	• Universal distension of hepatocytes by glycogen and fat
	• Lipid vacuoles are large and prominent
	Long-term consequences:
	• Growth impaired
	• Puberty frequently delayed
	• Gout starts around puberty
	• Increased risk of pancreatitis
	• Hepatic adenomas
	• Hepatomas
	• Heart failure secondary to pulmonary hypertension
	• Osteoporosis
	• Renal disease common
	
	• Type Ib glycogen storage:
	  ○ Additional findings of neutropenia and impaired neutrophil function
	  ○ Ulceration of oral and intestinal mucosa common
	  ○ Inflammatory bowel disease reported
		Main aim to prevent hypoglycaemia
		Dietary therapy:
		• Nocturnal nasogastric infusion of glucose
		• Orally administered uncooked corn starch
		Careful control of glucose during illness and perioperatively essential
		Allopurinol to reduce the levels of uric acid
		Liver transplantation:
		• Only if other treatments fail, or
		• If there has been malignant transformation of an adenoma
		Kidney transplantation in renal failure
		Management of bleeding tendency
		Type Ib:
		• Granulocyte and granulocyte-macrophage colony-stimulating factors to correct neutropenia

(Continued)

Table 30.5 (Continued)

	Clinical features	Treatment

Type III glycogen storage disease	Deficiency of glycogen debranching enzyme:
	• Impairs release of glucose from glycogen but does not affect glucose released from gluconeogenesis
	• Type IIIa involves both liver and muscle (most patients)
	• Type IIIb: only the liver is affected
	Clinical features:
	• Hepatomegaly
	• Growth retardation
	• Hypoglycaemia
	• Hyperlipidaemia
	• High liver transaminases
	• Fasting ketosis
	• Liver-related symptoms improve with age and disappear after puberty
	• Overt liver cirrhosis occurs rarely
	• Neuromuscular involvement, slowly progressive weakness and distal muscle wasting
	Liver histology:
	• Universal enlargement of hepatocytes by glycogen
	• Presence of fibrosis (non-progressive in most cases)
		Dietary management is less demanding than in type I:
		• Symptomatic if hypoglycaemia is present:
		  ○ Frequent meals high in carbohydrates with corn starch supplements or
		  ○ Nocturnal gastric drip feedings
		• Diet high in protein during the daytime plus overnight protein enteral infusion may be of some benefit in patients with myopathy

Type IV glycogen storage disease	Branching enzyme deficiency:
	• Accumulation of glycogen with unbranched, long outer chains
	• Unbranched glycogen is significantly less soluble than normal glycogen
	Clinical features:
	• Progressive liver cirrhosis with portal hypertension and death often occurs before the age of 5 years (minority not progressive)
	• Typically presents in the first year of life
	• Hepatosplenomegaly
	• Failure to thrive
	• Hypoglycaemia is rare
	Histology:
	• Diffuse interstitial fibrosis
	• Wide fibrous septa
	• Abnormally large hepatocytes with stores of coarsely clumped material (glycogen and aggregations of amylopectin-like material)
		No specific treatment:
		• Maintenance of normoglycaemia and adequate nutrient intake:
		  ○ Improves liver function
		  ○ Improves muscle strength
		  ○ May extend the time for growth
		• Liver transplantation for progressive hepatic failure may be effective

Type VI glycogen storage disease	Deficiency in liver phosphorylase or defects in one of the four subunits of phosphorylase kinase:	Symptomatic

Type VI glycogen storage disease

Deficiency in liver phosphorylase or defects in one of the four subunits of phosphorylase kinase:
- Heterogeneous group of diseases
- Phenotypes cannot easily be distinguished clinically

Clinical features:
- Relatively benign
- Usually presenting with hepatomegaly and growth retardation in early childhood
- Hypoglycaemia and hyperlipidaemia mild

X-linked phosphorylasekinase deficiency most common:
- Classical presentation at age 1–5 years:
  o Protuberant abdomen due to hepatomegaly
  o Fasting hyperketosis
  o Mild elevation of cholesterol, triglycerides, AST and ALT
- Clinical symptoms tend to disappear gradually with age
- Most achieve normal final height

Autosomal phosphorylase kinase deficiencies:
- Early childhood
- Hepatomegaly
- Growth retardation

Symptomatic
- High-carbohydrate diet and frequent feedings for hypoglycaemia
- Most patients require no specific treatment

Prognosis is usually good

Adult patients have minimal hepatomegaly and normal stature

Glycogen synthase deficiency

Different from other glycogen storage diseases:
- Decreased glycogen stores
- Present in early infancy
  o Fasting hypoglycaemia
  o Hyperketonaemia
  o No hepatomegaly or hyperlipidaemia
- Hyperglycaemia and a rise in blood lactate concentration may occur after meals (glucose is preferentially converted to lactate in the absence of glycogen synthesis)

Glucagon effect:
- During fasting, administration of glucagon has no effect on blood glucose, lactate or alanine concentrations

After a meal, glucagon causes a rise in glucose and a fall in lactate and alanine

Symptomatic:
- Frequent feedings to alleviate hypoglycaemia
- Protein-containing preferred to meals rich in carbohydrate:
  o Glycogen synthesis is compromised and excess glucose is converted to lactate

Investigations

- **Mandatory**:
  - Blood tests show marked conjugated hyperbilirubinaemia.
  - Ultrasound investigation or other forms of imaging can confirm the diagnosis.
- **Further testing**:
  - Radioisotope scans of the liver.
  - Liver biopsy.

Management

If the intrahepatic biliary tree is unaffected, surgical reconstruction of the extrahepatic biliary tract (hepatoportoenterostomy) is possible (Kasai procedure). If the atresia is complete, liver transplantation is the only option. A third of patients will have inadequate bile flow following the Kasai procedure and will require liver transplantation.

Postoperative breast feeding is encouraged when possible because breast milk contains both lipases and bile salts to aid in lipid hydrolysis and micelle formation. Theoretically, breast milk may also protect against cholangitis.

Prognosis

With advances in surgical technique over recent years, most infants with biliary atresia now survive. Access to transplant has also improved. Previously only whole livers from deceased donors of a similar size could be used. Now split liver transplants allow part of a deceased adult donor liver to be used and part of a living adult donor's liver can also be used.

 KEY POINTS

- Hereditary haemochromatosis:
  - Commonest genetic disease in Caucasians.
  - Autosomal dominant inherited mutations of the HHC gene (HFE) cause a defect in iron handling that leads to iron overload.
  - Extrahepatic manifestations include diabetes mellitus, cardiac manifestations, hypogonadotropic hypogonadism, porphyria cutanea tarda (PCT) and Yersinia enterocolitica infection.
  - Venesection is the mainstay of treatment.
- Wilson's disease:
  - Autosomal recessive disorder causing a defect in hepatic copper excretion.
  - Presentation highly variable: acute hepatitis; chronic liver disease; fulminant liver disease; progressive neurological disorder; psychiatric illness.
  - The hallmark is a low caeruloplasmin. Urinary copper excretion increases.
  - The mainstay of treatment is chelation therapy.
- Alpha-1-antitrypsin deficiency:
  - Liver disease mediated by accumulation of aggregated alpha-1-antitrypsin within the hepatocyte endoplasmic reticulum
  - A single gene located on chromosome 14 encodes alpha-1-antitrypsin.
  - Most common genetic cause of liver disease in infants and children.
  - Adult-onset liver disease is phenotypically variable.
  - Orthotopic liver transplantation is curative for both liver disease and the alpha-1-antitrypsin deficiency.
- Alagille's syndrome is characterised by cholestasis in conjunction with cardiovascular, facial, ocular, skeletal and neurodevelopmental abnormalities.
- The porphyrias are disorders of haem biosynthesis classified as either hepatic or erythropoietic:
  - Two presentations: photosensitive skin features and acute relapsing–remitting neurological features.
  - Blood, urine and stool porphyrins used to diagnose and classify.
  - Erythropoietic protoporphyria associated with progression to cirrhosis; liver transplant has been used successfully.
- Biliary atresia divided into two distinct groups: isolated biliary atresia; and associated situs inversus or polysplenia/asplenia:
  - If the intrahepatic biliary tree is unaffected, surgical reconstruction of the extrahepatic biliary tract is possible (Kasai procedure).
  - If the atresia is complete, liver transplantation is the only option.

SELF-ASSESSMENT QUESTION

(The answer to this question is given on p. 270)

A 32-year-old man is incidentally found to have elevated liver tests during an insurance medical. ALT 98, ALP 87, bilirubin 32, albumin 36, INR 1.0, platelets 152. He is screened for underlying causes, including hereditary liver disease.

Regarding the possibility of hereditary liver disease in this man, which of the following statements is most true?

(a) The screening test that should be performed for hereditary haemochromatosis are the HFE genes C282Y and H63D.

(b) Compound heterozygosity for C282Y and H63D alone would explain the liver test abnormalities.

(c) Hereditary haemochromatosis is the commonest genetic disease in Caucasians with a prevalence of around 1 in 300.

(d) Investigation for the presence of an elevated caeruloplasmin and serum copper would be the screening test of choice in Wilson's disease.

(e) Alpha-1-antitrypsin deficiency is very unlikely to be the cause of significant liver disease in the absence of pulmonary disease.

Part IV

Study Aids
and Revision

Gastrointestinal history check-list

Dysphagia	**Duration** (months = malignancy)
	Progressive (malignancy or benign stricture) or **intermittent** (other causes)
	Worse with liquids (functional, dysmotility), **solids** (benign or malignant stricture, webs) or **both** (dysmotility, neurological cause)
	Timing in relation to swallow (instant = pharyngeal or neuromuscular causes, or few seconds later)
	Nasal aspiration (pharyngeal or neuromuscular causes)
	Cough (nocturnal = dysmotility; instantly after swallowing = pharyngeal or neuromuscular causes)
	Weight loss (malignancy >> benign stricture, dysmotility)
	Associated features (e.g. systemic sclerosis, neurological disorders, past history of reflux suggesting benign stricture)
Abdominal pain	**Onset** (sudden = vascular/infection/obstruction; gradual = inflammatory/neoplastic/functional)
	Frequency/duration (intermittent vs constant)
	Location, radiation or referral (visceral poorly localised/somatic well localised, radiation and referral pattern may define organ involved)
	Character and nature (may define organ involved)
	Exacerbating and relieving features (association with food – timing/type of food, relief with passage of flatus = rectal sensitivity, effect of different medicines, stress)
	Associated symptoms (bowel habit, vomiting, abdominal distension, haematuria, haematochezia, haematemesis, malaena, weight loss, fevers)
GI bleed	**Haematemesis** (cause proximal to jejunum)
	Melaena (cause usually proximal to left colon)
	Visibly red blood loss (distal colon)
	On tissue only (anal disease)
	Associated mucus (IBD, colorectal cancer, villous adenoma, solitary rectal ulcer syndrome)
	Abdominal pain (see above)

Gastroenterology and Hepatology: Lecture Notes, Second Edition. Stephen Inns and Anton Emmanuel.
© 2017 John Wiley & Sons, Ltd. Published 2017 by John Wiley & Sons, Ltd.
Companion website: www.lecturenoteseries.com/gastroenterology

	Signs of chronic liver disease (varices)
	Signs of circulatory compromise (varices)
	Fever, sweating (Crohn's disease, intra-abdominal TB, infectious gastroenteritis)
	Drug history (especially NSAIDs, anticoagulants, alcohol, smoking)
	Weight loss (malignancy)
Diarrhoea	**Watery** (secretory small intestinal causes – infectious or neoplastic – or microscopic colitis), **steatorrhoea-like** (pancreatic or small intestinal disease) or **other**
	Nocturnal diarrhoea (organic cause) or **daytime only** (IBS)
	Weight loss (malignancy > IBD, malabsorption, hyperthyroidism)
	Relationship to pain (eased by bowel opening = diverticular disease, IBD stricture or IBS; unrelated = ischaemic colitis, drug-induced, hypolactasia)
	Family history (IBD, coeliac disease, colorectal cancer)
	Drug history (especially antibiotics, iron, NSAIDs, PPIs)
	Recent travel (infectious diarrhoea)
	Past history (surgical, radiation, systemic disease)
	Incontinence (complication of diarrhoea)
Constipation	**Urge frequency** (daily = normal transit; less than daily = slow transit)
	Bowel frequency (to confirm constipation)
	Stool consistency (to confirm constipation)
	Rectal evacuation difficulty (need to strain, incomplete emptying, perineal or anal digitation – all suggest pelvic floor dysfunction)
	Rectal prolapse (a cause and exacerbator of constipation)
	Diet (encourage more fibre in normal transit, avoid excess in slow transit)
	Drug history (especially anticholinergics, iron, opiates; eating behaviour)
	Past history (eating disorder, abdominal surgery (adhesions), pelvic or anal surgery (local pain causing constipation), neurological disorders, hypothyroidism, hypercalcaemia)
Jaundice	**Prehepatic** (haemolytic; unconjugated hyperbilirubinaemia, normal urine, normal stool; reduced serum haptoglobin, features of haemolysis on blood film)
	Hepatic (unconjugated or mixed hyperbilirubinaemia; dark urine, normal stool; acute or chronic liver disease, Gilbert's, neonatal jaundice)
	Posthepatic (obstructive/cholestatic; conjugated hyperbilirubinaemia; dark urine, pale stool, severe itch; extrahepatic [cholelithiasis, head of pancreas mass] vs intrahepatic biliary disease [sclerosing cholangitis, primary biliary cirrhosis])

Abdominal examination routine

1 Approach the patient's right-hand side and introduce yourself
2 Ensure patient is in a good position – lying comfortably on one pillow, with the abdomen exposed
3 General inspection (should take <60 s if examiner does not stop you):
   - Look around the bed (drip stands, diet sheets)
   - Survey the patient (scratch marks, gynaecomastia, reduced body hair)
   - Hands:
     - Clubbing (Crohn's disease, cirrhosis)
     - Dupuytren's contracture (alcoholic liver disease)
     - Palmar erythema (cirrhosis)
     - Leuconychia (cirrhosis, Crohn's disease)
     - Liver flap (examiner may stop you, but you should offer to examine for this)
       Ask patient to extend elbows and cock wrists back towards the face
       Then ask patient to fan fingers out gently
       You are looking for a bird's-wing flap at the wrist
   - Eyes:
     - Anaemia – expose lower eyelid
     - Jaundice – look at conjunctiva
   - Lips:
     - Cyanosis (liver disease)
     - Parotid swelling (alcoholic liver disease)
     - Pigmentation (Peutz–Jegher's)
     - Telangiectasia (hereditary haemorrhagic telangiectasia)
     - Ulcers (Crohn's disease)
   - Anterior chest wall:
     - Cervical lymphadenopathy (lymphoma, gastric cancer, Virchow's node)
     - Palpate for gynaecomastia
4 Inspect abdomen (should take <15 s, if examiner does not stop you):
   - Prominent abdominal vessels
   - Scars (do not forget nephrectomy scars posteriorly!)
   - Stoma (an ileostomy is generally in the left iliac fossa and smaller than a colostomy, which is often – but not always – on the right side)
   - Distension:
     - Generalised (ascites)
     - Localised (upper abdo, periumbilical, suprapubic, flanks, iliac fossae)
   - Pulsation
5 Palpate abdomen:
   - Enquire about areas of pain
   - Assess direction of flow (best assessed in veins *below* umbilicus):
     - Cranially in inferior vena cava
     - Away from the umbilicus in portal hypertension
   - Superficial palpation in a systematic fashion (traditionally in an anticlockwise spiral from the right iliac fossa, ending in the umbilicus):
     - Use pulps – not tips – of fingers
   - Internal organ palpation:
     - Begin at the right iliac fossa again:
       Liver: work upwards to right upper quadrant
       Spleen: work diagonally to left upper quadrant
     - Next to left and right flank for the kidneys, by bimanual palpation:
       Right hand under patient and left hand on top for left kidney; left hand under patient and right hand on top for right kidney
       Keep upper hand still and firmly pressed down, while lower hand 'ballotts' the kidney
   - *If* any organs are felt:
     - Ask patient to take a deep breath in to assess for movement with respiration
     - Assess edge of the mass – contour, texture
     - Assess if you can 'get above' the mass (kidney)
     - Assess if it is separate to the costal margin (kidney)

○ Offer to assess for inguinal lymph nodes and hernia orifices

6 Percuss abdomen – the principle of percussion is to move from resonant to dull:

○ Percuss down from lower right chest until upper border of liver dullness is reached, then repeat from lower abdomen upwards

○ Repeat the process for the spleen

○ Shifting dullness:
  – First check for stony dullness in flanks – if absent (rare), there is gross ascites and no need to continue; alternatively
  – Start percussing in the midline and gradually move laterally to patient's left until the note becomes stony dull; now ask patient to roll on to their left (facing away you) and allow 15 s for the fluid to settle before percussing towards the flank and listening for the note of dullness that will now represent the peritoneal reflection (rolling and percussing in the opposite direction is also valid and practised by many)

7 Auscultate abdomen:
  ○ Offer to listen to:
    – Bowel sounds
    – Liver venous hum (acute hepatitis)
    – Renal artery bruit

8 Complete examination:
  ○ Offer to:
    – Examine external genitalia
    – Undertake a rectal examination
    – Examine stool

Rectal examination routine

1 Try to put patient at ease, and explain the procedure
2 Place patient in left lateral position (underwear off or at knees), with a drape over them
3 Part the buttocks and inspect for:
  ○ Excoriation
  ○ External haemorrhoids
  ○ Anal fissure
  ○ Skin tags
  ○ Fistulous openings
  ○ Anal warts
4 Insert a well-lubricated finger into the anus, taking note of:
  ○ Anal tone at rest and on voluntary squeeze
  ○ Any rectal mass (polyp, cancer, stool)
  ○ Prostate size and texture in men
5 Withdraw finger and observe the nature of material on the glove
6 Clean the anus, and offer the patient tissues and privacy to dress

Common OSCE cases

It is essential to look for features of other diseases, to help identify causes.

Hepatomegaly	Common causes: • Cirrhosis • Right heart failure • Lymphoma • Myeloproliferative disorder (i.e. polycythaemia rubra vera, chronic myeloid leukaemia, myelofibrosis) • Malignancy (irregular edge to liver)
Hepatosplenomegaly	If also anaemic, diagnosis may be: • Cirrhosis with portal hypertension • Lymphoma • Myeloproliferative disorder • Tropical disorders (malaria, kala-azar) If lymphadenoapthy present, diagnosis may be: • Chronic lymphocytic leukaemia • Lymphoma
Splenomegaly	Massive – most commonly: • Myeloproliferative disorder; moderately enlarged – as above • Cirrhosis with portal hypertension • Lymphoma; slightly enlarged – as above • Infections – infectious mononucleosis, infectious hepatitis, bacterial endocarditis
Enlarged kidney(s)	Bilateral: • Polycystic kidney disease • Amyloidosis • Bilateral hydronephrosis Unilateral • Hydronephrosis • Renal carcinoma
Isolated ascites	Usually with features of chronic liver disease or hepatomegaly, but may be isolated. Look for signs of paracentesis and of causes other than liver disease (heart failure, intra-abdominal malignancy, operative scars)
Chronic liver disease	Have a list of causes and complications of cirrhosis at your fingertips

Surgical sieve

When asked for a list of causes for a condition, always state the most common and clinically important first. Following this the use of a list of categories, commonly referred to as a surgical sieve, can be very useful as an aide mémoire. A frequently used mnemonic for this is 'A VINDICATED PI':

Anoxic
Vascular
Inflammatory
Neoplastic
Degenerative
Intoxication
Congenital
Autoimmune
Trauma
Endocrine
Dietary
Psychiatric
Iatrogenic

Part V

Self-Assessment: Answers

Self-assessment: answers

Chapter 1

The correct answer is C.

This patient is describing the pain of biliary colic. While it is localising to an area of the abdomen, the site is diffuse and the description is not that of peritonitis. The scapular pain is likely to be referred pain rather than an indication of extra-abdominal disease. The pain follows a crescendo–decrescendo pattern and she cannot get comfortable with it, a description that is typical of colic from a hollow viscus. Midgut pain tends to localise to the central abdomen and pancreatic pain radiates to the centre of the back rather than the shoulder blade.

Chapter 2

The correct answer is B.

The presence of pale stool might indicate biliary obstruction, however dark urine is typical of both hepatitis and obstruction-related jaundice. Wilson's disease is very unlikely to present for the first time in a 66-year-old; patients typically present between the age of 6 and 20 years. Generally jaundice is visible at bilirubin levels above 35 micromol/L. When enquiring about potential drug-related causes of liver dysfunction, a drug history going back several weeks should be taken as some drugs, particularly antibiotics, can cause problems weeks after the last dose. Liver biopsy is not usually indicated in acute hepatitis, whereas ultrasound is a useful and safe first investigation to investigate the liver architecture and vascular system, biliary system and for any consequences of liver disease.

Chapter 3

The correct answer is B.

Serum ferritin is the most useful laboratory marker of iron-deficiency anaemia that is readily available. While an increased serum total iron binding capacity, decreased serum transferrin and decreased serum iron are also typical, they are non-specific as to the cause of anaemia. In addition, the red cell distribution width (RDW) can be useful, with increasing RDW being equivalent to the anisocytosis seen on the blood film of patients with iron-deficiency anaemia (IDA). IDA results from dietary deficiency alone only after adherence to a strict vegan diet for a period of 2 to 3 years. Although IDA is historically associated with lesions of the colon, upper GI tract lesions are also commonly found. Combined upper and lower GI endoscopy is therefore generally indicated. Synchronous lesions of the upper and lower GI tract are not uncommon. Radiological techniques may show larger lesions, but have low sensitivity for the full range of small bowel lesions. Thus wireless capsule endoscopy is generally considered the first-line investigation for the small bowel in IDA.

Chapter 4

The correct answer is D.

Marked malnutrition is strongly associated with psychiatric and cognitive disturbance. Multiple mechanisms for this exist, including glucose handling and the effects of micronutrient deficiencies such as zinc deficiency. Psychological treatment will not be effective in this patient until her malnutrition is

Gastroenterology and Hepatology: Lecture Notes, Second Edition. Stephen Inns and Anton Emmanuel.
© 2017 John Wiley & Sons, Ltd. Published 2017 by John Wiley & Sons, Ltd.
Companion website: www.lecturenoteseries.com/gastroenterology

addressed. Vitamin A deficiency affects vision, whereas folate and vitamin B complex deficiencies affect nerve and blood cell function. Thiamine deficiency is worsened by carbohydrate refeeding, as cellular thiamine utilisation is increased. Thiamine should be given to all patients suspected to be at risk of refeeding syndrome at least 30 minutes before refeeding commences. Profound disturbances of glucose, water, potassium, phosphate and magnesium handling occur with refeeding and all must be carefully monitored for and treated aggressively. Finally, tube feeding is only appropriate if oral intake is unsafe or insufficient to ensure an adequate intake; oral feeding should always be attempted first.

Chapter 5

The correct answer is B.

This is antibiotic-associated diarrhoea and while *C. difficile* is not the only organism implicated, the suspicion should be high. In an unwell patient with short-lived diarrhoea, colonoscopy or flexible sigmoidoscopy is not indicated immediately. Instead, early diagnostic endeavours should focus on excluding infectious causes. *C. difficile* is a commensal organism and only causes disease when it produces toxin (A or B); its presence alone is not diagnostic of disease. *Campylobacter* typically causes dysentery, whereas *C. difficile* is associated with watery diarrhoea. Loperamide is not generally indicated in acute infection and may even promote life-threatening ileus. Finally, **IV** vancomycin is not indicated in infectious diarrhoea; conversely, **oral** vancomycin is very effective against *C. difficile*.

Chapter 6

The correct answer is A.

Diagnostic colonoscopy is extremely safe and in most series was associated with a perforation rate of less than 0.1%. The risk is higher with polypectomy and increases with polyp size, as does the risk of haemorrhage. Colonoscopy and CT colonography have supplanted barium enema in modern practice. While CT colonography is a useful diagnostic test, particularly in high-risk patients, it is not as sensitive to small lesions as is colonoscopy and, unlike colonoscopy, does not allow the collection of tissue samples or removal of suspicious lesions. Antibiotics are only used in patients with high-risk valvular lesions or prosthetic valves.

Chapter 7

The correct answer is D.

Black, tarry stool (melaena) suggests that the source of bleeding is proximal to the caecum;

haematemesis suggest a source proximal to the jejunum. The mortality associated with significant upper GI bleeding is high and can be predicted using scoring systems that take account of haemodynamic factors and comorbidities, such as the Rockall pre-endoscopic score. In a patient with haemodynamic compromise, fluid resuscitation is the highest priority. Endoscopy should be undertaken once the patient is haemodynamically stable. Tranexamic acid has been used for upper GI bleeding, but studies have failed to show a mortality benefit. Proton pump inhibitors given as an IV infusion have been shown to reduce transfusion requirement and length of hospital stay in high-risk upper GI bleeding.

Chapter 8

The correct answer is E.

The suspicion here is that the patient has Boerhaave's syndrome as a result of the vigorous vomiting induced by the preparation fluid ingestion, perhaps in the presence of small bowel stricturing from Crohn's disease. Urgent endoscopy would risk worsening any oesophageal perforation. The fact that the vomiting started soon after ingestion of a large volume of fluid suggests the possibility of a small bowel stricture. A colonic stricture would be very unlikely to result in presentation in this way. Presuming that the suspicion of Boerhaave's syndrome proves to be correct, even with prompt treatment the mortality rate is still very high at around 25%. A plain chest X-ray may well show pneumomediastinum and pleural effusion, thus confirming the diagnosis.

Chapter 9

The correct answer is A.

The King's College Criteria, which are used as a guide to considering transplantation, are subtly different for paracetamol-induced acute liver failure compared to other causes. In this situation the only isolated marker of poor prognosis is pH <7.3. A combination of INR >6.5, creatinine >300 micromol/l and grade 3 or 4 encephalopathy is otherwise required. This patient fulfils all of the prognostic criteria. While extracorporeal liver support might be useful as a bridge to liver transplantation, it is not a replacement for it. The commonest cause of death in acute liver failure is intracranial hypertension and brain herniation. Infection develops in up to 80% of patients with acute liver failure and because of the relative immunodeficiency associated with the condition, they may not demonstrate the classical signs of sepsis.

Chapter 10

The correct answer is C.

A BMI over 30 is associated with a 2- to 3-fold increase in the risk of a severe clinical course in acute pancreatitis. Ranson's criteria are a useful tool for stratifying risk at 48 hours. Only some of the Ranson criteria can be completed at admission. Amylase is elevated in several non-pancreatic diseases and is not diagnostic of pancreatitis; instead, a clinical syndrome consistent with pancreatitis in the setting of an elevated amylase is required. Lipase has a superior sensitivity and specificity to amylase. Treatment of pain usually requires opiate analgesia and, while morphine is generally avoided because of concerns that it might exacerbate pancreatitis by increasing sphincter of Oddi tone, no definitive human study supports this.

Chapter 12

The correct answer is B.

The presentation is typical of achalasia. The long time course makes oesophageal cancer less likely. Dysphagia to solids and liquids is more typical of achalasia, whereas strictures tend to permit a liquid diet until very advanced. Oesophageal manometry is the investigation of choice and endoscopy and barium swallow are most useful to rule out differential diagnoses. The typical features of achalasia on barium swallow are a 'bird's beak' appearance of the distal oesophagus with proximal dilatation and aperistalsis. The oesophagus is typically dilated in achalasia, despite the absence of a fixed lower oesophageal stricture.

Chapter 13

The correct answer is C.

While familial gastric cancer is rare, a family history is always useful to determine whether a patient is at increased risk. This is particularly true for people of Māori descent, where multiple families with frequent gastric carcinomas have been identified. Although gastritis is a pathological, not endoscopic, diagnosis, the classical description in *H. pylori* infection is of a predominantly antral gastritis, whereas autoimmune gastritis is often confined to the gastric body. In a young Māori the diagnosis of gastric cancer should immediately trigger careful examination of the family tree and consideration of mutation testing. C-kit mutation testing is useful in gastrointestinal stromal tumours, but not with adenocarcinoma. Gastric ulcers are usually re-examined endoscopically after 8 to 12 weeks to ensure healing and rule out underlying gastric carcinoma.

Chapter 14

The correct answer is D.

Lynch syndrome predisposes to small bowel adenocarcinoma, although it remains a rare malignancy. Given her new symptoms, structural examination of the small bowel is indicated, both to rule out neoplasia and to examine for underlying structural disease. In view of the description of intermittent obstructions, progressive deterioration in ileostomy function with flatulence and bloating and response to antibiotics, it seems likely that she might have small bowel bacterial overgrowth. Coeliac disease should be excluded, but the best test would be IgA tissue transglutaminase or anti-endomysial antibodies, not HLA status. Presuming that bacterial overgrowth is present, then the action of the small intestinal bacteria will result in metabolism of B_{12} but leave folate absorption unaffected. Intestinal failure is unlikely to result unless <100 cm of the small bowel is retained.

Chapter 15

The correct answer is B.

IBD is a polygenic disease, and most patients have multiple genetic mutations contributing to their disease. Thus no one mutation is seen in all patients. The *CARD15/NOD2* gene is linked to Crohn's disease and the clinical situation here most fits with ulcerative colitis. Thiopurine methyl transferase levels are very useful in guiding thiopurine dose. Inflammation of the terminal ileum is typical of Crohn's disease, but does occur in 17% of ulcerative colitis patients and is called backwash ileitis. Corticosteroids are used for induction of remission, but have no role in maintenance of remission. 5-aminosalicylic acid should generally be administered orally and rectally for the greatest efficacy in extensive colitis.

Chapter 16

The correct answer is D.

Hereditary non-polyposis colorectal cancer (HNPCC), or Lynch syndrome, is the most common familial cause of colorectal cancer and in this patient, who has *not* been shown to have multiple colonic polyps, it is the most likely cause. Familial adenomatous polyposis (FAP) is caused by mutation of the APC gene on chromosome 5; HNPCC is caused by mutations of mismatch repair genes. Prophylactic colectomy is not generally recommended in HNPCC, but is considered in FAP. In this situation, where HNPCC is strongly suspected, any tumour should be tested for microsatellite instability and, if it is present, family screening for mismatch repair gene mutations should be considered. Gardner's syndrome is the variant of FAP associated with osteomas.

Chapter 17

The correct answer is E.

Prolapse is often not visible until a patient strains, thus it may not be seen on routine digital rectal examination. Perhaps the best way to detect prolapse, where it is suspected, is to ask the patient to sit on the toilet and strain, and then come in immediately following to observe the anus briefly. While somewhat undignified, this technique is acceptable to patients if explained carefully and gives the best chance of identifying a problem that can be very troubling for the individual. Second-degree haemorrhoids are, by definition, spontaneously reducing. Rectal prolapse is very common, affecting up to 1% of the population over 65 years of age.

Chapter 18

The correct answer is A.

Between episodes of acute pancreatitis, and increasingly as the pancreas atrophies, the amylase is not elevated and so is generally not of great diagnostic use. Ca 19-9, when initially positive, may be useful in following the response to treatment of a pancreatic cancer, but it is not helpful in diagnosis. 24-hour faecal fat collection is generally not used to confirm exocrine failure. A low level of faecal elastase in the right clinical setting is sufficient. Proton pump inhibitors can be used to improve the effectiveness of pancreatic supplements, by preventing their breakdown by acid, but are not particularly effective for exocrine failure on their own. Diabetes management in chronic pancreatitis is complicated by the loss of glucagon-producing cells, resulting in an increased propensity for hypoglycaemia. Given that the survival of such patients is limited, the aim should be adequate, not aggressive, control of glucose and avoidance of hypoglycaemia.

Chapter 19

The correct answer is D.

Charchot's triad consists of RUQ pain, jaundice and *fever*. She may have cholangitis developing, but in the absence of fever it is difficult to make this diagnosis. Transabdominal ultrasound is very specific for cholelithiasis, but not very sensitive (27–49%).

Cholecystectomy is protective for recurrent choledocholithiasis, although it does still occur, either because of retained stones in the bile ducts at surgery or *de novo* stone formation in the bile ducts. MRCP is definitely indicated in this case if the cause is not obvious at ultrasound. It is much more sensitive than ultrasound (overall >90%) in detecting bile duct stones. While it is likely that recurrent choledocholithiasis or sphincter of Oddi dysfunction is the cause of this episode, there is not enough evidence of this to proceed directly to endoscopic sphincterotomy, with its significant risk of causing pancreatitis and perforation.

Chapter 20

The correct answer is A.

The mainstay of therapy for hepatic encephalopathy is non-digestible disaccharides such as lactulose. Non-absorbable antibiotics were historically used to detoxify the colon and reduce the production of nitrogenous metabolites, and are increasingly being used again in the form of rifaximin, but do not replace lactulose as the mainstay of therapy. Spontaneous bacterial peritonitis can be diagnosed if the *neutrophil count* is greater than 250/mm³. Third-generation cephalosporins are best used for the empirical therapy of spontaneous bacterial peritonitis. Generally grade 1 varices do not require prophylactic therapy. If it is believed that they have bled then secondary prophylaxis is indicated. When ascites results from portal hypertension it is caused by transudation and has a relatively low protein content. This is evidenced by a widening of the serum to ascites albumin gradient to greater than 11 g/L.

Chapter 21

The correct answer is D.

The King's College Criteria are used to estimate risk in fulminant hepatitis. The Child–Turcotte–Pugh score comprises bilirubin, albumin, INR, ascites and encephalopathy. The score described in this case is the MELD score. *Chronic* rejection is characterised by vanishing bile ducts. Acute cellular rejection is common in the first 2 weeks after transplantation. Hepatitis B infection frequently recurs in the tranplant liver and prophylaxis with hepatitis B immunoglobulin (with or without antiviral treatment) is usually given.

Chapter 23

The correct answer is B.

While no one test can be used to differentiate alcoholic from non-alcoholic liver disease, the ratio of

ALT:AST can be useful. The relatively low ALT in alcoholic liver disease relates in part to dietary deficiency of pyridoxal phosphate (vitamin B_6). While the GGT is elevated in alcoholic liver disease, it is also elevated in many other liver diseases and cannot be considered specific for alcoholism. It is not uncommon for patients to under-report their alcohol intake. When alcoholism is suspected, techniques such as the CAGE questionnaire and seeking a collateral history from family and friends of the patient can help to determine objectively whether there is a problem. Even on liver biopsy the differentiation between alcoholic liver disease and NAFLD is not straightforward. Generally liver biopsy should be reserved as a tool to stage the degree of fibrosis if significant liver damage is suspected.

Chapter 24

The correct answer is D.

Hepatitis A causes a self-limiting acute hepatitis, not chronic liver disease, and is not relevant in this case. Caucasians resident in the UK fall into a low prevalence category for hepatitis B and the commonest modes of transmission are sexual or percutaneous transmission in adulthood. Hepatitis E causes outbreaks of acute hepatitis in developing countries. Hepatitis D causes superinfection or coinfection with hepatitis B. The sequencing of the hepatitis C virus genome has opened multiple new targets for therapy and will revolutionise the treatment of hepatitis C. Loss of HBeAg can be associated with development of the precore mutation. This is associated with a worse prognosis than infection with wild-type virus strains.

Chapter 25

The correct answer is D.

In this patient using stable doses of azathioprine in the long term, azathioprine-related liver injury is very unlikely. While azathioprine-related liver injury is idiosyncratic, it tends to occur early in the course of therapy. The liver test abnormality seen with azathioprine tends to be of a mixed pattern. Antibiotic-related liver injury can develop at any point in the course of treatment, but commonly develops 3 to 4 weeks after cessation of therapy, particularly with certain antibiotics including amoxycillin clavulanate. Azathioprine does not interact with amoxycillin clavulanate; it is metabolised by the enzymes thiopurine methyl transferase and xanthine oxidase and its levels are markedly altered by concomitant administration of allopurinol. Antibiotics are one of the commoner causes of DILD and in this case it is likely that the liver test abnormalities are a result of the administration of amoxycillin clavulanate.

Chapter 26

The correct answer is E.

The strongly positive ANA and SMA in this young woman make autoimmune hepatitis the most likely diagnosis. This can be triggered by exposure to a number of drugs, including nitrofurantoin. The absence of anti-liver kidney microsomal antibody 1 makes classic, or type 1, autoimmune hepatitis more likely than type 2. Primary biliary cirrhosis is generally associated with modest elevations of the serum aminotransferases and ANA but positive antimitochondrial antibodies, unlike in this case. The hallmark pathological feature of autoimmune hepatitis is an interface hepatitis.

Chapter 27

The correct answer is C.

Unfortunately, hepatocellular carcinoma is not an uncommon consequence of HBV infection, even in the absence of cirrhosis. This is in contrast to most other diseases associated with HCC, where cirrhosis is generally present prior to the development of HCC. If HCC is suspected, then biopsy should not be undertaken because of the risk of seeding the tumour along the biopsy tract. In most situations a diagnosis can be reached using a combination of imaging modalities. Hepatocellular adenoma occurs in women of childbearing age and is associated with oral contraceptive use. Often stopping the oral contraceptive will result in shrinkage of the tumour. Oestrogen-containing therapies should be avoided in patients with this condition. Haemangiomas of the liver are a common incidental finding and require no treatment. A single metastatic lesion in the liver is most commonly due to adenocarcinoma of the bowel and is resectable in 20% of cases, with 5-year survival of up to 38%.

Chapter 28

The correct answer is B.

In this case ischaemic hepatitis is most likely given the description of a probably cardiac event resulting in profound hypotension and the onset of very marked liver test abnormalities 24 hours after this, despite the finding of normal liver tests soon after the event. Where massive elevations or the aminotransferases are found during an inpatient episode, more than 50% of the time it is due to ischaemic hepatitis. There may be congestive hepatopathy, but on its own this tends to result in low-grade liver test abnormalities and ascites is typical with more severe congestion. Budd–Chiari syndrome can present with fulminant hepatitis, but it is very uncommon; the most common presentations of Budd–Chiari syndrome are subacute and chronic. Portal vein thrombosis is not associated with marked abnormalities of the liver tests and hepatic veno-occlusive disease may be more likely in patients with advanced age and comorbidities, although it is generally a consequence of hepatopoietic stem cell transplantation.

Chapter 29

The correct answer is D.

The physiological changes of pregnancy share many similarities with the changes caused by chronic liver disease, including those listed here. The liver test changes of intrahepatic cholestasis of pregnancy are not those normally expected with cholestasis, with marked elevation of transaminases, up to 10 times normal being the hallmark. The ALP is not useful as it is mildly elevated in late pregnancy normally. Hypoglycaemia typically occurs early in acute fatty liver of pregnancy and, along with the presence of hyperammonaemia, coagulopathy, polydipsia and polyuria, is useful in diferentiating AFLP from HELLP. Haemolytic anaemia resulting from microangiopathy, and resulting in deformation of the red cells seen on blood film, is typical of HELLP, which it seems this woman may well have. Steroids are indicated in HELLP as they promote maturity of the foetal lungs and ameliorate HELLP.

Chapter 30

The correct answer is C.

When screening for haemochromatosis, the first-line tests are the ferritin and transferrin saturation. The more expensive genetic tests are used as second-line confirmatory tests. Compound heterozygosity for the common hereditary haemochromatosis gene mutations is not associated with iron overload disease on its own. It may act as a cofactor leading to fibrosis in conditions such as porphyria cutanea tarda. Hereditary haemochromatosis is the most common genetic disease among Caucasians, with a prevalence of approximately that stated in the case. Carrier frequency is as high as 1 in 9 in some populations, which would predict an even higher prevalence than that stated, emphasising the complex genotype–phenotype association. Caeruloplasmin is the carrier molecule for plasma copper and is reduced with the copper overload of Wilson's disease. Onset of pulmonary disease in the most severe phenotype of alpha-1-antitrypsin deficiency (PiZZ) occurs after age 40 in non-smokers; liver disease often occurs prior to this.

Index

Note: Page references in *italics* refer to Figures; those in **bold** refer to Tables

Gastroenterology and Hepatology: Lecture Notes, Second Edition. Stephen Inns and Anton Emmanuel.
© 2017 John Wiley & Sons, Ltd. Published 2017 by John Wiley & Sons, Ltd.
Companion website: www.lecturenoteseries.com/gastroenterology